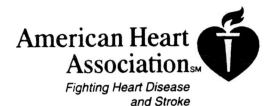

American Heart
Association_SM

*Fighting Heart Disease
and Stroke*

Monograph Series

THE VULNERABLE
ATHEROSCLEROTIC PLAQUE

Understanding, Identification, and Modification

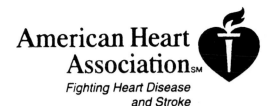

American Heart
Association SM
*Fighting Heart Disease
and Stroke*

Monograph Series

THE VULNERABLE
ATHEROSCLEROTIC PLAQUE
Understanding, Identification, and Modification

Edited by

Valentin Fuster, MD, PhD

*Richard Gorlin, MD/Heart Research Foundation Professor of Cardiology
Director, Zena and Michael A. Weiner Cardiovascular Institute
Dean for Academic Affairs
Mount Sinai School of Medicine
New York, NY*

Co-edited by

The Members of the American Heart Association
Vascular Lesions Committee

**J. Fredrick Cornhill, DPHIL
Robert E. Dinsmore, MD
John T. Fallon, MD, PhD
William Insull, Jr., MD
Peter Libby, MD
Steven Nissen, MD
Michael E. Rosenfeld, PhD
William D. Wagner, PhD**

**Futura Publishing
Company, Inc.**
Armonk, NY

Library of Congress Cataloging-in-Publication Data

The vulnerable atherosclerotic plaque : understanding, identification,
    and modification / edited by Valentin Fuster.
        p.   cm. — (American Heart Association monograph series)
    Includes bibliographical references and index.
    ISBN 0-87993-406-9 (alk. paper)
    1. Atherosclerotic plaque.   2. Coronary artery disease–
–Pathophysiology.   I. Fuster, Valentin.   II. Series.
    [DNLM: 1.   Coronary Arteriosclerosis—physiopathology.
    2.   Coronary Arteriosclerosis—diagnosis.   3.   Coronary
Arteriosclerosis—therapy.
    WG 300 V991   1998]
    RC692.V85   1995
    616.1'3607—dc21
    DNLM/DLC
    for Library of Congress   98-17362
                                                                    CIP

Copyright © 1999
Futura Publishing Company, Inc.

Published by
Futura Publishing Company, Inc.
135 Bedford Road
Armonk, New York 10504

LC #: 98-17362
ISBN #: 0-87993-406-9

Historical Perspective:

The Vascular Lesions Committee of The American Heart Association

The Importance of Its Existence and Mission

The Committee on Vascular Lesions of the American Heart Association was first appointed as an ad hoc committee to the American Society for the Study of Arteriosclerosis a few years before this society became a part of the American Heart Association as the Council on Arteriosclerosis in 1959. The main organizer and first Chairman of the Committee on Vascular Lesions was Russell Holman. The initial purpose of the Committee was to develop standardized methods to quantitate atherosclerotic lesions in the arteries of individuals at autopsy. The result of this work was published in 1960.[1] After this, Robert Wissler served briefly as chairman of the Committee, followed by Henry McGill, who turned the attention of the Committee to the problem of how to further refine the measurement of atherosclerosis severity in a way that would make it possible to compare the results from one laboratory to another or from one time period to another in a given autopsy service. These activities lead to two important publications in 1968.[2,3]

In the 1970s, the Committee considered the important problem of how to develop quantitative pathological information from the arteries of individuals who succumb while participating in large-scale studies such as the National Diet Heart Study. Although valuable suggestions were developed, the critical study was never undertaken as a national objective. Nevertheless, the efforts did lead to the development of useful tools which were first applied in the International Atherosclerosis Project. This study[4] had a strong interaction with the Committee on Lesions throughout its existence, headed as it was by Henry McGill.

Following this, under the leadership of Tom Clarkson, the Committee turned its attention to the relatively neglected subject of the arterial mesenchyme and its role in arteriosclerosis. This led to a national conference on the arterial mesenchyme and arteriosclerosis that resulted in a unique monograph with the same title.[5]

The multicenter PDAY research program was first proposed to the Committee on Lesions in 1974. It was the strong endorsement of that committee, followed by the support of the Executive Committee of the AHA Council on Arteriosclerosis and the encouragement and support given to the concept of the program by Drs. McGill and Strong, which led Dr. Wissler to undertake the 10-year effort to plan and develop this unique study of the Pathobiological Determinants of Atherosclerosis in Youth, which is now in its 10th year of highly innovative and informative work.[6,7]

In the early 1980s, the Committee turned its attention to the numerous methods that were then being developed in many disciplines to quantify the progress or the effects of treatment on atherosclerotic lesions in living subjects. It organized the first concerted effort to bring theses disciplines together, to compare their results, and to start using the same terminology. This meeting led to two publications.[8,9]

This was followed by an intensive series of committee meetings in which the pathogenesis of atherosclerosis was considered in depth. A national conference on The Pathobiology of the Human Atherosclerotic Plaque was held in 1986. The proceedings were published in 1990, and were edited by Seymour Glagov, William P. Newman, and Sheldon A. Schaffer.[10]

More recently, based on a better understanding of the vascular wall, the Committee has developed a classification of atherosclerotic lesions. This effort has lead to a series of three reports. The first provided a definition of the arterial intima and its atherosclerosis prone regions.[11] The second publication defined initial lesions, fatty streaks, and intermediate lesions of atherosclerosis.[12] The third report was just published and it describes the different types of advanced atherosclerotic lesions and provides a histopathological classification of all human atherosclerotic lesion types that will be of value for understanding the clinical manifestations of these diseases and the contributions of the evolving diagnostic modalities of imaging.[13]

Since 1996 the Committee has comprised a group of experts from various disciplines (ie, pathology, imaging, clinical, vascular biology). This variety of disciplines is critical for the main mission of the Committee, which is to focus on the vascular wall of humans.

1. Through the multidisciplinary membership of the Committee, there is a drive toward a better understanding of the pathogenesis and pathological-clinical implications of atherosclerosis, particularly in relation to the stabilization of lesions, their thrombogenicity, and vascular reactivity. This will provide the basis for the enhancement of new modalities of diagnostic imaging, prevention, and treatment of

atherosclerosis. Such knowledge and understanding is being reviewed every 2 years in the form of an expert scientific meeting, as well as in other creative forums.

2. To disseminate such knowledge and promote its use, the scientific meeting held every 2 years is summarized in a book, in a manner of a statement.[14] The present statement, entitled *The Vulnerable Atherosclerotic Plaque: Understanding, Identification, and Modification*,[15] is the second of these documents, and this meeting has also been recorded on CD-ROM.

3. To identify the critical questions that must be addressed in order to increase our knowledge of atherosclerosis and of the consequences of treatment modalities including the positive and negative results of direct interventions on lesions, the Committee meets twice a year for critical discussions.

In summary, the drive toward a better understanding of the factors influencing the natural history of plaques, of the correlation of vascular lesions and clinical syndromes, including their underlying pathogenesis, and of the utility of new methods of imaging for the evaluation of atherosclerotic disease will lead to better modalities of both prevention and treatment. These problems and perspectives should be disseminated by an interdisciplinary group. In addition, critical new questions should be identified for appropriate evaluation and dissemination. The multidisciplinary Committee on Vascular Lesions is the ideal group to accomplish this goal.

References

1. Holman RL, Brown WB, Gore I, et al. An index for the evaluation of arteriosclerotic lesions in the abdominal aorta. A report by the Committee on Lesions of the American Society for the Study of Arteriosclerosis. *Circulation* 1960;22:1137–1143.
2. McGill HC, Brown WB, Gore I, et al. Grading human atherosclerotic lesions using a panel of photographs. Report of the Committee on Grading Lesions, Council on Arteriosclerosis, American Heart Association. *Circulation* 1968; 37:455–459.
3. McGill HC, Brown WB, Gore I, et al. Grading stenosis in the right coronary artery. Report of the Committee on Grading Lesions, Council on Arteriosclerosis, American Heart Association. *Circulation* 1968;37:460–463.
4. Guzman MA, McMahan CA, McGill HC, et al. Selected methodologic aspects of International Atherosclerotic Project. *Lab Invest* 1968;18:479–497.
5. Wagner WD, Clarkson TB eds: *Arterial Mesenchyme and Arteriosclerosis*. New York: Plenum Press; 1974.
6. Pathobiological Determinants in Youth (PDAY) Research Group. Natural

history of aortic and coronary atherosclerotic lesions in youth: Findings from the PDAY Study. *Arterioscler Thromb* 1993;13:1291–1298.

7. Wissler RW. New insights into the pathogenesis of atherosclerosis as revealed by PDAY. *Arteriosclerosis* 1994;108(suppl):S3–S20.

8. Chandler AB, Bond MG, Insull W Jr, et al. Quantitative evaluation of atherosclerosis. *Arteriosclerosis* 1983;3(2):183–186.

9. Bond MG, Insull W Jr, Glagov S, et al eds: *Clinical Diagnosis of Atherosclerosis: Quantitative Methods of Evaluation.* New York: Springer-Verlag; 1983.

10. Glagov S, Newman WP III, Schaffer SA eds: *Pathobiology of the Human Atherosclerotic Plaque.* New York: Springer-Verlag; 1990.

11. Stary HC, Blankenhorn DH, Chandler AB, et al. A definition of the intima of human arteries and of its atherosclerosis-prone regions. A report from the Committee on Vascular Lesions of the Council on Arteriosclerosis, American Heart Association. *Circulation* 1992;85:391–405.

12. Stary HC, Chandler AB, Glagov S, et al. A definition of initial, fatty streak and intermediate lesions of atherosclerosis. A report from the Committee on Vascular Lesions of the Council on Arteriosclerosis, American Heart Association. *Circulation* 1994;89:2462–2478.

13. Stary HC, Chandler AB, Dinsmore MD, et al. Definitions of advanced types of atherosclerotic lesions and the histological classification of atherosclerosis. A report from the Committee on Vascular Lesions of the Council on Arteriosclerosis, American Heart Association. *Circulation* 1995;92: 1355–1374.

14. Fuster V ed: *Syndromes of Atherosclerosis: Correlations of Clinical Imaging and Pathology.* Armonk, NY: Futura Publishing Company, Inc.; 1996.

15. Fuster V ed: *The Vulnerable Atherosclerotic Plaque: Understanding, Identification, and Modification.* Armonk, NY: Futura Publishing Company, Inc.; 1998.

Contributors

Pierre Amarenco, MD   Professor of Neurology, Pierre and Marie Curie University; Department of Neurology, Lariboisiere Hospital, Paris, France

Juan Jose Badimon, PhD   Director, Cardiovascular Biology Research Laboratory, Zena and Michael A. Weiner Cardiovascular Research Institute, Associate Professor of Medicine, Mount Sinai School of Medicine

Lina Badimon, PhD   Professor, Department of Molecular Pathology and Therapeutics, Consejo Superior de Investigaciones Cietilicas, Barcelona, Spain

Hisham S. Bassiouny, MD   Associate Professor of Vascular Surgery, Department of Surgery and Pathology, The University of Chicago, Chicago, IL

Greg Bearman, PhD   National Aeronautics and Space Administration's Jet Propulsion Laboratory at the California Institute of Technology, Santa Barbara, CA

Sophie Biz, MS   Graduate Student, School of Mechanical Engineering, Georgia Institute of Technology, Atlanta, GA

Mark E. Brezinski, MD, PhD   Department of Electrical Engineering and Computer Science, Massachusetts Institute of Technology, Cambridge, MA; Cardiac Unit, Massachusetts General Hospital, Boston, MA

Ward Casscells, MD   Theodore and Maureen O'Driscoll Levy Professor of Medicine, Chief of Cardiology, Hermann Hospital and University of Texas, Houston Medical School; Associate Director, Cardiology Research, Texas Heart Institute/St. Luke's Episcopal Hospital, Houston, TX

Fred Clubb, Jr., PhD, DVM   Chief of Comparative Cardiovascular Services, The Texas Heart Institute at St. Luke's Episcopal Hospital, Houston, TX; Adjunct Professor, Department of Pathology, College of Veterinary Medicine, Texas A&M University, College Station, TX

Ariel Cohen, MD   Professor of Cardiology, Pierre and Marie Curie University; Department of Cardiology, Saint-Antoine Hospital, Paris, France

Søren Dalager-Pederson, MS   Research Associate, Departments of Cardiology, Cardiothoracic and Vascular Surgery, and MR Center, Aarhus University Hospital (SKS), Aarhus, Denmark

Mark David, MD   Fellow in Cardiology, Hermann Hospital; Department of Internal Medicine, Division of Cardiology, University of Texas, Houston Medical School; The Texas Heart Institute at St. Luke's Episcopal Hospital, Houston, TX

Linda L. Demer, MD, PhD   Associate Professor of Medicine and Physiology, Chief, Division of Cardiology, UCLA School of Medicine, Los Angeles, CA

J. Micah Downing, PhD   Research Physicist, Noise and Vibration Branch, US Air Force Research Laboratory, Wright Patterson Air Force Base, Ohio

Robert R. Edelman, MD   Director, Magnetic Resonance Imaging, Beth Israel-Deaconess Medical Center; Professor of Radiology, Harvard Medical School, Boston, MA

Rosalind P. Fabunmi, PhD   Research Fellow in Medicine, Brigham and Women's Hospital, Boston, MA

Erling Falk, MD, PhD   Research Professor, Department of Cardiology, Research Unit, Aarhus University Hospital (SKS), Aarhus, Denmark

John T. Fallon, MD, PhD   Chief of Cardiovascular Pathology, The Cardiovascular Institute, Professor of Medicine and Pathology, The Mount Sinai School of Medicine, New York, NY

Zahi A. Fayad, PhD   Assistant Professor of Radiology and Medicine, The Cardiovascular Institute, The Mount Sinai School of Medicine, New York, NY

James G. Fujimoto, PhD   Professor, Department of Electrical Engineering and Computer Science, Massachusetts Institute of Technology, Cambridge, MA

Valentin Fuster, MD, PhD   Richard Gorlin, MD/Heart Research Foundation Professor of Cardiology, Director, Zena and Michael A. Weiner Cardiovascular Institute, Dean for Academic Affairs, Mount Sinai School of Medicine, New York, NY

Peter Ganz, MD   Director of Cardiovascular Research, Cardiac Catheterization Laboratory, Brigham and Women's Hospital; Associate Professor of Medicine, Harvard Medical School, Boston, MA

Seymour Glagov, MD   Professor of Pathology, Department of Surgery and Pathology, The University of Chicago, Chicago, IL

Catherine A. Goudet, PhD   Georgia Institute of Technology, Atlanta, GA

Alan D. Guerci, MD   Executive Vice President for Medical Affairs, St. Francis Hospital, Roslyn, NY

John R. Guyton, MD   Associate Professor of Medicine, Assistant Professor of Pathology, Division of Endocrinology, Metabolism, and Nutrition, Department of Medicine, and the Sarah W. Stedman Center for Nutritional Studies, Duke Medical Center, Durham, NC

Ian N. Hamilton, Jr., MD   Assistant Professor of Surgery, Department of Surgery, Chattanooga Unit, University of Tennessee College of Medicine, Chattanooga, TN

Larry H. Hollier, MD   Franz W. Sichel Professor of Surgery, Chairman, Department of Surgery, The Mount Sinai Medical Center, New York, NY

Scott Kinlay, MBBS, PhD   Research Fellow in Cardiology, Brigham and Women's Hospital and Harvard Medical School, Boston, MA

David N. Ku, MD, PhD   Professor of Mechanical Engineering, School of Mechanical Engineering, Georgia Institute of Technology; Professor of Surgery, Emory University, Atlanta, GA

Richard T. Lee, MD   Assistant Professor of Medicine, Vascular Medicine and Atherosclerosis Unit, Cardiovascular Division, Department of Medicine, Brigham and Women's Hospital, Harvard Medical School, Boston, MA

Peter Libby, MD   Chief, Cardiovascular Medicine, Brigham and Women's Hospital; Mallinckrodt Professor of Medicine, Harvard Medical School, Boston, MA

Steven E. Nissen, MD   Vice Chairman, Department of Cardiology, Director, Clinical Cardiology, Director, Coronary Intensive Care Unit, Cleveland Clinic, Cleveland, OH

Farhad Parhami, PhD   Assistant Professor of Medicine, Division of Cardiology, UCLA School of Medicine, Los Angeles, CA

Gerard Pasterkamp, MD, PhD   Department of Cardiology and Department of Functional Anatomy, Utrecht University Hospital; Interuniversity Cardiology Institute of the Netherlands; Fellow of the Catharijne Foundation, Utrecht, the Netherlands

Erik Morre Pederson, MD, PhD   Research Fellow, Departments of Cardiothoracic and Vascular Surgery and MR Center, Aarhus University Hospital (SKS), Aarhus, Denmark

Steffen Ringgaard, MSc   Research Associate, Departments of Cardiothoracic and Vascular Surgery and MR Center, Aarhus University Hospital (SKS), Aarhus, Denmark

Luis Rohde, MD, MSc   Research Fellow, Vascular Medicine and Atherosclerosis Unit, Cardiovascular Division, Department of Medicine, Brigham and Women's Hospital, Harvard Medical School, Boston, MA

Yasuhiro Sakaguchi, MD   Assistant Professor of Pathology, Nara Medical University, Nara, Japan

Andrew P. Selwyn, MD   Professor of Medicine, Harvard Medical School; Director, Cardiac Catheterization Laboratory, Brigham and Women's Hospital, Boston, MA

Meir Shinnar, MD, PhD   Director of Cardiovascular MRI, The Cardiovascular Institute, Associate Professor of Medicine and Radiology, Department of Medicine, The Mount Sinai School of Medicine, New York, NY

James F. Southern, MD, PhD   Pathologist, Cardiac Unit, Massachusetts General Hospital, Boston, MA

Guillermo J. Tearney, PhD   Department of Electrical Engineering and Computer Science, Massachusetts Institute of Technology, Cambridge, MA; Cardiac Unit, Massachusetts General Hospital, Boston, MA

Jean-François Toussaint, MD, PhD   Service de Physiologie et Radioisitopes, Hospital Broussais, Paris, France

E. Murar Tuzcu, MD   Medical Director, Intravascular Ultrasound Laboratory, Section of Interventional Cardiology, Department of Cardiology, The Cleveland Clinic Foundation, Cleveland, OH

Yasumi Uchida, MD   Professor, Clinical Physiology and Cardiovascular Center, Toho University Hospital at Sakura, Sakura, Japan

Shankar Vallabhajosula, PhD   Professor of Radiopharmacy/Radiology, Department of Radiology, Division of Nuclear Medicine, New York Hospital-Cornell University Medical College, New York, NY

Ray Vito, PhD   Professor of Mechanical Engineering, School of Mechanical Engineering, Georgia Institute of Technology, Atlanta, GA

William D. Wagner, PhD   Professor of Comparative Medicine, Wake Forest University School of Medicine, Winston-Salem, NC

David Waters, MD, FRCP(C), FACC   Director of Cardiology, Hartford Hospital, Hartford, CT; Director of Cardiology, The University of Connecticut Health Center, Professor of Medicine, The University of Connecticut School of Medicine, Farmington, CT

James T. Willerson, MD   Professor and Chairman, Department of Internal Medicine, University of Texas, Houston Medical School; Chief of Medicine, Hermann Hospital; Chief of Medicine, Lyndon B. Johnson General Hospital; Director of Cardiology Research, The Texas Heart Institute at St. Luke's Episcopal Hospital, Houston, TX

Khalid Ziada, MD   Interventional Fellow, Section of Interventional Cardiology, Department of Cardiology, The Cleveland Clinic Foundation, Cleveland, OH

Contents

Chapter 1

Coronary Artery Disease:
Plaque Vulnerability, Disruption, and Thrombosis

Søren Dalager-Pedersen, MS,
Erik Morre Pedersen, MD, PhD,
Steffen Ringgaard, MSc,
and Erling Falk, MD, PhD

Introduction

Coronary atherosclerosis starts early in life. Coronary lesions are present in most young adults, particularly in Western countries, but usually it takes decades to evolve the mature plaques responsible for ischemic heart disease (IHD). Proliferation of smooth muscle cells (SMC), matrix synthesis, and lipid accumulation may narrow the arterial lumen gradually and lead to myocardial ischemia and anginal pain but survival is good if thrombotic complications can be prevented. It is thrombosis, superimposed on mature plaques, that may turn an otherwise benign disease into a life-threatening condition, being mainly responsible for the acute coronary syndromes of unstable angina, myocardial infarction, and sudden coronary death.[1,2] Therefore, for event-free survival, the vital question is not why atherosclerosis develops, but rather why some plaques remain thrombus-resistant and innocuous while other plaques, after years of indolent growth, become thrombus-prone and life-threatening. In this context, plaque vulnerability and thrombogenicity have emerged as being much more important than plaque size and stenosis severity. Plaques containing a core of soft lipid-rich atheromatous "gruel" are particularly dangerous because they are unstable and vulnerable to rupture, whereby the highly thrombogenic

From: Fuster, V (ed). *The Vulnerable Atherosclerotic Plaque: Understanding, Identification, and Modification.* Armonk, NY: Futura Publishing Company, Inc.; © 1999.

gruel is suddenly exposed to the flowing blood.[3-6] Plaque disruption, or fissuring, with thrombosis superimposed is the most frequent cause of the acute coronary syndromes.[1-3]

Mature Uncomplicated Plaques

In patients with IHD, the coronary arteries are diffusely involved with confluent atherosclerotic plaques. The composition, vulnerability, and thrombogenicity of individual plaques vary greatly without any obvious relation to the well-known risk factors for clinical disease[7-10] other than a recently reported association between serum cholesterol and plaque vulnerability in men who died suddenly of IHD.[11] Calcification of coronary plaques increases with age and the overall plaque burden[12-14] but not with the degree of luminal obstruction.[12] Interestingly, culprit lesions responsible for unstable angina[12] and myocardial infarction[15] are less calcified, indicating that calcium actually might stabilize plaques against disruption and thrombosis.

Importantly, there is no simple relation among plaque type, plaque size, and stenosis severity,[16] which highlights the problem in identifying vulnerable plaques by focusing only on their flow-limiting potential.[17] Besides, even advanced plaques may not compromise the lumen at all, due to compensatory vascular enlargement (remodeling).[18-20a]

Atherosclerosis: Atherosis + Sclerosis

As the name *atherosclerosis* implies, mature plaques typically consist of two main components: *atheromatous* "gruel," which is lipid-rich and soft, and *sclerotic* tissue, which is collagen-rich and hard (Fig. 1). Although the sclerotic component is usually the most voluminous, constituting greater than 70% of an average stenotic coronary plaque,[21,22] it is a relatively benign component because collagen secreted by SMC probably stabilizes plaques, protecting them against disruption. In contrast, the soft atheromatous gruel destabilizes plaques, making them vulnerable to rupture with high risk of subsequent thrombus formation.[23] Accordingly, a significant atheromatous component is usually present in culprit lesions responsible for the thrombus-mediated acute coronary syndromes.[24,25]

The atheromatous core within a plaque lacks supporting collagen[25] and is rich in extracellular lipids (predominantly cholesterol and its esters),[26,27] avascular,[28,29] hypocellular (macrophage foam cells are, however, frequently present at the periphery of the core),[29-31] and usually soft like gruel. It is generally believed that macrophage foam cell

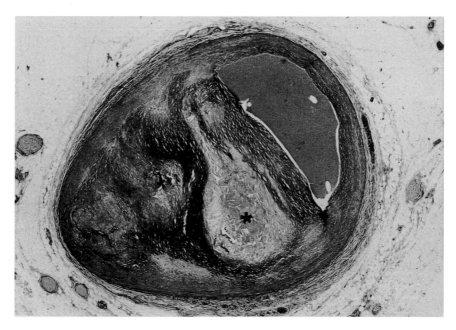

Figure 1. Microscopic view of a cross-sectioned coronary artery containing a mature atherosclerotic plaque. A mature plaque consists typically of two main components: atheromatous gruel and sclerotic tissue. The atheromatous component (asterisk) is lipid-rich and soft, which is why it is dangerous; lipid destabilizes plaques, making them vulnerable to rupture, the most frequent cause of coronary thrombosis.

necrosis or apoptosis, possibly due to the cytotoxic effect of oxidized low-density lipoprotein (LDL) taken up by macrophages via their scavenger receptors, plays an important role in extracellular lipid accumulation and core formation.[32–35] Insudated lipoproteins trapped and retained within the extracellular space without first being taken up and subsequently released by macrophages may, however, also contribute to extracellular lipid accumulation, core formation, and core enlargement.[36,37]

Vulnerable Plaques

A small subset of mature uncomplicated plaques is unstable and rupture-prone. There are three major determinants of a plaque's vulnerability to rupture: (1) the size and consistency of the atheromatous core;

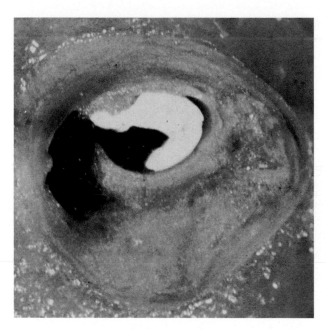

Figure 2. Macroscopic view of a cross-sectioned coronary artery containing a disrupted plaque. The fibrous cap is ruptured at the shoulder of the plaque. Blood has penetrated into the soft gruel through the disrupted surface (plaque hemorrhage) and a nonocclusive thrombus is projecting into the lumen. The lumen contains white radiographic contrast medium injected postmortem.

(2) the thickness of the fibrous cap covering the core; and (3) inflammation and repair within the cap (Figures 2 and 3). Cap "fatigue" may also play a role, as long-term repetitive cyclic stresses can weaken a material and increase its vulnerability to fracture, ultimately leading to sudden and unprovoked (ie, untriggered) mechanical failure and disruption.

Core Size and Consistency

The size of the atheromatous core is critical for the stability of individual plaques. Gertz and Roberts[28] reported the composition of plaques in 5-mm segments from 17 infarct-related arteries examined postmortem and found much larger atheromatous cores in the 39 segments with plaque rupture than in the 229 segments with intact surface (32% and 5% to12% of plaque area, respectively). By studying aortic plaques, Davies et al[38] found a similar relation between core size and plaque rupture and they identified a critical threshold; intact aortic plaques containing a core occupying more than 40% of the plaque area were considered particularly vulnerable and at high risk of rupture and thrombosis.

The consistency of the core, which probably also is important for the stability of a plaque, depends on temperature and lipid composition. The core gruel usually has a consistency like toothpaste at room temperature postmortem and it is even softer at body temperature in vivo.[26,27] Liquid cholesteryl esters soften the gruel, while crystalline cholesterol has the opposite effect.[26,27] Based on animal experiments,[26,39] lipid-lowering therapy in humans is expected to deplete plaque lipid with an overall reduction in the liquid and mobile cholesteryl esters and a relative increase in the solid and inert crystalline cholesterol, theoretically resulting in a stiffer and more stable plaque.[40]

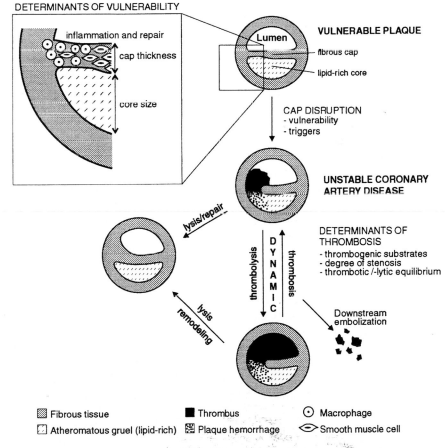

Figure 3. Schematic of plaque vulnerability, disruption, and thrombosis.

Cap Thickness

The thickness, cellularity, matrix, strength, and stiffness of fibrous caps vary widely. Cap thinning and reduced collagen content increase a plaque's vulnerability to rupture.[41] Caps of eccentric plaques are often thinnest and most heavily foam cell infiltrated at their shoulder regions, where they most frequently rupture.[42] Collagen is important for the tensile strength of tissues, and ruptured aortic caps contain fewer SMC (the collagen-synthesizing cell in plaques) and less collagen than intact caps.[38,43] The cause of this potentially dangerous lack of SMC in disrupted caps is not completely understood, but SMC could vanish as the result of apoptotic cell death,[44] which has recently been shown to occur in fibrous caps and thus could lead to plaque destabilization, disruption, and thrombosis.[32,34,45]

Cap Inflammation and Repair

Disrupted fibrous caps are usually heavily infiltrated by macrophage foam cells (Fig. 2),[46–48] and recent observations have revealed that such rupture-related macrophages are activated, indicating ongoing inflammation at the site of plaque disruption.[49] For eccentric plaques, the shoulder regions are sites of predilection for both active inflammation (endothelial activation and macrophage infiltration) and disruption,[42,50] and mechanical testing of aortic fibrous caps indicate that foam cell infiltration indeed weakens caps locally, reducing their tensile strength.[51] van der Wal et al[49] identified superficial macrophage infiltration in plaques beneath all 20 coronary thrombi examined, whether the underlying plaque was disrupted or just eroded, although a more recent study of coronary thrombi responsible for sudden coronary death could not confirm that observation.[52] By evaluation with immunohistochemical technique, van der Wal et al[49] found that macrophages and adjacent T lymphocytes (SMC were usually lacking at rupture sites) were activated, indicating ongoing disease activity. Comparable results were obtained by the same group in a study of atherectomy specimens showing an inverse relation between the extent of inflammatory activity in plaque tissues of culprit lesions and the clinical stability of the ischemic syndrome.[53] However, there was considerable overlap between groups, indicating that not all patients with clinically stable angina have histologically stable plaques.[53] These observations confirmed a previous study of atherectomy specimens from culprit lesions responsible for stable angina, unstable rest angina, or non–Q-wave infarction.[54] Culprit lesions responsible for the acute coronary syndromes contained significantly more macrophages than did lesions responsible for stable angina pectoris (14% versus 3% of plaque tissue occupied by macrophages).[54]

Macrophages are capable of degrading extracellular matrix by phagocytosis or by secreting proteolytic enzymes such as plasminogen activators and a family of MMPs (matrix metalloproteinases: collagenases, gelatinases, and stromeolysins), which may weaken the fibrous cap, predisposing it to rupture.[45,55] The MMPs are secreted in a latent zymogen form requiring extracellular activation, after which they are capable of degrading virtually all components of the extracellular matrix. The MMPs and their cosecreted tissue inhibitors of metalloproteinases, TIMP-1 and TIMP-2, are critical for cell migration, tumor invasion and metastasis, and vascular remodeling.[55] Collagen is the main component of caps, responsible for their tensile strength; and human monocyte-derived macrophages grown in culture are capable of degrading collagen of aortic fibrous caps during incubation.[56] Simultaneously, they express MMP-1 (interstitial collagenase) and induce MMP-2 (gelatinolytic) activity in the culture medium.[56]

Besides macrophages, a wide variety of cells may produce MMPs.[55] Activated mast cells may secrete powerful proteolytic enzymes (such as tryptase and chymase) that can activate pro-MMPs secreted by other cells (eg, macrophages), and mast cells are actually present in shoulder regions of mature plaques and at sites of disruption, but at very low density.[57,58] Neutrophils are also capable of destroying tissue by secreting proteolytic enzymes but neutrophils are rarely found in intact plaques.[49] Neutrophils may occasionally be found in disrupted plaques beneath coronary thrombi, probably entering these plaques shortly after disruption,[49] and they may also migrate into the arterial wall shortly after reperfusion of occluded arteries in response to ischemia/reperfusion.[59]

Cap Fatigue

When a material is exposed to a steady load that does not cause immediate fracture, the material may weaken if the load is applied repeatedly. Ultimately, this repetitive stress may lead to sudden fracture of the tissue due to fatigue. This is analogous to the breaking of a paper clip that has been weakened by repeated bending.[60] Cyclic stretching, compression, bending, flexion, shear, and pressure fluctuations may fatigue and weaken a fibrous cap, causing spontaneous rupture (ie, untriggered). If fatigue plays a role, lowering the frequency (heart rate) and magnitude (flow- and pressure-related) of loading should reduce the risk of plaque disruption. This could partly explain the beneficial effect of β-blockers after myocardial infarction (reduction of reinfarction).[61]

Plaque Disruption

Disruption of vulnerable plaques is not an infrequent event. It is followed by a variable amount of luminal thrombosis and/or hemorrhage into the soft gruel, causing rapid growth of the lesion (Figures 2 and 3).[62] Autopsy data indicate that 9% of "normal" healthy persons are walking around with disrupted plaques (without superimposed thrombosis) in their coronary arteries, increasing to 22% in persons with diabetes or hypertension.[63] Further, one or more disrupted plaques, with or without superimposed thrombosis, are usually present in coronary arteries of patients dying of IHD.[46,64] As mentioned, disruption of the plaque surface occurs most often where the cap is thinnest, most heavily infiltrated by macrophages and, therefore, weakest—namely at the cap's shoulders.[3,42] The weak shoulder regions are, however, also points where biomechanical and hemodynamic forces acting on plaques often are concentrated.[42,65] Thus, the risk of plaque disruption is related to both *intrinsic* plaque features (actual vulnerability) and *extrinsic* stresses imposed on plaque (rupture triggers). The former predisposes a plaque to rupture (discussed above), while the latter may precipitate it if the plaque is vulnerable (discussed below). As the presence of a vulnerable plaque is a prerequisite for plaque disruption, vulnerability is probably more important than triggers in determining the risk of a future heart attack. If there are no vulnerable plaques present in the coronary arteries, there is no rupture-prone substrate for a potential trigger to work on.

Triggers of Plaque Disruption

Coronary plaques are constantly stressed by a variety of biomechanical and hemodynamic forces that may precipitate or "trigger" disruption of vulnerable plaques.[3,60,66] Plaque disruption may occur from the lumen into the plaque due to increase in luminal blood pressure, or the cap may rupture from the plaque into the lumen due to increase in intraplaque pressure. This could be caused by, for example, vasospasm, bleeding from vasa vasorum, plaque edema, and/or collapse of compliant stenoses.

Blood Pressure

The luminal pressure induces both circumferential tension (tensile stress) in and radial compression of the vessel wall. The circumferential wall tension caused by the blood pressure is given by Laplace's law, which relates luminal pressure and radius to wall tension: the higher the blood pressure and the larger the luminal diameter, the more tension develops in the wall.[66] If components within the wall (eg, soft gruel) are unable to bear the imposed load, the stress is redistributed to adjacent structures (eg, fibrous cap over gruel), where it may be critically concentrated.[41,42,65] As previously mentioned, the consistency of the gruel may be important for stress distribution within plaques; the stiffer the gruel, the more stress it can bear and correspondingly less is redistributed to the adjacent fibrous cap.[40] Calcification may also play a role in making the plaque more stable, as previously mentioned.[12] It is important to note that the thickness of the fibrous cap is most critical for the peak circumferential stress: the thinner the fibrous cap, the higher the stress that develops in it.[41] For fibrous caps of the same tensile strength, caps covering mildly or moderately stenotic plaques are probably more prone to rupture than are caps covering stenotic plaques, because the former have to bear a greater circumferential tension (according to the law of Laplace).[41]

Pulse Pressure

The propagating pulse wave causes cyclic changes in lumen size and shape with deformation and bending of plaques, particularly the "soft" ones. Eccentric plaques typically bend at their edges, ie, at the junction between the stiff plaque and the more compliant plaque-free vessel wall.[60] Changes in vascular tone also cause bending of eccentric plaques at their edges. Cyclic bending may, in the long term, weaken these points, leading to unprovoked "spontaneous" fatigue disruption, while a sudden accentuated bending may trigger rupture of a weakened cap.

Heart Contraction

The coronary arteries are tethered to the surface of the beating heart and they undergo cyclic longitudinal deformations by axial bending (flexion) and stretching, particularly the left anterior descending coronary artery.[67] Angiographically, the angle of flexion was recently found to correlate with subsequent lesion progression, but the coefficient of correlation was low.[67] Like circumferential bending, a sudden accentuated longitudinal flexion may trigger plaque disruption, while long term cyclic flexion may fatigue and weaken the plaque.

Spasm

Plaque rupture and vasospasm do frequently coexist, but the former most likely gives rise to the latter rather than vice versa.[68-70] Onset of myocardial infarction is uncommon during or shortly after drug-induced spasm of even severely diseased coronary arteries,[71,72] indicating that spasm infrequently precipitates plaque disruption and/or luminal thrombosis.

Capillary Plaque Bleeding

Bleeding and/or transudation (edema) into plaques from thin-walled new vessels originating from vasa vasorum and frequently found at the plaque base[64,73] could theoretically increase the intra-plaque pressure with resultant cap rupture from the inside.[74] Although frequently found,[64] it is difficult to imagine how a small capillary bleeding at the base of an advanced plaque may disrupt a fibrous cap against the much higher luminal pressure.

Fluid Dynamic Stress

High blood velocity within stenotic lesions may shear the endothelium away, but whether high wall shear stress alone may disrupt a stenotic plaque is questionable.[28] The absolute stresses induced by wall shear are usually much smaller than the mechanical stresses imposed by blood and pulse pressures[60] but are not directly comparable, as the wall shear stresses act tangentially to the endothelium while blood and pulse pressures act radially and circumferentially on the plaque surface.

Triggering of Disease Onset

Onset of acute coronary syndromes does not occur at random.[75] Myocardial infarction occurs at increased frequency in the morning, particularly within the first hour after awakening, on Mondays, during winter months and on colder days the year around, during emotional stress, and during vigorous exercise.[75-80] The pathophysiological mechanisms responsible for the nonrandom and apparently often triggered onset of myocardial infarction are unknown but probably related to: (1) *plaque disruption*, likely due to surges in sympathetic activity with a sudden increase in blood pressure, pulse rate, heart contraction, and coronary blood flow; (2) *thrombosis*, occurring on previously disrupted or intact plaques when the systemic thrombotic tendency is high because of platelet activation, hypercoagulability, and/or impaired fibrinolysis; and (3) *vasoconstriction*, generalized or occurring locally around a coronary plaque.

Plaque Thrombosis

Coronary thrombosis is the result of a dynamic interaction between the arterial wall and the flowing blood. About 75% of thrombi responsible for acute coronary syndromes are precipitated by plaque disruption whereby thrombogenic material is exposed to the flowing blood (Fig. 2).[2] Superficial plaque erosion without frank disruption, ie, no deep injury, is found beneath the remaining 25% of thrombi,[11,49,52] usually in combination with a severe atherosclerotic stenosis. There are three major determinants for the thrombotic response to plaque disruption/erosion: (1) character and extent of exposed thrombogenic plaque materials (local thrombogenic substrates); (2) degree of stenosis and surface irregularities (local flow disturbances); and (3) thrombotic—thrombolytic equilibrium at the time of plaque disruption/erosion (systemic thrombotic tendency) (Fig. 3).

Local Thrombogenic Substrates

Information on the thrombogenicity of the individual plaque components is still rather limited and it remains unclear which components or factors within the plaque are the primary initiators of the thrombotic response and which pathway(s) is (are) involved. The current opinion seems to be that the lipid-rich atheromatous gruel is the most thrombogenic plaque component, based primarily on an ex vivo study of platelet deposition on human plaque specimens exposed to flowing blood in a perfusion chamber.[4] In contrast, another study that used cryostat sections of human coronary arteries identified collagen types I and/or III as being the most reactive plaque component toward platelets.[81] The lipid-rich and soft atheromatous gruel is derived from insudated and retained serum lipids, necrotic and disintegrated cells (preferentially macrophage foam cells), and degraded extracellular matrix. It contains free cholesterol (hard crystals), cholesteryl esters (soft droplets), lipoprotein(a), phospholipids, cellular debris, and collagen degradation products. Recent studies indicate that the component responsible for the high thrombogenicity of the gruel is macrophage-derived tissue factor.[4,5,82] By use of immunohistochemical techniques, tissue-factor protein has been identified in lipid-filled macrophages (foam cells) as well as extracellularly within the atheromatous core of human carotid plaques,[5,82,83] and tissue factor content is actually increased in plaques that are responsible for unstable compared to stable angina.[84] Furthermore, not only tissue factor protein (antigen) but also its activity (by use of a factor Xa generation assay) were recently shown to be significantly higher in culprit lesions obtained by coronary atherectomy from patients with unstable angina and myocardial infarction than in those from patients with stable angina.[85] Tissue factor expressed by activated macrophages and SMCs could also be critical for the thrombotic response associated with superficial plaque erosion without frank disruption.[49,52]

Local Flow Disturbances

The severity of stenosis and surface irregularities at the site of plaque disruption influences the thrombotic response. The tighter the stenosis and the rougher the surface, the more platelets are activated and deposited.[4,46,86,87] A platelet thrombus may indeed form and grow within a severe stenosis where the blood velocity and shear forces are highest,[88] probably due to shear-induced platelet activation.[89]

Systemic Thrombotic Tendency

Thrombogenic factors such as platelet hyperaggregability, hypercoagulability, and impaired fibrinolysis are associated with increased risk of thrombus-mediated coronary events.[90] A transient or persistent hypercoagulable state, probably partly mediated by activated monocytes in the peripheral blood, can be identified in many patients with acute coronary syndromes.[91,92] The importance of the actual thrombotic-thrombolytic equilibrium at the time of plaque disruption is clearly documented by the protective effect of antiplatelet agents and anticoagulants against myocardial infarction and coronary death in patients with IHD.[90]

Dynamics of Thrombosis

The thrombotic response to plaque disruption is dynamic; thrombosis/rethrombosis and thrombolysis/embolization occur simultaneously in many patients with acute coronary syndromes, with or without concomitant vasospasm, causing intermittent flow obstructions.[2] The initial flow obstruction is usually caused by platelet aggregation, but fibrin is important for subsequent stabilization of the early and fragile platelet thrombus. Therefore, both platelets and fibrin play a role in the evolution of a persisting coronary thrombus.

Identification of Vulnerable And Active Plaques

Coronary angiography may reveal advanced lesions, plaque disruption, luminal thrombosis, and calcification, but other qualitative features cannot be assessed by this imaging technique. For identification of early lesions and nonstenotic vulnerable plaques at high risk of becoming culprits, visualization of the vessel wall and the plaque itself rather than the lumen is necessary. This may be partly accomplished by intravascular ultrasound[93–96] and angioscopy,[69,97–102] which can reveal important plaque and surface features not seen angiographically.[99,100] Magnetic resonance imaging (MRI) has shown great potential for plaque characterization in peripheral arteries and coronary arteries in vitro[103–105] and, recently, noninvasively in the carotid bifurcation in vivo.[106,107] MRI of coronary plaques might also be possible in the future, although it remains an immense technical challenge due to the relatively small size of coronary arteries and their movement during respiration and heart contraction. However, the use of ECG gating, navigator gating,[108] and dedicated surface coils or intravascular receiver coils[109,110] holds promise for the future. For clinical application in coronary artery disease, MRI must visualize the entire coronary artery tree (ie, 3-D acquisition with thin slices)[111] rather than just selected thick slices (eg, 3 to 5 mm)[106,107] from different coronary segments of interest. Otherwise, vulnerable plaques will easily be missed. MR diffusion imaging[112,113] and spectroscopy,[114,115] as well as near infrared spectroscopy[116,117] and scintigraphy,[118–122] may also be future modalities capable of improving the in vivo identification and characterization of coronary plaques.

Actively progressing atherosclerosis and vulnerable high-risk plaques are characterized by increased endothelial permeability with insudation of plasma constituents; lipoprotein accumulation; endothelial activation with expression of adhesion molecules; monocyte recruitment; macrophage retention and cell activation within lesions; denudation and ulceration of plaque surfaces with platelet adhesion/aggregation/degranulation; activation of coagulation; and ongoing fibrinolysis—features that might be visualized in living persons by appropriate imaging techniques. However, even a simple blood sample may prove to be useful in the identification of ongoing disease activity, revealing signs of inflammation[123] and activation of endothelial cells,[124] leukocytes,[91,125,126] platelets,[127] coagulation,[92,128,129] and fibrinolysis.[128–133]

Clinical Manifestations

The occurrence and course of coronary atherosclerosis and IHD are largely unpredictable.[17] For individuals with the same number and degree of stenoses evaluated angiographically, some live for years without any symptoms while others are severely handicapped by angina pectoris, experience acute coronary syndromes, or die suddenly and unexpectedly. Plaque composition, rather than plaque size or stenosis severity, is most important for event-free survival in IHD.[1-3]

Stable Angina

Hangartner et al[134] categorized the plaque type in 54 men with stable angina and found that 60% of the plaques were fibrous and 40% were lipid-rich. More interestingly, all the plaques were fibrous in 15% of the patients and not a single plaque with a large lipid pool was found in as many as one third of the patients. Apparently, many patients with stable angina lack the appropriate pathoanatomic substrate for plaque disruption and may, consequently, be at low risk of an acute coronary syndrome. It should be noted, however, that in the same patient, individual plaques usually differ significantly, and the composition of one plaque does not predict the composition of a nearby plaque in the same artery.

Silent Plaque Disruption

Plaque disruption itself is asymptomatic, and also the associated rapid plaque growth is usually clinically silent. Silent plaque disruption is probably the most important mechanism responsible for the unpredictable, sudden, and nonlinear progression of coronary lesions frequently observed angiographically.[135]

Acute Coronary Syndromes

Following plaque disruption, hemorrhage into the plaque, luminal thrombosis, and/or vasospasm may cause sudden flow obstruction, giving rise to new or changing symptoms. The culprit lesion is frequently "dynamic," causing intermittent flow obstruction, and the clinical presentation and the outcome depend on the severity and duration of myocardial ischemia. A nonocclusive or transiently occlusive thrombus most frequently underlies primary unstable angina with pain at rest and non–Q-wave infarction (often but not always subendocardial), while a more stable and occlusive thrombus is most frequently seen in Q wave infarction (often but not always transmural)—overall modified by vascular tone and collateral flow.[1] The lesion responsible for out-of-hospital cardiac arrest or sudden death is often similar to that of unstable angina: a disrupted plaque with superimposed nonocclusive thrombosis.[1,64,90]

Conclusions

Atherosclerosis without thrombosis is in general a benign disease. However, acute thrombosis frequently complicates the course of coronary atherosclerosis, causing unstable angina, myocardial infarction, and sudden death. The mechanism responsible for the sudden conversion of a stable disease to a life-threatening condition is usually plaque disruption with superimposed thrombosis. The risk of plaque disruption depends more on plaque vulnerability and thrombogenicity than on plaque size or stenosis severity; *plaque vulnerability* predisposes the plaque to rupture, and *rupture triggers* may precipitate it. The challenge of today is to identify and treat the dangerous vulnerable plaques responsible for the life-threatening acute heart attacks—to find and treat only angina-producing stenotic lesions is no longer enough. Culprit lesion-based interventions usually eliminate anginal pain but do not substantially improve the long-term outcome because myocardial infarction and death depend more on coexisting non-symptomatic vulnerable plaques than on stenotic angina-producing lesions. For prevention and treatment, a systemic approach that addresses all coronary plaques will prove to be most rewarding. Such an approach includes lipid-lowering therapy, which prevents clinical events despite the fact that most of the stenotic lesions remain unchanged.[136–140] The reduction in clinical events is, however, associated with a significant retardation in plaque progression as observed angiographically, which could reflect plaque stabilization[45,139,141] due to gradual depletion of soft lipid and matrix-degrading macrophages. However, the beneficial effect on clinical events does not occur rapidly; there is a risky lag period of several months. Therefore, research in progress focuses on how an *acutely unstable* coronary plaque can be stabilized and passivated rapidly, eg, by inhibition of matrix metalloproteinase and tissue factor expression and activity.

References

1. Fuster V, Badimon L, Badimon J, Chesebro JH. The pathogenesis of coronary artery disease and the acute coronary syndromes. *N Engl J Med* 1992; 326:242–250 and 310–318.

2. Falk E. Coronary thrombosis: Pathogenesis and clinical manifestations. *Am J Cardiol* 1991;68(suppl B):28B–35B.
3. Falk E, Shah PK, Fuster V. Coronary plaque disruption. *Circulation* 1995; 92:657–671.
4. Fernandez-Ortiz A, Badimon JJ, Falk E, et al. Characterization of the relative thrombogenicity of atherosclerotic plaque components: Implications for consequences of plaque rupture. *J Am Coll Cardiol* 1994;23:1562–1569.
5. Moreno PR, Bernardi VH, López-Cuéllar J, et al. Macrophages, smooth muscle cells, and tissue factor in unstable angina. Implications for cell-mediated thrombogenicity in acute coronary syndromes. *Circulation* 1996; 94:3090–3097.
6. Toschi V, Gallo R, Lettino M, et al. Tissue factor modulates the thrombogenicity of human atherosclerotic plaque. *Circulation* 1997;95:594–599.
7. Kragel AH, Roberts WC. Composition of atherosclerotic plaques in the coronary arteries in homozygous familial hypercholesterolaemia. *Am Heart J* 1991;121:210–211.
8. Gertz SD, Malekzadeh S, Dollar AL, et al. Composition of atherosclerotic plaques in the four major epicardial coronary arteries in patients   90 years of age. *Am J Cardiol* 1991;67:1228–1233.
9. Dollar AL, Kragel AH, Fernicola DJ, et al. Composition of atherosclerotic plaques in coronary arteries in women <40 years of age with fatal coronary artery disease and implications for plaque reversibility. *Am J Cardiol* 1991;67:1223–1227.
10. Mautner SL, Lin F, Roberts WC. Composition of atherosclerotic plaques in the epicardial coronary arteries in juvenile (type I) diabetes mellitus. *Am J Cardiol* 1992;70:1264–1268.
11. Burke AP, Farb A, Malcom GT, et al. Coronary risk factors and plaque morphology in men with coronary disease who died suddenly. *N Engl J Med* 1997;336:1276–1282.
12. Mintz GS, Pichard AD, Popma JJ, et al. Determinants and correlates of target lesion calcium in coronary artery disease: A clinical, angiographic and intravascular ultrasound study. *J Am Coll Cardiol* 1997;29:268–274.
13. Rumberger JA, Simons B, Fitzpatrick LA, et al. Coronary artery calcium area by electron- beam computed tomography and coronary atherosclerotic plaque area. A histopathologic correlative study. *Circulation* 1995;92: 2157–2162.
14. Wexler L, Brundage B, Crouse J, et al. Coronary artery calcification: Pathophysiology, epidemiology, imaging methods, and clinical implications. A statement for Health Professionals from the American Heart Association. *Circulation* 1996;94:1175–1192.
15. Khurana S, Schreiber TL, Nino CL, et al. Does coronary calcification influence plaque stability? *Circulation* 1994;90(suppl I):I–438.
16. Mann JM, Davies MJ. Vulnerable plaque. Relation of characteristics to degree of stenosis in human coronary arteries. *Circulation* 1996;94:928–931.
17. Tavazzi L, Volpi A. Remarks about postinfarction prognosis in light of the experience with the Gruppo Italiano per lo Studio della Sopravvivenza nell'Infarto miocardico (GISSI) trials. *Circulation* 1997;95:1341–1345.
18. Glagov S, Weisenberd E, Zarins C, et al. Compensatory enlargement of human atherosclerotic coronary arteries. *N Engl J Med* 1987;316:1371–1375.
19. Ge J, Erbel R, Zamorano J, et al. Coronary artery remodeling in atherosclerotic disease: An intravascular ultrasound study in vivo. *Coron Artery Dis* 1993;4:981–986.

20. Losordo DW, Rosenfield K, Kaufmann J, et al. Focal compensatory enlargement of human atherosclerotic coronary arteries in response to progressive atherosclerosis: In vivo documentation using intravascular ultrasound. *Circulation* 1994;89:2570–2577.
20a. Mintz GS, Kent KM, Pichard AD, et al. Contribution of inadequate arterial remodeling to the development of focal coronary artery stenoses. An intravascular ultrasound study. *Circulation* 1997;95:1791–1798.
21. Kragel AH, Reddy SG, Wittes JT, Roberts WC. Morphometric analysis of the composition of atherosclerotic plaques in the four major epicardial coronary arteries in acute myocardial infarction and in sudden coronary death. *Circulation* 1989;80:1747–1756.
22. Kragel AH, Reddy SG, Wittes JT, Roberts WC. Morphometric analysis of the composition of coronary arterial plaques in isolated unstable angina pectoris with pain at rest. *Am J Cardiol* 1990;66:562–567.
23. Falk E. Why do plaques rupture? *Circulation* 1992;86(suppl III): III–30–III–42.
24. Falk E. Morphologic features of unstable atherosclerotic plaques underlying acute coronary syndromes. *Am J Cardiol* 1989;63(suppl E):114E–120E.
25. Davies MJ. A macro and micro view of coronary vascular insult in ischemic heart disease. *Circulation* 1990;82(suppl II):II–38–II–46.
26. Small DM. Progression and regression of atherosclerotic lesions. Insights from lipid physical biochemistry. *Arteriosclerosis* 1988;8:103–129.
27. Lundberg B. Chemical composition and physical state of lipid deposits in atherosclerosis. *Atherosclerosis* 1985;56:93–110.
28. Gertz SD, Roberts WC. Hemodynamic shear force in rupture of coronary arterial atherosclerotic plaques. *Am J Cardiol* 1990;66:1368–1372.
29. Friedman M. The coronary thrombus: Its origin and fate. *Hum Pathol* 1971; 2:81–128.
30. Guyton JR, Klemp KF. The lipid-rich core region of human atherosclerotic fibrous plaques. Prevalence of small lipid droplets and vesicles by electron microscopy. *Am J Pathol* 1989;134:705–717.
31. Stary HC. Evolution and progression of atherosclerotic lesions in coronary arteries of children and young adults. *Arteriosclerosis* 1989;9(suppl I): I–19–I–32.
32. Geng Y-J, Libby P. Evidence for apoptosis in advanced human atheroma. *Am J Pathol* 1995;147:251–266.
33. Ball RY, Stowers EC, Burton JH, et al. Evidence that the death of macrophage foam cells contributes to the lipid core of atheroma. *Atherosclerosis* 1995;114:45–54.
34. Björkerud S, Björkerud B. Apoptosis is abundant in human atherosclerotic lesions, especially in inflammatory cells (macrophages and T cells), and may contribute to the accumulation of gruel and plaque instability. *Am J Pathol* 1996;149:367–380.
35. Witztum JL. The oxidation hypothesis of atherosclerosis. *Lancet* 1994;344: 793–795.
36. Wight TN. Cell biology of arterial proteoglycans. *Arteriosclerosis* 1989;9: 1–20.
37. Guyton JR, Klemp KF. Development of the atherosclerotic core region: Chemical and ultrastructural analysis of microdissected atherosclerotic lesions from human aorta. *Arterioscler Thromb* 1994;14:1305–1314.
38. Davies MJ, Richardson PD, Woolf N, et al. Risk of thrombosis in human atherosclerotic plaques: Role of extracellular lipid, macrophage, and smooth muscle cell content. *Br Heart J* 1993;69:377–381.

39. Wagner WD, St.Clair RW, Clarkson TB, Connor JR. A study of atherosclerosis regression in Macaca mulatta: III. Chemical changes in arteries from animals with atherosclerosis induced for 19 months and regressed for 48 months at plasma cholesterol concentrations of 300 or 200 mg/dL. *Am J Pathol* 1980;100:633–650.

40. Loree HM, Tobias BJ, Gibson LJ, et al. Mechanical properties of model atherosclerotic lesion lipid pools. *Arterioscler Thromb* 1994;14:230–234.

41. Loree HM, Kamm RD, Stringfellow RG, Lee RT. Effects of fibrous cap thickness on peak circumferential stress in model atherosclerotic vessels. *Circ Res* 1992;71:850–858.

42. Richardson PD, Davies MJ, Born GVR. Influence of plaque configuration and stress distribution on fissuring of coronary atherosclerotic plaques. *Lancet* 1989;ii:941–944.

43. Burleigh MC, Briggs AD, Lendon CL, et al. Collagen types I and III, collagen content, GAGs and mechanical strength of human atherosclerotic plaque caps: Span-wise variations. *Atherosclerosis* 1992;96:71–81.

44. Majno G, Joris I. Apoptosis, oncosis and necrosis: An overview of cell death. *Am J Pathol* 1995;146:3–15.

45. Libby P. Molecular bases of the acute coronary syndromes. *Circulation* 1995;91:2844–2850.

46. Falk E. Plaque rupture with severe pre-existing stenosis precipitating coronary thrombosis. Characteristics of coronary atherosclerotic plaques underlying fatal occlusive thrombi. *Br Heart J* 1983;50:127–134.

47. Friedman M. The coronary thrombus: Its origin and fate. *Hum Pathol* 1971; 2:81–128.

48. Constantinides P. Plaque fissures in human coronary thrombosis. *J Atheroscler Res* 1966;6:1–17.

49. van der Wal AC, Becker AE, van der Loos CM, Das PK. Site of intimal rupture or erosion of thrombosed coronary atherosclerotic plaques is characterized by an inflammatory process irrespective of the dominant plaque morphology. *Circulation* 1994;89:36–44.

50. Poston RN, Haskard DO, Coucher JR, et al. Expression of intercellular adhesion molecule-1 in atherosclerotic plaques. *Am J Pathol* 1992;140: 665–673.

51. Lendon CL, Davies MJ, Born GVR, Richardson PD. Atherosclerotic plaque caps are locally weakened when macrophages density is increased. *Atherosclerosis* 1991;87:87–90.

52. Farb A, Burke AP, Tang AL, et al. Coronary plaque erosion without rupture into a lipid core: A frequent cause of coronary thrombosis in sudden coronary death. *Circulation* 1996;93:1354–1363.

53. van der Wal AC, Becker AE, Koch KT, et al. Clinically stable angina pectoris is not necessarily associated with histologically stable atherosclerotic plaques. *Heart* 1996;76:312–316.

54. Moreno PR, Falk E, Palacios IF, et al. Macrophage infiltration in acute coronary syndromes: Implications for plaque rupture. *Circulation* 1994;90: 775–778.

55. Matrisian LM. The matrix degrading metalloproteinases. *Bioessays* 1992; 14:455–463.

56. Shah PK, Falk E, Badimon JJ, et al. Human monocyte-derived macrophages induce collagen breakdown in fibrous caps of atherosclerotic plaques. Potential role of matrix-degrading metalloproteinases and implications for plaque rupture. *Circulation* 1995;92:1565–1569.

57. Kaartinen M, Penttilä A, Kovanen PT. Accumulation of activated mast cells in the shoulder region of human coronary atheroma, the predilection site of atheromatous rupture. *Circulation* 1994;90:1669–1678.
58. Kovanen PT, Kaartinen M, Paavonen T. Infiltrates of activated mast cells at the site of coronary atheromatous erosion or rupture in myocardial infarction. *Circulation* 1995;92:1084–1088.
59. Kloner RA, Giacomelli F, Alker KJ, et al. Influx of neutrophils into the walls of large epicardial arteries in response to ischemia/reperfusion. *Circulation* 1991;84:1758–1772.
60. MacIsaac AI, Thomas JD, Topol EJ. Toward the quiescent coronary plaque. *J Am Coll Cardiol* 1993;22:1228–1241.
61. Fitzgerald JD. By what means might beta blockers prolong life after acute myocardial infarction? *Eur Heart J* 1987;8:945–951.
62. Davies MJ, Thomas AC. Plaque fissuring: The cause of acute myocardial infarction, sudden ischaemic death, and crescendo angina. *Br Heart J* 1985; 53:363–373.
63. Davies MJ, Bland JM, Hangartner JRW, et al. Factors influencing the presence or absence of acute coronary artery thrombi in sudden ischaemic death. *Eur Heart J* 1989;10:203–208.
64. Davies MJ, Thomas A. Thrombosis and acute coronary-artery lesions in sudden cardiac ischemic death. *N Engl J Med* 1984;310:1137–1140.
65. Cheng GC, Loree HM, Kamm RD, et al. Distribution of circumferential stress in ruptured and stable atherosclerotic lesions. A structural analysis with histopathological correlation. *Circulation* 1993;87:1179–1187.
66. Lee RT, Kamm RD. Vascular mechanics for the cardiologist. *J Am Coll Cardiol* 1994;23:1289–1295.
67. Stein PD, Hamid MS, Shivkumar K, et al. Effects of cyclic flexion of coronary arteries on progression of atherosclerosis. *Am J Cardiol* 1994;73: 431–437.
68. Bogaty P, Hackett D, Davies G, Maseri A. Vasoreactivity of the culprit lesion in unstable angina. *Circulation* 1994;90:5–11.
69. Etsuda H, Mizuno K, Arakawa K, et al. Angioscopy in variant angina: Coronary artery spasm and intimal injury. *Lancet* 1993;342:1322–1324.
70. Zeiher AM, Schächinger V, Weitzel SH, et al. Intracoronary thrombus formation causes focal vasoconstriction of epicardial arteries in patients with coronary artery disease. *Circulation* 1991;83:1519–1525.
71. Bertrand ME, LaBlanche JM, Tilmant PY, et al. Frequency of provoked coronary arterial spasm in 1089 consecutive patients undergoing coronary arteriography. *Circulation* 1982;65:1299–1306.
72. Kaski JC, Tousoulis D, McFadden E, et al. Variant angina pectoris. Role of coronary spasm in the development of fixed coronary obstructions. *Circulation* 1992;85:619–626.
73. Zhang Y, Cliff WJ, Schoefl GI, Higgins G. Immunohistochemical study of intimal microvessels in coronary atherosclerosis. *Am J Pathol* 1993;143: 164–172.
74. Barger AC, Beeuwkees R. Rupture of coronary vaso vasorum as a trigger of acute myocardial infarction. *Am J Cardiol* 1990;66(suppl G):41G–43G.
75. Muller JE, Abela GS, Nesto RW, Tofler GH. Triggers, acute risk factors and vulnerable plaques: The lexicon of a new frontier. *J Am Coll Cardiol* 1994;23:809–813.
76. Mittleman MA, Maclure M, Tofler GH, et al. Triggering of acute myocardial infarction by heavy physical exertion: Protection against triggering by regular exertion. *N Engl J Med* 1993;329:1677–1683.

77. Willich SN, Lewis M, Löwel H, et al. Physical exertion as a trigger of acute myocardial infarction. *N Engl J Med* 1993;329:1684–1690.
78. Mittleman MA, Maclure M, Sherwood JB, et al. Triggering of acute myocardial infarction onset by episodes of anger. *Circulation* 1995;92: 1720–1725.
79. Muller JE, Mittleman A, Maclure M, et al. Triggering myocardial infarction by sexual activity. Low absolute risk and prevention by regular physical exertion. *JAMA* 1996;275:1405–1409.
80. Leor J, Poole WK, Kloner RA. Sudden cardiac death triggered by an earthquake. *N Engl J Med* 1996;334:413–419.
81. van Zanten GH, de Graaf S, Slootweg PJ, et al. Increased platelet deposition on atherosclerotic coronary arteries. *J Clin Invest* 1994;93:615–632.
82. Wilcox JN, Harker LA. Molecular and cellular mechanisms of atherogenesis: Studies of human lesions linked with animal modelling. In: Bloom AL, Forbes CD, Thomas DP, Tuddenham EGD eds: *Haemostasis and Thrombosis.* London: Churchill Livingstone; 1994:1139–1152.
83. Wilcox JN, Smith KM, Schwartz SM, Gordon D. Localization of tissue factor in the normal vessel wall and in the atherosclerotic plaque. *Proc Natl Acad Sci U S A* 1989;86:2839–2843.
84. Moreno PR, Bernardi VH, López-Cuéllar J, et al. Macrophages, smooth muscle cells, and tissue factor in unstable angina. Implications for cell-mediated thrombogenicity in acute coronary syndromes. *Circulation* 1996; 94:3090–3097.
85. Ardissino D, Merlini PA, Ariëns R, et al. Tissue-factor antigen and activity in human coronary atherosclerotic plaques. *Lancet* 1997;349:769–771.
86. de Cesare NB, Ellis SG, Williamson PR, et al. Early reocclusion after thrombolysis is related to lesion length and roughness. *Coron Artery Dis* 1993; 4:159–166.
87. Folts J. An in vivo model of experimental arterial stenosis, intimal damage, and periodic thrombosis. *Circulation* 1991:83(suppl IV):IV–3–IV–14.
88. Badimon L, Badimon JJ. Mechanism of arterial thrombosis in non-parallel streamlines: Platelet thrombi grow on the apex of stenotic severely injured vessel wall. *J Clin Invest* 1989;84:1134–1144.
89. Ruggeri ZM. Mechanisms of shear-induced platelet adhesion and aggregation. *Thromb Haemost* 1993;70:119–123.
90. Fuster V, Lewis A. Connor Memorial Lecture: Mechanisms leading to myocardial infarction: Insights from studies of vascular biology. *Circulation* 1994;90:2126–2146.
91. Jude B, Agraou B, McFadden EP, et al. Evidence for time-dependent activation of monocytes in the systemic circulation in unstable angina, but not in acute myocardial infarction or in stable angina. *Circulation* 1994;90: 1662–1668.
92. Merlini PA, Bauer KA, Oltrona L, et al. Persistent activation of coagulation mechanism in unstable angina and myocardial infarction. *Circulation* 1994; 90:61–68.
93. Nissen SE, Gurley JC, Grines CL, et al. Intravascular ultrasound assessment of lumen size and wall morphology in normal subjects and patients with coronary artery disease. *Circulation* 1991;84:1087–1099.
94. Roelandt JRTC, di Mario C, Pandian NG, et al. Three-dimensional reconstruction of intracoronary ultrasound images. Rationale, approaches, problems, and directions. *Circulation* 1994;90:1044–1055.
95. Hodgson JM, Reddy KG, Suneja R, et al. Intracoronary ultrasound imag-

ing: Correlation of plaque morphology with angiography, clinical syndrome, and procedural results in patients undergoing coronary angioplasty. *J Am Coll Cardiol* 1993;21:35–44.

96. Ge J, Erbel R, Gerber T, et al. Intravascular ultrasound imaging of angiographically normal coronary arteries: A prospective in vivo study. *Br Heart J* 1994;71:572–578.

97. Baptista J, de Feyter P, di Mario C, et al. Stable and unstable anginal syndromes: Target lesion morphology prior to coronary interventions using angiography, intra-coronary ultrasound, and angioscopy. *Eur Heart J* 1994;15(abstract suppl):321.

98. Nesto RW, Sassower MA, Manzo KS, et al. Angioscopic differentiation of culprit lesions in unstable versus stable coronary artery disease. *J Am Coll Cardiol* 1993;21(suppl A):195A.

99. Tabata H, Mizuno K, Arakawa K, et al. Angioscopic identification of coronary thrombus in patients with postinfarction angina. *J Am Coll Cardiol* 1995;25:1282–1285.

100. Uchida Y, Nakamura F, Tomaru T, et al. Prediction of acute coronary syndromes by percutaneous coronary angioscopy in patients with stable angina. *Am Heart J* 1995;130:195–203.

101. Thieme T, Wernecke KD, Meyer R, et al. Angioscopic evaluation of atherosclerotic plaques: Validation by histomorphologic analysis and association with stable and unstable coronary syndromes. *J Am Coll Cardiol* 1996;28:1–6.

102. Waxman S, Sassower MA, Nesto RW. Characterization of the culprit lesion underlying thrombus: Insights from angioscopy. *Circulation* 1995;92(suppl I):I–353.

103. Toussaint JF, Southern JF, Fuster V, Kantor HL. T_2-weighted contrast for NMR characterization of human atherosclerosis. *Aterioscler Thromb Vasc Biol* 1995;15:1533–1542.

104. Martin AJ, Gotlieb AI, Henkelman, RM. High-resolution MR imaging of human arteries. *J Magn Reson Imaging* 1995;5:93–100.

105. Yuan C, Mitsumori LM, Reinecke D, et al. Magnetic resonance imaging techniques which identify and distinguish between lipid- and calcium-rich regions of human coronary atherosclerotic plaques. *Proceedings 1997 ISMRM Fifth Annual Meeting*. Abstract 790.

106. Yuan C, Murakami JW, Hayes CE, et al. Phased-array magnetic resonance imaging of the carotid artery bifurcation: Preliminary results in healthy volunteers and a patient with atherosclerotic disease. *J Magn Reson Imaging* 1995;5(5):561–565.

107. Toussaint JF, LaMuraglia GM, Southern JF, et al. Magnetic resonance images lipid, fibrous, calcified, hemorrhagic, and thrombotic components of human atherosclerosis in vivo. *Circulation* 1996;94:932–938.

108. McConnel MV, Goldfarb JW, Manning WJ, Edelman RR. High-resolution black-blood coronary MR imaging using navigator gating. *Proceedings 1997 ISMRM Fifth Annual Meeting*. Abstract 797.

109. Ataler E, Bottomley PA, Ocali O, et al. High resolution intravascular MRI and MRS by using a catheter receiver coil. *Magn Reson Med* 1996;36:596–605.

110. Quick HH, Zimmermann GG, Erhart P, et al. 'In vivo' high resolution intravascular imaging with a single loop receiver coil. *Proceedings 1997 ISMRM Fifth Annual Meeting*.

111. Luk Pat GT, Gold GE, Hu BS, Nishimura DG. High-resolution 3D imaging

of atherosclerotic plaque. *Proceedings 1997 ISMRM Fifth Annual Meeting.* Abstract 791.
112. Shinnar M, Fallon JT, Wehrli S, et al. Diffusion weighted MRI better characterizes atherosclerotic plaque and thrombus. *Circulation* 1996;94(suppl I):I-345.
113. Toussaint JF, Southern JF, Fuster V, Kantor HL. Water diffusion properties of human atherosclerosis and thrombosis measured by pulse field gradient nuclear magnetic resonance. *Arterioscler Thromb Vasc Biol* 1997;17: 542–546.
114. Toussaint JF, Southern JF, Fuster V, Kantor HL. 13C-NMR spectroscopy of human atherosclerotic lesions: Relation between fatty acid saturation, cholesteryl ester content , and luminal obstruction. *Arterioscler Thromb* 1994;14:1951–1957.
115. Lo W, Shehan M, Appleberg M, et al. Distinction of complex necrotic and simple carotid plaques by 1H MRS. *Proceedings 1997 ISMRM Fifth Annual Meeting.* Abstract 1293.
116. Baraga JJ, Feld MS, Rava RP. In situ optical histochemistry of human artery using near infrared Fourier transform Raman spectroscopy. *Proc Natl Acad Sci U S A* 1992;89:3473–3477. 117. Manoharan R, Baraga JJ, Rava RP, et al. Biochemical analysis and mapping of atherosclerotic human artery using FT-IR microspectroscopy. *Atherosclerosis* 1993; 103(2): 181–193.
118. Vallabhajosula S, Paidi M, Badimon JJ, et al. Radiotracers for low density lipoprotein biodistribution studies in vivo: Technetium-99m low density lipoprotein versus radioiodinated low density lipoprotein preparations. *J Nucl Med* 1988;29:1237–1245.
119. Lees AM, Lees RS, Schoen FJ, et al. Imaging human atherosclerosis with ^{99m}Tc-labeled low density lipoproteins. *Arteriosclerosis* 1988;8:461–470.
120. Lupatelli G, Fedeli L, Fiacconi M, et al. Scintigraphic detection of atherosclerosis by means of radiolabeled lipoproteins. *Thromb Haemorrh Disorders* 1991;3;sh2:61–65.
121. Lees RS, Lees AM. Radiopharmaceutical imaging of active atherosclerosis. *Atherosclerosis* 1994;109(suppl):352.
122. Miller DD, Rivera FJ, Garcia OJ, et al. Imaging of vascular injury with ^{99m}Tc-labeled monoclonal antiplatelet antibody S12: Preliminary experience in human percutaneous angioplasty. *Circulation* 1992;85:1354–1363.
123. Liuzzo G, Biasucci LM, Gallimore JR, et al. The prognostic value of C-reactive protein and serum amyloid A protein in severe unstable angina. *N Engl J Med* 1994;331:417–424.
124. Wada H, Mori Y, Kaneko T, et al. Elevated plasma levels of vascular endothelial cell markers in patients with hypercholesterolemia. *Am J Hematol* 1993;44:112–116.
125. Leatham EW, Bath PMW, Tooze JA, Camm AJ. Increased monocyte tissue factor expression in coronary disease. *Br Heart J* 1995;73:10–13.
126. Biasucci LM, D'Onofrio G, Liuzzo G, et al. Neutrophil activation in unstable angina and acute myocardial infarction is possible marker of inflammation and of disease activity. *Eur Heart J* 1994;15(abstract suppl):472.
127. Lam JY, Latour JG, Lesperance J, Waters D. Platelet aggregation, coronary artery disease progression and future coronary events. *Am J Cardiol* 1994; 73:333–338.
128. Meade TW, Ruddock V, Stirling Y, et al. Fibrinolytic activity, clotting factors, and long- term incidence of ischaemic heart disease in the Northwick Park Heart Study. *Lancet* 1993;342:1076–1079.

129. Herren T, Stricker H, Haeberli A, et al. Fibrin formation and degradation in patients with arteriosclerotic disease. *Circulation* 1994;90:2679–2686.
130. Fowkes FG, Lowe GD, Housley E, et al. Cross-linked fibrin degradation products, progression of peripheral artery disease, and risk of coronary heart disease. *Lancet* 1993;342:84–86.
131. Jansson JH, Olofsson BO, Nilsson TK. Predictive value of tissue plasminogen activator mass concentration on long-term mortality in patients with coronary artery disease: A 7–year follow-up. *Circulation* 1993;88: 2030–2034.
132. Ridker PM, Vaughan DE, Stampfer MJ, et al. Endogenous tissue-type plasminogen activator and risk of myocardial infarction. *Lancet* 1993;341: 1165–1168.
133. Ridker PM, Hennekens CH, Cerskus A, Stampfer MJ. Plasma concentration of cross-linked fibrin degradation product (D-dimer) and the risk of future myocardial infarction among apparently healthy men. *Circulation* 1994;90:2036–2240.
134. Hangartner JRW, Charleston AJ, Davies MJ, Thomas AC. Morphological characteristics of clinically significant coronary artery stenosis in stable angina. *Br Heart J* 1986;56:501–508.
135. Bruschke AVG, Kramer JR, Bal ET, et al. The dynamics of progression of coronary atherosclerosis studied in 168 medically treated patients who underwent coronary arteriography three times. *Am Heart J* 1989;117: 296–305.
136. Group SSSS. Randomized trial of cholesterol lowering in 4444 patients with coronary heart disease: The Scandinavian Simvastatin Survival Study (4S). *Lancet* 1994;344:1383–1389.
137. Shepherd J, et al, for the West of Scotland Coronary Prevention Study Group. Prevention of coronary heart disease with pravastatin in men with hypercholesterolemia. *N Engl J Med* 1995;333:1301–1307.
138. Sacks FM, et al, for the Cholesterol and Recurrent Events Trial Investigators. The effect of pravastatin on coronary events after myocardial infarction in patients with average cholesterol levels. *N Engl J Med* 1996;335: 1001–1009.
139. Blankenhorn DH, Hodis HN. Arterial imaging and atherosclerosis reversal. *Arterioscler Thromb* 1994;14:177–192.
140. Simoons ML, Vos J, Deckers JW, de Feyter PJ. Clinical perspective. Coronary artery disease: Prevention of progression and prevention of events. *Eur Heart J* 1995;16:729–733.
141. Brown BG, Zhao XQ, Sacco DE, Albers JJ. Lipid lowering and plaque regression: New insights into prevention of plaque disruption and clinical events in coronary disease. *Circulation* 1993;87:1781–1791.

Chapter 2

Pathobiology of Symptomatic Carotid Atherosclerosis

Hisham S. Bassiouny, MD,
Yasuhiro Sakaguchi, MD, Catherine A. Goudet, PhD,
Ray Vito, PhD, and Seymour Glagov, MD

Introduction

It is estimated that approximately 40% to 50% of retinal and hemispheric ischemic events are related to embolic debris and thrombi originating from atherosclerotic plaque and involving the carotid bifurcation.[1] In recent years investigations have focused on better understanding of the pathobiology of plaque formation at the carotid bifurcation, and its natural history. Biomechanical forces have been shown to play a role in the induction and localization of early intimal atherosclerotic lesions. However, the role of such physical forces in plaque progression and disruption remains to be elucidated. It is yet clear, that unless plaques exhibit histopathological features that connote structural vulnerability, plaque fatigue and disruption is unlikely.

Critically stenotic carotid plaques are morphologically complex. The clinical recognition and detection of those morphological features which connote plaque instability and predisposition to disruption and symptoms is a desired goal. Insight into these microanatomic features can be gained by detailed examination of excised endarterectomy plaques from symptomatic and asymptomatic patients.

In this chapter, several features of carotid plaque induction and

This work was supported by grants from the National Heart, Lung, and Blood Institute of the United States Public Health Service (HL 15062 SCOR - Atherosclerosis and R01-HL55296-01) and Grant-In-Aide from the American Heart Association.

From: Fuster, V (ed). *The Vulnerable Atherosclerotic Plaque: Understanding, Identification, and Modification.* Armonk, NY: Futura Publishing Company, Inc.; © 1999.

evolution are discussed. First, the role of biomechanical forces in early plaque formation at the carotid bifurcation is described. With plaque progression, the artery wall exhibits reactive defense mechanisms designed to isolate the plaque, preserve lumen size and configuration, and restore artery wall structure. The adaptive modeling responses to the developing plaque are presented. Finally, the morphological features associated with carotid plaque disruption and symptoms and the location of peak stress in relation to the distribution of plaque components is reviewed.

Biomechanical Forces and Localization of Carotid Atherosclerosis

The pathogenesis of the carotid atherosclerosis has been inferred from observations into the morphology of human plaques,[2–4] from the study of experimental animals models, and from the reactions of artery cells in culture. Recent increased attention to the geometric, microanatomic (artery wall), and mechanical (hemodynamic) microenvironment in which human plaques develop has added significant insights into the tissue processes associated with artery reactions and adaptations to plaque formation and to questions dealing with plaque stability.[3,5–7] The sequence of events leading to plaque formation is complex and probably variable in relation to the degree and duration of exposure to each of the clinical risk factors, and more than likely, it includes the interaction of several processes. There is now abundant evidence that the endothelial cell is not merely a protective barrier against thrombus formation. Endothelial cells are active mediators of many aspects of artery wall function. It is also clear that the initiating events in plaque formation are not precipitated by focal ulcerations of the lumen surface or by desquamations of endothelial cells.[8] Instead, focal activation of endothelial cells by circulating vasoactive and/or toxic materials engenders modifications in endothelial function.[9] These result in alterations of permeability; in oxidative modification of the low-density lipoprotein (LDL) particle; in the liberation of chemoattractants, mitogens, and growth factors that determine migration and proliferation of smooth muscle cells, expression of surface adhesion molecules for leukocytes, disturbances of the antithrombogenic function, as well as of factors such as nitric oxide and endothelin-1, which regulate smooth muscle tone in the underlying media. These modifications are reflected in the early intimal lesion in the form of lipid accumulation in extracellular interstices and within both macrophages and smooth muscle cells in the form of foam cells.[3] Smooth muscle cell accumulation and fibrogenesis are prominent features. In addition to smooth muscle cells,[3] macrophages and lymphocytes also participate in lesion formation and in the modification of plaque composition by elaboration of growth factors, cytokines, and proteolytic enzymes. These features, as well as evidence of cell necrosis, apoptosis, and stratification of lesion components, indicate that both destructive and defensive modeling healing processes are occurring.

Plaques tend to develop in locations where wall shear stress is relatively low and changes direction in the course of the cardiac cycle.[10,11] In model studies[12] as well as in color Doppler images in humans (Fig. 1), such regions are demonstrably sites of increased residence time for circulating particles; that is, particles tend to remain in these regions over several cardiac cycles, exposing such sites to increased contact with atherogenic agents compared with regions where wall shear stress is elevated and unidirectional. Because flow reversal at such regions occurs during the downstroke of systole, increased heart rate, over time, is likely to be an additional indirect clinical risk factor for plaque induction.[13,14]

In the Framingham Study heart rate was a recognized independent risk factor in human cardiovascular events and mortality.[15] Experimentally, animals subjected to repeated psychosocial stress demonstrate differences in cardiovascular responsiveness and heart rate. Animals with a high heart rate have more extensive coronary and carotid atherosclerosis than less responsive animals.[16,17] Conversely, lowering the heart rate by means of sinoatrial node ablation or drugs reduces both coronary and carotid atherosclerosis.[14,18] It is proposed that the frequency of shear stress oscillation, which is heart rate dependent, enhances plaque localization in regions of the arterial tree, where flow reversal during end systole is a characteristic feature of the flow velocity profile. With increasing heart rate there is a relative increase in time spent in systole per minute relative to diastole because of the shortening of diastolic time. In regions of the arterial tree such as the infrarenal aorta and the outer wall of the carotid bifurcation, where systolic hemodynamic events such as flow reversal and shear stress oscillation occur, high heart rate is associated with longer periods of zero, negative, and low shear stress levels. Evidence has been presented that regions of relatively low wall shear stress are regions of increased endothelial permeability, whereas areas subjected to high shear stress are less permeable. Oscillation in shear stress direction may perturb intercellular junctions, thereby increasing permeability of the endothelial monolayer and favoring ingress of atherogenic particles.

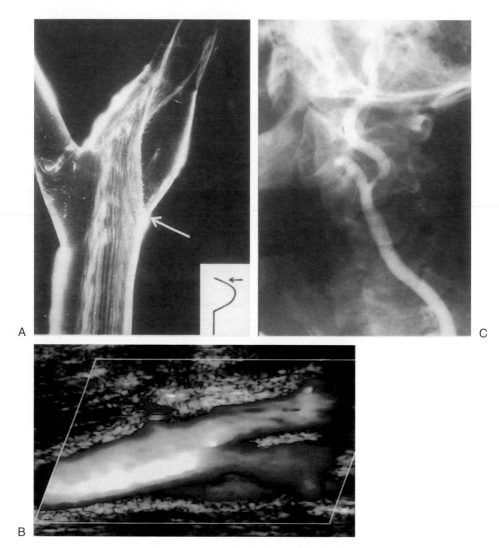

Figure 1. A. Model flow study of carotid bifurcation. **B.** During the ascending phase of systole, flow departs from its laminar profile along with the outer wall of this carotid sinus, creating a recirculation region where wall shear stress is relatively low. In vivo color duplex imaging of a normal carotid bifurcation demonstrates this zone of flow reversal (blue area). **C.** The susceptible human carotid bifurcation sinus region for plaque formation.

Adaptive and Modeling Reactions to Plaque

Artery wall stability depends on the maintenance of normal or otherwise acceptable levels of wall shear stress and tensile stress. Wall shear stress is a direct function of blood flow and viscosity and varies inversely with the third power of the radius. When flow is increased for long periods of time, artery radius increases until the original baseline wall shear stress is restored. For mammalian arteries this value is approximately 15 dynes/cm.[3,19–21] When flow is decreased, the radius decreases also, resulting in restoration of baseline wall shear stress. As regards tensile stress, artery wall thickness is determined by blood pressure and artery radius in accordance with the law of Laplace. In simplified form, for arteries with thin walls compared to radius, wall tension is proportional to the product of pressure and radius and tensile stress is equal to wall tension divided by the wall thickness. In mammalian development, the thickness of the walls of homologous arteries of similar structure is proportional to the wall tension such that tensile stress is maintained at a baseline level. In the event of reduced flow, and therefore of reduced wall shear stress, thickening of the intima may serve to narrow the lumen, thereby increasing flow and restoring baseline wall shear stress. In the event of adjustments to long-term increases in flow, the increased radius results in an increase in wall tension. Tensile stress may be restored to baseline levels or to levels consistent with wall stability by thickening of the wall and/or by changes in structure and composition of the media. There is evidence, however, both from animal experimental models[22] and from human vessels,[23–25] that the intima may participate in these adaptations.

As a plaque enlarges, the artery usually enlarges, often preserving a patent and adequate lumen despite the presence of a large and advanced complex lesion.[26,27] The nature of this compensatory reaction is not entirely clear but is closely associated with outward bulging of the artery wall beneath the evolving plaque (Fig. 2). This effect is noted at nearly all stages of plaque formation, and the uninvolved wall opposite the plaque may remain largely unchanged. As with the formation of atherosclerosis-related aneurysms, the changing wall contour[26,28] beneath the plaque may result from erosion by metalloproteinases liberated from smooth muscle cells and/or macrophages and accumulated in the lipid core.[29] The limits of compensatory enlargement and outward bulging beneath the lesion may be related to progression of plaque density and rigidity and resistance to proteolysis related to changes in plaque and wall composition and to calcification.

Thus, several morphological manifestations of putative artery defense against the development of stenosis and flow instability are noted as plaques progress. The lumen tends to remain circular and of regular

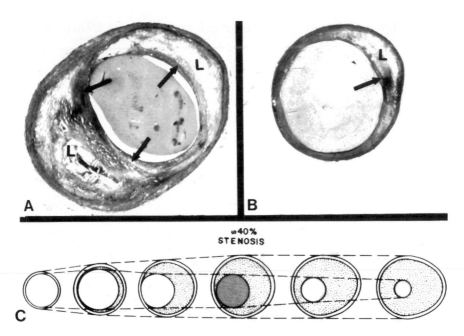

Figure 2. In relation to the modeling and remodeling processes described, arteries appear to enlarge initially as plaques form, tending to preserve a lumen in adequate cross section, even in the presence of relatively large intimal plaques. **A.** Postmortem sections of the left anterior descending coronary artery taken at the same level in two individuals. The lumen cross-sectional area (L) is approximately the same for each individual, although the lesion area is vastly different. If the artery on the left had not enlarged to compensate for the large plaque that formed, the lumen would have been totally occluded. That artery enlargement is a consequence of plaque formation is indicated by the fact that in any given artery segment, lumen cross-sectional area is often similar for involved and uninvolved segments. Enlargement occurs only where plaques are forming. **B.** Diagram of artery enlargement with plaque formation based on a study of the human left main coronary artery. Although plaque formation may be arrested at any stage, lumen stenosis appears to be evidence on the average when 40;pc or more of the potential lumen area (as defined by the area encompassed by internal elastic lamina), is occupied by plaque. Plaque enlargement is mainly associated with outward bulging of the artery wall beneath the lesion. Reprinted with permission.

contour as the eccentric lesion is effectively sequestered by fibrosis and outward bulging of the underlying artery wall. The fibrous cap isolates the lesion from the circulation and its structure suggests an adaptive modeling reaction which results in what appears to be the neoformation of a supportive media-like structure. Both the outward compensatory bulging process and possibly-flow related processes which may cause dilation of the preserved wall opposite the plaque tend to preserve an adequate lumen in the face of advancing disease.

The sequence of morphological features set forth above is an idealized representation of the characteristic intimal changes associated with plaque formation. It should be noted however that deviations and modifications of these transitions are frequent. Atherosclerotic lesions may stabilize and persist with little subsequent change at any of the advanced stages outlined above, ie, plaques do not necessarily or inevitably evolve to more complex types. Furthermore, advanced lesions beyond the atheroma stage may contain regions that are characteristic of earlier or later types. Such features are usually due to focal alterations associated with plaque regression, with healing reactions following plaque disruptions, or with secondary plaque formation.

Morphological and Cellular Features That Underlie Carotid Plaque Disruption

Much of our information about the composition and complication of advanced plaques is derived from the examination of highly stenotic endarterectomy specimens. Although tight stenoses correspond to large, complex plaques, it should be emphasized that images of lumen diameter on angiograms provide information regarding comparative degrees of lumen narrowing but do not provide an accurate appraisal of lesion cross-sectional area, volume, or composition.[25-27] This limitation is due to the compensatory enlargement of arteries where plaques form, as noted above, to changes in lumen size due to modifications of plaque modeling and composition, to the occurrence of plaque disruptions and ulcerations, to erosions of the underlying media, and to the formation and organization of thrombi. Focal irregularities and depressions at the lumen surface do not necessarily portend the presence of current ulcerations, as examination of many endarterectomy specimens and corresponding angiograms indicate that these may be regions of healing where previous thrombi or ulcerations may have occurred.

Although severe atherosclerotic disease at the carotid bifurcation frequently presents clinically as transient ischemic attacks or stroke, marked degrees of stenosis can be detected in the absence of such symptoms. Tissue vibrations created by turbulent flow distal to tight stenoses may be detected as *bruits* on physical examination and flow velocity profiles characteristic of stenoses can be detected using duplex Doppler methods. Angiography and magnetic resonance imaging may also provide information on lumen configuration. As noted above, tight stenoses are associated with the presence of large complex plaques, which tend to be complicated by ulceration, calcification, hematoma, and thrombus formation even when manifest symptoms are not present clinically.[30-31] Preemptive excision of such lesions and comparison with those removed because of retinal or cerebrovascular clinical events have permitted studies that provide insights into the nature of the morphological changes associated with symptoms.

Table 1

Symptomatic and Asymptomatic Carotid Endarterectomies
with Critical Stenosis (>80%)

	Lipid related		
	DNA (ng/mg)	Cholesterol (μg/mg)	Lipase (μM/mim/g)
Sympt	182 ± 28	82 ± 18	56 ± 15
Asympt	206 ± 50	77 ± 13	73 ± 28
	Connective tissue related		
	Collagen (μg*/mg)	Collagenase (cpm/hr/g)	Elastase (cpm/hr/g)
Sympt	10 ± 1	190 ± 37	350 ± 50
Asympt	11 ± 1	285 ± 84	519 ± 84

* = hydroxyproline

Chemical and Structural Composition of Critical Symptomatic and Asymptomatic Carotid Stenoses

Determination of the chemical composition of highly stenotic lesions has failed to reveal any significant differences between symptomatic and asymptomatic plaques (Table 1). Specimens with little or only moderate stenosis that are not associated with evidence of clinical symptomatology may be obtained at autopsy and compared with findings in stenotic endarterectomy specimens.[25,31-33] In view of the axial variation in lesion composition and complication, such correlations require detailed sequential sampling. Our own studies are based on sections of the entire bifurcation taken at 0.5-cm intervals, ie, on 6 to10 sections of each specimen. We have compared the morphological evidences of plaque complication in endarterectomy specimens of highly stenotic plaques (terectomy plaques associated with clinical symptoms were compared with those without clinical symptoms and with the moderately stenotic plaques. One or more of the complicating features was noted in most of the specimens. Evidence of a necrotic core was present in 58% of the highly stenotic specimens and in only 12% of those with little or moderate narrowing. Ulceration was evident in 53% of the highly stenotic specimens but in only 6% of the moderately stenotic samples. Hematoma, usually within an associated necrotic core, or evidence of previous hemorrhage or hematoma in the form of collections of siderophages was noted in 73% of the highly stenotic, but in only 41% of the moderately narrowed asymptomatic plaques. Calcification was a common finding, noted in 84% of the tight stenoses and 53% of the moderately narrowed arteries. These differences were significant at the $P<0.05$ to $P<0.01$ level for each finding. Thus, plaques associated with tight stenoses were more complicated than those associated with moderate stenoses.

When only the asymptomatic highly stenotic plaques were compared with the asymptomatic moderately stenotic postmortem specimens, the comparisons gave similar results. Necrotic core was evident in 50% of those with tight stenosis and in 12% of those with little or moderate stenosis. Ulceration was present in 43% of the highly stenotic and only 6% of the moderately stenotic plaques. Hematoma was evident in 86% of the tightly stenotic and 41% of the moderately stenotic plaques. Calcification was present in 71% of the tightly stenotic and in 53% of the moderately stenotic plaques. There were no significant differences between highly stenotic symptomatic and highly stenotic asymptomatic plaques with respect to the incidence of these complications.

These results indicate that carotid plaque complexity and predisposition to potential complications, ie, disruption, thrombosis, hemorrhage, and embolic events, are related to plaque burden and degree of luminal stenosis. Conversely, evidence is presented[34,35] which indicates that coronary plaque disruption and superimposed thrombosis may be independent of the degree of luminal stenosis occurring in soft lipid-laden plaques producing moderate stenoses. This contrast between carotid and coronary plaques may be related to differences in the susceptibility of each respective vascular bed to the various atherogenic risk factors and to differences in the imposed biomechanical factors. For example, coronary plaques are subjected to cyclical bending and flexing forces by virtue of the epicardial course of the coronary arteries, while the carotid bifurcation is spared from such solid mechanical stress.

Plaque Component Spatial Distribution and Clinical Outcome

Atherosclerotic plaque disruption is considered a salient feature critical to the development of clinical ischemic manifestations in both the coronary and carotid circulation.[36–38] Although the structural features of advanced atherosclerotic plaques as well as the biomechanical forces imposed on them have been extensively studied, the relevance of particular features of plaque morphology to fibrous cap erosion and plaque complications such as thrombosis, embolization, and intraplaque has yet to be determined. As noted above, carotid plaques associated with symptomatic and asymptomatic critical stenosis have similar morphological and chemical features. Morphological complexity appears to be related to the plaque size, regardless of symptoms.[31]

Conversely, other investigators have observed that carotid artery plaques in symptomatic patients contained more soft cholesterol amorphous debris and hemorrhage and less collagenous material when compared to those in asymptomatic patients.[39–41] Recognized limitations inherent to the aforementioned studies are a lack of precise quantitation of the individual components of the plaque and inconsistencies with regards to the selected sampling site.

As previously mentioned, the presence of inflammatory cell infiltration has been associated with or proposed as a major factor in unstable, symptom-producing carotid and coronary plaques,[42–44] and is related to degradation of the fibrous cap and plaque neoformation. A variety of biomechanical factors have also been postulated to play a role in plaque disruption. These include mechanical stresses associated with hemodynamic wall shear or pressure fluctuations.[45–48] While advanced symptomatic and asymptomatic carotid plaques contain similar fibrous, necrotic, and calcific components, we have postulated that the spatial distribution of these individual components in relation to the lumen and the extent of inflammatory cell infiltration, in particular macrophage foam cell in the abluminal fibrous cap, could connote plaque neoformation and discriminate between symptomatic and asymptomatic potential. We have examined a large number of symptomatic and asymptomatic aortic plaques with similar degrees of stenosis removed at endarterectomy.[49] In view of the relationship between plaque complexity, ie, the presence of a diversity of plaque components, and plaque size or degree of stenosis, histologic sections from the most stenotic region of these plaques, with respect to the relative quantity and location of the various plaque components and the proximity of these elements to each other and the lumen surface, were evaluated (Fig. 3). The degree of macrophage infiltration in and about the fibrous cap as a measure of likely plaque neoformation was also measured.

Indications for operation were symptomatic disease in 59 instances (including hemispheric transient ischemic attack in 29, stroke in 19, and amaurosis fugax in 11) and angiographic asymptomatic stenosis greater than 70% in 40. Plaques removed after remote symptoms beyond 6 months were excluded. Histologic sections from the most stenotic region of the plaque were examined by use of computer-assisted morphometry. The percent-area of plaque cross section occupied by necrotic lipid core with or without associated plaque hematoma, by calcification, and the distance from the lumen and/or fibrous cap of each of these features, was determined. The presence of foam cells, macrophages, and/or inflammatory cell collections within, upon, or just beneath the fibrous cap was taken as an additional indication of plaque neoformation.

Mean percent angiographic lumen diameter reduction was 82 ± 11 and 79 ± 13 for the asymptomatic and symptomatic groups, respec-

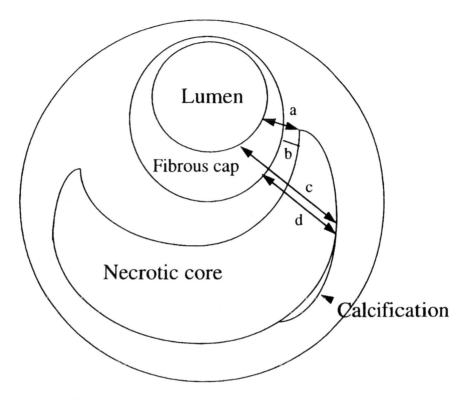

Figure 3. Computer-assisted morphometric analysis of plaque cross sections. Individual plaque components are contour-traced and distance between each component and fibrous cap and lumen were measured. a and b = distance between necrotic core and fibrous cap or lumen; c and d = distance between calcification and fibrous cap or lumen. Reprinted from Reference 49, with permission.

tively ($P<0.05$). The necrotic core was twice as close to the lumen in symptomatic plaques than in asymptomatic plaques (0.27 ± 0.3 versus 0.5 ± 0.5, respectively; $P<0.01$) (Table 2). Percent-area of necrotic core or calcification was similar for both groups (22% versus 26% and 7% versus 6%, respectively) (Table 3). There was no significant relationship to symptom production of either the distance of calcification from the lumen or of the percent-area occupied by the lipid necrotic core or calcification. The number of macrophages infiltrating the region of the fibrous cap was three times greater in symptomatic plaques compared to asymptomatic plaques. Regions of fibrous cap disruption or ulceration were more commonly observed in symptomatic than in asymptomatic plaques (32% versus 20%). None of the demographic or clinical

Table 2

Distance of Plaque Components from Fibrous Cap and Lumen

	All patients (n = 99)	Symptomatic (n = 59)	Asymptomatic (n = 40)	P
N1 (mm)	0.2 ± 0.3	0.05 ± 0.2	0.20 ± 0.3	0.01
N2 (mm)	0.4 ± 0.7	0.27 ± 0.3	0.50 ± 0.5	0.01
C1 (mm)	0.5 ± 0.9	0.55 ± 1.1	0.05 ± 0.3	NS
C2 (mm)	0.8 ± 1.0	0.78 ± 1.3	0.27 ± 1.0	NS

N1 = Distance between necrotic core and fibrous cap; N2 = distance between necrotic core and lumen; C1 = distance between calcification and fibrous cap; C2 = distance between calcification and lumen. Values expressed as mean ± SD.

atherosclerosis risk factors distinguished between symptomatic and asymptomatic plaques.[49]

It is evident from these findings that the proximity of the necrotic core to the overlying fibrous cap and lumen rather than its absolute or percent cross-sectional area is a striking feature of symptomatic plaques. In symptomatic plaques (Fig. 4), the necrotic core was twice as close to the lumen as in asymptomatic plaques (Fig. 5), while the degree or location of calcification had little effect. Thus, the spatial relationship among the matrix and necrotic components appears to be most important in defining likely plaque stability rather than content of these elements. These findings likely represent the dynamic equilibrium which exists among factors that favor fibrogenesis versus those that induce matrix degradation.[50]

Symptomatic plaques also appear to a greater degree of macrophage infiltration in and about the fibrous cap and have been associated

Table 3

Plaque Component Area

	All patients (n = 99)	Symptomatic (n = 59)	Asymptomatic (n = 40)	P
Plaque area (mm^2)	35% ± 12%	35% ± 11%	35% ± 13%	NS
Percent stenosis	81% ± 12%	79% ± 13%	82% ± 11%	NS
Percent necrotic core	21% ± 18%	22% ± 16%	26% ± 18%	NS
Percent calcification	7% ± 11%	7% ± 10%	6% ± 10%	NS
Percent fibrous cap	10% ± 6%	11% ± 6%	10% ± 6%	NS

Values expressed as mean ± SD of mean.

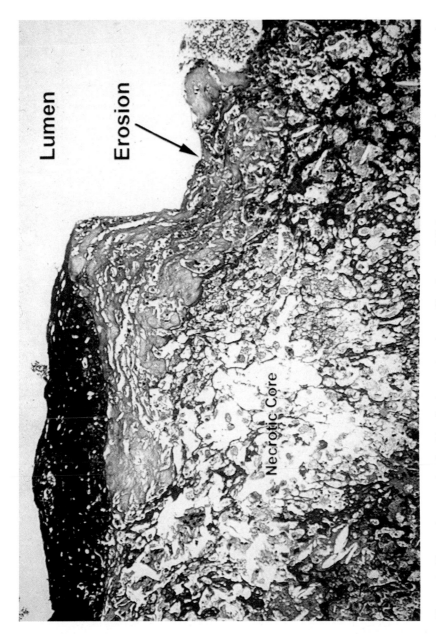

Figure 4. Photomicrograph of a histologic section (magnification × 25) in a symptomatic plaque representing fibrous cap thinning and erosion with exposure of the necrotic core to the lumen.

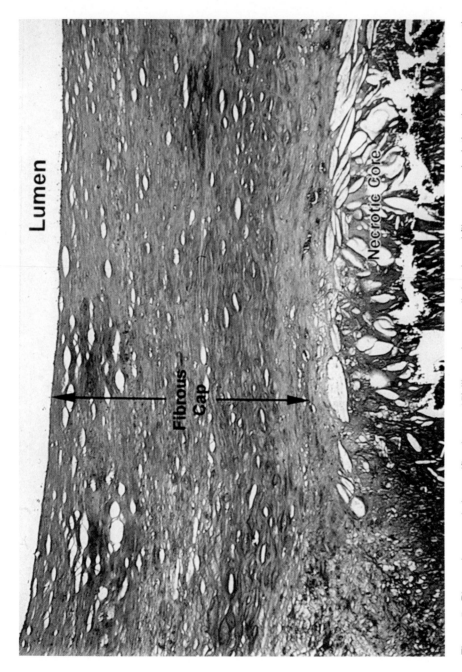

Figure 5. Photomicrograph (magnification × 15) illustrating a well-developed fibrous cap isolating the plaque necrotic core from the lumen in an asymptomatic plaque.

with fibrous cap thinning and erosion, implicating an ongoing induction of plaque formation and/or an inflammatory or immune mediated response as a factor in plaque instability. Other investigators have also noted that ruptured plaques are infiltrated by foam cells, especially in regions where the fibrous cap is thinnest. [37,38,43,44,51]

Foam cells derived from mononuclear phagocytes in atherosclerotic plaques are known to elaborate a number of matrix metalloproteinases such as interstitial collagenase, gelatinase and stromelysin, all of which are capable of degrading collagen, elastin, and proteoglycans.[52-55] Such processes could lead to thinning of the fibrous cap and disruption, particularly if potent mechanical stresses are present. We are currently investigating the contribution of macrophage infiltration and apoptosis to the relative activity of metalloproteinases and tissue inhibitors of metalloproteinases. Preliminary results indicate that the apoptotic rate is proportional to the number of infiltrating macrophages and related to symptomatic disease and position of the necrotic core within the plaque. Macrophage infiltration and apoptosis may modulate lesion progression and necrosis by the release of injurious free radicals and other mitogenic and tissue necrosis factors.[56-59]Activated macrophages may also induce a prothrombotic effect by inhibiting tissue plasminogen activators and thereby enhancing the thrombotic complications associated with complex atherosclerotic plaques.[60]

It is interesting to note that plaque complications such as intraplaque hematoma and surface thrombosis, although characteristic of large advanced plaques, did not discriminate between symptomatic and asymptomatic plaques and appeared to represent events probably secondary to plaque fissuring or disruption of the fibrous cap.

Relation Between Plaque Component Distribution and Location of Peak Stress

The potential role of biomechanical forces in the induction of structural fatigue of plaque constituents and the localization of plaque neoformation and inflammatory cell responses is under study. Marked elevation of wall shear stress occurs within a stenosis associated with large plaques. Although high shear may inhibit plaque formation,[61] changes in flow dynamics associated with marked stenoses, including wall vibration, flutter, and cyclical collapse,[62] could induce disruptions within plaques, lumen ulcer formation, and associated surface irregularities. Vito and others[63,64] have emphasized the relationship between plaque composition and the location of peak stress.

Conditions under which mechanical factors induce disruptions in susceptible fragile plaques are not well understood. The use of finite element analysis in the study of stress distribution in plaque cross sections from carotid bifurcation endarterectomy specimens has revealed that stresses are greatest within the fibrous cap. In addition, proximity of the necrotic lipid core or macrophages to the fibrous cap, particularly to thinned regions of the cap, significantly increases both the peak stress and the stress gradient. Movement of the lipid core closer to the fibrous cap has been demonstrated to increase the maximum stress by more than 60%, while the presence of discrete calcifications increased the peak stress by up to 70% and displaced its focus to within the plaque. Thus, the distribution of plaque constituents, particularly the necrotic core and calcification regions, appears to determine both the location and the magnitude of the peak stress within the plaque and therefore the propensity for plaque rupture.

Conclusions

In conclusion, the spatial distribution of individual carotid plaque components in relation to the lumen, rather than overall plaque composition, is an important determinant of plaque disruption and symptoms. In particular, proximity of the necrotic core to the lumen and carotid plaque neoformation are strong markers associated with clinical ischemic events. Further fibrous cap thinning and erosion is observed with macrophage infiltration and apoptosis. This inflammatory response induces matrix degradation and appears to play a role in plaque rupture, embolic, and thrombotic events.

Identification of high-risk stenoses prone to disruption will require (1) detailed 3-D reconstruction of carotid plaques from histology and ultrasound to better define the relationship of the individual plaque components to the lumen in vivo; and (2) investigation of the solid mechanical properties of plaques in relation to structure to map the distribution of peak stenoses within the different components of the plaque.

References

1. Pressin MS, Duncan GW, Mohr JP, Poskanzer DC. Clinical and angiographic features of carotid transient ischemic attacks. *N Engl J Med* 1977; 296:358.
2. Stary HC. Changes in components and structure of atherosclerotic lesions developing from childhood to middle age in coronary arteries. *Basic Res Cardiol* 1994;89(suppl I):17.
3. Stary HC, Blankenhorn DH, Chandler AB, et al. A definition of initial, fatty streak and intermediate lesions of arteriosclerosis. *Circulation* 1994;89:2462.
4. Stary HC, Chandler AB, Dinsmore RE, et al. A definition of advanced types

of atherosclerotic lesions and a histological classification of atherosclerosis. *Arterioscler Thromb Vasc Biol* 1995;15(9):1512–1531.

5. Glagov S, Zarins CK, Giddens DP. Mechanical factors in the pathogenesis, localization and evolution of atherosclerotic plaques. In: Camilleri JP, Berry CL, Fiessinger J-N, et al eds: *Diseases of the Artery Wall*. London: Springer-Verlag; 1989:217.

6. Glagov S, Zarins CK, Giddens DP, et al. Establishing the hemodynamic determinants of human plaque configuration, composition and complication. In: Yoshida Y, Yamaguchi CG, Caro S, et al eds: *Role of Blood Flow in Atherogenesis*. New York: Springer-Verlag; 1988:3–10.

7. Glagov S, Zarins CK, Giddens DP, et al. Hemodynamics and atherosclerosis: Insights and perspectives gained from studies of human arteries. *Arch Pathol Lab Med* 1988;112:1018.

8. Taylor KE, Glagov S, Zarins CK. Preservation and structural adaptation of endothelium over experimental foam cell lesions: A quantitative ultrastructural study. *Arteriosclerosis* 1989;9:881.

9. Ross R. The pathogenesis of atherosclerosis: A perspective for the 1990s. *Nature* 1993;362:801.

10. Ku DN, Zarins CK, Giddens DP, et al. Pulsatile flow and atherosclerosis in the human carotid bifurcation: Positive correlation between plaque localization and low and oscillating shear stress. *Arteriosclerosis* 1985;5:292.

11. Zarins CK, Giddens DP, Bjaradaj BK, et al. Carotid bifurcation atherosclerosis: Quantitative correlation of plaque localization with flow velocity profiles and wall shear stress. *Circ Res* 1983;53:502.

12. Ku DN, Giddens DP. Pulsatile flow in a model carotid bifurcation. *Arteriosclerosis* 1983;3:31.

13. Beere PA, Glagov S, Zarins CK. Experimental atherosclerosis at the carotid bifurcation of the cynomolgus monkey: Localization, compensatory enlargement and the sparing effect of heart rate. *Arterioscler Thromb* 1992;12:1245.

14. Beere PA, Glagov S, Zarins CK. Retarding effect of lowered heart rate on coronary atherosclerosis. *Science* 1984;226:180.

15. Kannel W, Kannel C, Paffenbarge R, et al. Heart rate and cardiovascular mortality: The Framingham Study. *Am Heart J* 1987;113:1489–1494.

16. Kaplan JR, Clarkson TB. Social instability and coronary artery atherosclerosis in cynomolgus monkeys. *Neurosci Biobehav Rev* 1983;7:486–491.

17. Bassiouny H, Zarins C, Hovanessian A, et al. Heart rate and experimental carotid atherosclerosis. *Surg Forum Volume XLIII*, 1992.

18. Kaplan J, Manuck S, Adams M, et al. Inhibition of coronary atherosclerosis by propranolol in behaviorally predisposed monkeys fed an atherogenic diet. *Circulation* 1987;76:1364–1372.

19. Clark JM, Glagov S. Transmural organization of the arterial wall: The lamellar unit revisited. *Arteriosclerosis* 1985;5:19–34.

20. Kamiya A, Togawa T. Adaptive regulation of wall shear stress to flow change in the canine aortic artery. *Am J Physiol* 1990;239:H14–H21.

21. Zarins CK, Zatina MA, Giddens DP, et al. Shear stress regulation of artery lumen diameter in experimental atherogenesis. *J Vasc Surg* 1987;5:413–420 synthetic response with medial tension. Circulation Res 41:316–323, 1977.

22. Bassiouny HS, Lieber BB, Giddens DP, et al. Quantitative inverse correlation of wall shear stress with experimental intimal thickening. *Surgical Forum* 1988;39:328–330.

23. Zarins CK, Giddens DP, Bharadvaj BK, et al. Carotid bifurcation atheroscle-

rosis: Quantitative correlation of plaque localization with flow velocity profiles and wall shear stress. *Circ Res* 1983;53:502–514.

24. Masawa N, Glagov S, Zarins CK. Quantitative morphologic study of intimal thickening at the human carotid bifurcation. I. Axial and circumferential distribution of maximum intimal thickening in asymptomatic uncomplicated plaques. *Atherosclerosis* 1994;107:137–146.

25. Masawa N, Glagov S, Zarins CK. Quantitative morphologic study of intimal thickening at the human carotid bifurcation. II. The compensatory enlargement response and the role of the intima in tensile support. *Atherosclerosis* 1994;107:147–155.

26. Glagov S, Weisenberg E, Zarins CK, et al. Compensatory enlargement of human atherosclerotic coronary arteries. *N Engl J Med* 1987;316:1371–1375.

27. Zarins CK, Weisenberg E, Kolettis G, et al. Differential enlargement of artery segments in response to enlarging atherosclerosis plaques. *J Vasc Surg* 1988;7:386–394.

28. Ko C, Glagov S, Zarins CK. Structural basis for the compensatory enlargement of arteries during early atherogenesis. In: Gorgatti E ed: *Proceedings of the 3rd International Workshop on Vascular Hemodynamics (Bologna, 1991).* Centro Scientifico Editore; 1992:157–161.

29. Evans CH, Georgescu HI, Lin CW, et al. Inducible synthesis of collagenase by cells of aortic origin. *J Surg Res* 1991;42:328–330.

30. Hatsukami TS, Thackray BD, Primozich JF, et al. Echolucent regions in carotid plaque: Prelaminar analysis comparing three-dimensional histologic reconstructions to sonographic findings. *Ultrasound Med Biol* 1994; 20(8):743–749.

31. Bassiouny HS, Davis H, Masawa N, et al. Critical carotid stenosis: Morphological and chemical similarity between symptomatic and asymptomatic plaques. *J Vasc Surg* 1989;9:202–212.

32. Masawa N, Glagov S, Zarins CK. Quantitative morphologic study of intimal thickening at the human carotic bifurcation. I. Axial and circumferential distribution of maximum intimal thickening in asymptomatic uncomplicated plaques. *Atherosclerosis* 1994;107:137–146.

33. Glagov S, Masawa N, Bassiouny H, et al. Morphologic bases for establishing end-points for early plaque detection and plaque stability. *Int J Card Imaging* 1995;4:1–7.

34. Ambrose J, Nembaum D, Alexopoulos D. Angiographic progression of coronary artery disease and the development of myocardial infarction. *J Am Coll Cardiol* 1988;12:56.

35. Little WC, Constantinescu M, Applegate RJ, et al. Can coronary angiography predict the site of a subsequent myocardial infarction in patients with mild to moderate coronary artery disease? *Circulation* 1988;78:1157–1166.

36. Carr SA, Farb A, Pearce WH, et al. Atherosclerotic plaque rupture in symptomatic carotid artery stenosis. *J Vasc Surg* 1996;23:755–765.

37. Falk E. Why do plaques rupture? *Circulation* 1992;86:(suppl III):30–42.

38. Falk E, Shah PK, Fuster V. Coronary plaque disruption. *Circulation* 1995; 92:657–671.

39. Feely TM, Leen EJ, Colgan MP, et al. Histologic characteristics of the carotid artery plaque. *J Vasc Surg* 1991;13:719–724.

40. Seeger JM, Klingman N. The relationship between carotid plaque composition and neurologic symptoms. *J Surg Res* 1987;43:78–85.

41. Geroulakos G, Ramaswami G, Nicolaides A, et al. Characterization of symptomatic and asymptomatic carotid plaques using high-resolution real-time ultrasonography. *Br J Surg* 1993;80(10):1274–1277.

42. Hansson GK, Jonasson L, Seifert PS, et al. Immune mechanisms in athero-sclerosis. *Arteriosclerosis* 1989;9:567–578.
43. Mazzone A, De Servi S, Ricevuti G, et al. Increased expression of neutrophil and monocyte adhesion molecules in unstable coronary artery disease. *Circulation* 1993;88:358–363.
44. Moreno PR, Falk E, Palacios IF, et al. Macrophage infiltration in acute coronary syndromes: Implications for plaque rupture. *Circulation* 1994;90: 775–778.
45. Gertz SD, Robert WC. Hemodynamic shear forces in rupture of coronary arterial atherosclerotic plaque. *Am J Cardiol* 1990;66:1368–1372.
46. Loree HM, Kamm RD, Atkinson CM, et al. Turbulent pressure fluctuation on surface of model vascular stenosis. *Am J Physiol* 1991;261:H664–H650.
47. Binns RL, Ku DN. Effect of stenosis on wall motion: A possible mechanism of stroke and transient ischemic attack. *Arteriosclerosis* 1989;261: H644–H650.
48. Muller JE, Rofler GH, Stone PH. Circadian variation and triggers of onset of acute cardiovascular disease. *Circulation* 1989;79:733–743.
49. Bassiouny HS, Sakaguchi Y, Mikucki SA, et al. Juxtalumenal location of plaque necrosis and neoformation in symptomatic carotid stenosis. *J Vasc Surg* 1997;26:589–594.
50. Hennerici M, Trockel U, Rautenberg W, et al. Spontaneous progression and regression of small carotid atheroma. *Lancet* 1985;1(8443):1415–1419.
51. Lendon CL, Davies MJ, Born GVR, et al. Atherosclerotic plaques are locally weakened when macrophage density is increased. *Atherosclerosis* 1991;87: 87–90.
52. Welgus HG, Campbell EJ, Cury JD, et al. Differential susceptibility of type X collagen to cleavage by two mammalian interstitial collagenases and 72–KD a type IV collagenase. *J Biol Chem* 1990;265:13521–13527.
53. Chin JR, Murphy G, Werb Z. Stromelysin, a connective tissue degrading metalloendopeptidase secreted by stimulated rabbit synovial fibroblasts in parallel with collagenase. *J Biol Chem* 1985;260:12367–12376.
54. Henney AM, Wakekey PR, David MJ, et al. Location of stromelysin gene in atherosclerotic plaques using in situ hybridization. *Proc Nat Acad Sci U S A* 1991;88:8154–8158.
55. Brown DL, Hibbs MS, Kearney M, et al. Expression and cellular location of 92 Kda gelatinase in coronary lesions of patients with unstable angina. *J Am Coll Cardiol* 1994;Special Issue 123A. Abstract.
56. Galis ZS, Sukhova GK, Lark MW, et al. Increased expression of matrix metalloproteinases and matrix degrading activity in vulnerable regions of human atherosclerotic plaques. *J Clin Invest* 1994;94:2493–2503.
57. Tipping PG, Hancock WW. Production of tumor necrosis factor and interleukin-1 by macrophages from human atheromatous plaques. *Am J Pathol* 1993;142:1721–1728.
58. Clinton SK, Underwood R, Hayes L, et al. Macrophage colony-stimulating factor gene expression in vascular cells and in experimental and human atherosclerosis. *Am J Pathol* 1992;140:301–306.
59. Geng Y, Libby P. Evidence for apoptosis in advanced human atheroma: Colocalization with interleukin-b-converting enzyme. *Am J Pathol* 1995;147: 251–226.
60. Emeis JJ, Kooistra T. Interleukin and lipopolysaccharide induce an inhibitor of tissue-type plasminogen activator in vivo and in cultured endothelial cells. *J Exp Med* 1986;163:1260–1266.

61. Zarins CK, Bomberger RA, Glagov S. Local effects of stenoses: Increased flow velocity inhibits atherogenesis. *Circulation* 1981;64:221–227.
62. Cancelli C, Pedley TJ. A separated flow model for collapsible rube oscillations. *J Fluid Mech* 1985;157:375–404.
63. Vito RP, Whang MC, Giddens DP, et al. Stress analysis of the diseased arterial cross-section, ASME. *Adv Bioeng Proc* 1990;273–276.
64. Richardson PD, Davies MJ, Born GVR. Influence of plaque configuration and stress distribution and fissuring of coronary atherosclerotic plaque. *Lancet* 1989;2:941–944.

Chapter 3

The Vulnerable Plaque:
Aortic Disease

Ian N. Hamilton, Jr., MD
and Larry H. Hollier, MD

Introduction

An aortic atherosclerotic plaque may remain asymptomatic or cause devastating consequences. Complicated atherosclerotic aortic lesions may be responsible for damage to the aorta itself or to the organs and tissues supplied by the aorta and its branches. Injury to tissues supplied by the aorta may result from atheromatous or cholesterol embolization presenting as transient ischemic attack or stroke, renal or visceral microembolization, and cutaneous or lower extremity microembolization. Complicated atherosclerotic lesions may damage the aorta through the formation of intramural hematoma, limited aortic dissection, pseudoaneurysm formation, or aneurysmal degeneration. This chapter reviews the pathophysiology and treatment of complicated aortic atherosclerotic plaques.

Aortic Atherosclerosis

The term *atherosclerosis* was coined by Marchand in 1904 to denote the characteristics of arterial lesions consisting of a soft central atheroma (*porridge* or *gruel* in Greek) and an overlying firm (sclerotic) fibrous cap.[1] Atherosclerotic lesions are distinct, well-delineated focal changes of the intima of large elastic and medium-sized muscular distributing arteries. Conventionally, atherosclerotic lesions may be classified as early, advanced, or complicated.[1] It has been proposed that the compo-

From: Fuster, V (ed). *The Vulnerable Atherosclerotic Plaque: Understanding, Identification, and Modification.* Armonk, NY: Futura Publishing Company, Inc.; © 1999.

nents of the earliest lesion, the fatty streak, which itself is not clinically significant, are also responsible for the latter events leading to clinically significant atherosclerotic lesions.[2] Advanced lesions are the hallmark of atherosclerosis. These clinically important lesions project considerably above the intimal surface and may contain almost exclusively fibrous tissue or a central atheroma.[1] Complicated lesions are atherosclerotic plaques characterized by the presence of calcification, ulceration, thrombosis, or hemorrhage.[1] Calcification of an atherosclerotic plaque may be observed in the atheroma, the fibrous cap, or in both. When severely calcified, the tissue of the fibrous cap may crack, forming a fissure. On the other hand, ulceration results when a portion of the overlying fibrous cap is lost. In both circumstances, but especially in the presence of ulceration, the contents of the atheroma may be discharged through the intimal discontinuity into the aortic circulation in the form of atheromatous or cholesterol emboli. Ulcerated atherosclerotic lesions may also be the site for deposition of mural thrombi. Hemorrhage into an atherosclerotic plaque may result from rupture of thin-walled capillaries in the base of the lesion, rupture of adjacent vasa vasorum, or as a result of arterial (luminal) blood entering the substance of a preexisting ulceration or fissure of an atherosclerotic plaque.[1]

Pathophysiology and Treatment of the Complicated Aortic Atherosclerotic Plaque

Calcification, ulceration, thrombosis, and hemorrhage characterize the complicated atherosclerotic plaque. Complicated aortic plaques may be responsible for systemic embolization, aortic intramural hematoma formation, limited aortic dissection, pseudoaneurysm formation, aortic rupture, and aneurysmal degeneration.

Systemic Embolization

Complicated atherosclerotic lesions of the ascending aorta and aortic arch may be responsible for cerebral infarction. Similar lesions of the descending thoracic aorta may be responsible for visceral and renal ischemia. Lastly, complicated plaques in the infrarenal abdominal aorta may be responsible for diffuse microembolization to the lower trunk and extremities, with livido reticularis of the buttocks, thighs, legs, and feet.[3]

Risk Factors

Risk factors commonly found among patients suffering systemic embolization from an aortic source include greater than or equal to

60% carotid artery stenosis (16%),[4] diabetes mellitus (18% to 28%),[4,5] smoking (24% to 98%),[3,4] cerebral vascular disease (29% to 47%),[3,5] hypercholesterolemia (31% to 36%),[4,6] hypertension (48% to 64%),[5,6] male gender (49% to 73%),[4,6] coronary artery disease (58% to 75%),[3,6] and advanced age (65 to 74 years).[4,5] Additional risk factors include the performance of an invasive arteriographic study (27.8% of patients with visceral embolization)[3] and coumadin therapy (22% of patients with visceral embolization).[3]

When detected, aortic atherosclerotic plaques have been shown to be a stronger predictor of coronary artery disease than were conventional risk factors including age, male gender, smoking, diabetes mellitus, and hypertension.[6] Ascending aorta and aortic arch atheroma have also been demonstrated to be significant risk factors for cerebral ischemia independent of high-grade carotid artery stenosis.[4,5,7]

Lesion Location

In patients with coronary artery disease, transesophageal echocardiography has demonstrated the distribution of atherosclerotic plaques in the thoracic aorta to include, in the order of frequency, the descending thoracic aorta (90 of 97 patients), the aortic arch (77 of 97 patients), and the ascending aorta (36 of 97 patients).[6] The distribution of complicated atherosclerotic plaques in the same subset of patients with coronary artery disease was similar, with these high-risk lesions located most frequently in the descending thoracic aorta (56 of 97 patients), followed by the aortic arch (39 of 97 patients). There were no complicated plaques found in the ascending aorta in this study.[6] Similarly, in 18 patients with 29 aortic ulcers, thoracic and abdominal aortic imaging with computed tomography, magnetic resonance imaging, and aortography demonstrated that the most common sites of aortic ulceration were the distal descending thoracic aorta (31%), infrarenal aorta (25%), mid-descending thoracic aorta (17%), proximal descending thoracic aorta (14%), suprarenal aorta (10%), and aortic arch (3%).[8]

Cerebral Embolization

The etiology of extracranial cerebral ischemia includes embolization from or thrombosis of atherosclerotic lesions, embolization from cardiac sources, fibromuscular dysplasia, arteritides, aneurysm, radiation damage, trauma, hematologic disorders, hypertensive hemorrhage, and severe systemic hypertension.[9] Among atherosclerotic lesions, complicated plaques in the aortic arch have recently been shown to be an independent risk factor for systemic embolization similar to that of atrial fibrillation and severe atherosclerosis of the carotid arteries.[10] Necropsy studies that examine the proximal part of the arterial system including the thoracic aorta, carotid arteries, and major cerebral arteries have shown 40 of 120 consecutive specimens to have pathological evidence of arterial embolization.[10] Among 215 consecutive patients with a first stroke or transient ischemic attack, thoracic aortic atheroma as demonstrated by transesophageal echocardiography was found to be an independent risk factor for cerebral ischemia.[4] Furthermore, multivariate analysis demonstrated a statistically significant association between the degree of aortic atheroma and the occurrence of stroke. In addition, after adjusting for other accepted risk factors for stroke, including atrial fibrillation, hypertension, smoking, echocardiographically demonstrated cardiac source of embolism, as well as carotid vascular disease, both simple and complicated aortic atheroma remain significant independent risk factors for ischemic stroke or transient cerebral ischemia.[4] In an attempt to determine the risk of recurrent cerebral ischemia Amarenco and colleagues[7] followed 331 patients 60 years of age or older who were admitted to the hospital with brain infarction. Transesophageal echocardiography was serially performed for a period of 2.4 years. The patients were divided into three groups according to the thickness of the wall of the aortic arch wall (<1 mm, 1mm to 3.9 mm, and ≥4 mm), thus stratifying the lesion associated risk for embolization.[7] Aortic plaques greater than or equal to 4 mm in thickness (including the thickness of the aortic wall) were found to be independent predictors of recurrent brain infarction, after adjustment for the presence of carotid stenosis, atrial fibrillation, and peripheral arterial disease. These data were confirmed by DiTullio et al[5] when they used biplane transesophageal echocardiography to assess for the presence of aortic atheroma in 106 patients with acute ischemic stroke and in 114 stroke-free control subjects. They found proximal aortic atheromas greater than or equal to 0.5 cm in size to be an independent risk factor for ischemic stroke in patients aged 60 years or older. Additionally, ulcerated or mobile atheromas of the proximal aorta (mid or distal aortic arch) were also more frequent in stroke patients (12% versus 5%) than in control subjects.[5] Large aortic atheromas were independently associated with ischemic stroke even after adjustment for variables typically associated with stroke, such as age, atrial fibrillation, history of coronary artery disease, and diabetes.

The best therapeutic approach to patients with symptomatic proximal aortic atheromas is, as of yet, still undefined. Anticoagulation as a means for reducing the embolic potential of complicated aortic lesions has not been proven. In fact, the safety of anticoagulation in patients with complicated lesions has traditionally been questioned for fear that it might induce bleeding into the atheroma, lead to further ulceration, and increase the risk of embolization.[5] Anticoagulation may facilitate microembolization of cholesterol crystals by removing the thrombin coating from ulcerated atheromas.[3] The role of antiplatelet agents in this condition is also unclear, however the majority of stroke patients without compelling indications for formal anticoagulation are treated with long-term aspirin for secondary prevention of vascular events. Therefore, antiplatelet agents may be the most appropriate therapy for the prevention of subsequent embolization from complicated atheromatous aortic plaques as well.[4] Surgical removal of echocardiographically demonstrated atheromatous debris in the aortic arch has been described in patients with recurrent embolic symptoms and may be an option in selected good-risk patients.[4] Surgery could also be considered for highly mobile masses that appear to have a particularly great embolic potential as determined by real-time echocardiography. Experimental use of lipid-lowering agents and calcium antagonists has been shown to prevent progression or to induce regression of atheroma in coronary arteries, however, this has not been investigated in the human aorta.[4] It is tempting to speculate that complicated atherosclerotic lesions of the proximal aorta may soon be selectively treated with endovascular techniques including stents, stent grafts, and mechanical removal of masses or debris with significant embolic potential.

Visceral and Lower Extremity Embolization

Spontaneous peripheral and visceral embolization from diffuse aortic atherosclerotic disease has been termed *the shaggy aorta syndrome*.[3] Distinct from the focal embolization of thrombotic material originating from the atrium, laminated ventricular thrombus, and aortic or popliteal aneurysm, diffuse atheromatous embolization is a result of multiple and recurrent microembolizations arising from extensive atheromatous ulceration in the descending thoracic and abdominal aorta.

Pathological examination of the luminal surface of such an aorta reveals extensive atheromatous disease with advanced plaques, diffuse ulceration, and soft, loosely held debris with a paucity of actual thrombus. Originally, aortography demonstrated a spiculated and irregular appearance to the luminal surface of such a diffusely diseased aorta. However, the role of aortography in the precipitation of the diffuse embolic event has been realized. In patients with diffuse atheromatous ulcerations, a guide wire or catheter inserted through the femoral artery and passed retrograde into the abdominal and thoracic aorta has been responsible for dislodging extensive atheromatous debris as it creates a furrow along the wall of the diseased aorta.[3] More recently, computed tomography, including spiral and three-dimensional computed tomography scanning,[11] magnetic resonance imaging,[12] and three-dimensional transabdominal ultrasound,[13] have been used to noninvasively evaluate the aorta in patients at risk for embolic complications of conventional aortography.

The clinical features of the shaggy aorta syndrome may include peripheral embolization alone, visceral embolization alone, or both visceral and peripheral embolization.[3] Atheromatous embolization to the visceral vessels may cause renal failure, pancreatitis, or bowel infarction. This phenomenon is recognized by a rise in serum creatinine, by pancreatitis, and by intestinal embolization with the risk of sepsis and the development of multiorgan failure. In a 27-year review, 88 patients, each with a clinical course compatible with a diagnosis of shaggy aorta syndrome, were reviewed.[3] Fifty-two patients presented with diffuse microembolization to the lower trunk with livido reticularis of the buttocks, thighs, legs, and feet. This included multiple ischemic toes in those with lower extremity embolization. The remaining 36 patients had evidence of diffuse renal or visceral microembolization; all except two of these patients also had diffuse peripheral embolization. Prior to 1985, nine patients were treated nonoperatively. Three of these patients died within a week of presentation, due to multiorgan failure. An additional five patients died within 5 years, due to progressive renal and intestinal embolization. Only one patient remained alive at the time of publication with no treatment and with no evidence of recurrent embolization. There was an 88.8% mortality rate among those patients treated nonoperatively.

Surgical therapy was undertaken 28 times in 27 patients with an overall mortality of 33.3%. Six patients died following direct aortic operations. All of these patients had preexisting renal dysfunction as a result of atheroembolization preoperatively. An additional two patients died 4 months and 13 months postoperatively because of complications due to renal dysfunction. Two patients suffered recurrent embolization postoperatively.

As a result of this initial experience of direct aortic replacement in this high-risk subset of patients, treatment evolved to include axillo-bifemoral bypass with external iliac artery ligation in seven patients in the latter years of this review. Among this group of seven patients there was one operative death secondary to multisystem organ failure attributable to the original embolic event. No surviving patients developed recurrent peripheral or visceral emboli following axillo-bifemoral bypass with external iliac artery ligation. These patients were not maintained on any form of postoperative anticoagulation. Concomitant lumbar sympathectomy was performed in 20 patients in an attempt to improve cutaneous blood flow to the skin of the feet in those with gangrenous or pregangrenous toes. Only one patient required major lower extremity amputation; three patients underwent one or more toe amputations with complete healing.

Subsequent to this experience, axillo-bifemoral bypass with ligation of the external iliac arteries has been recommended as a safer alternative for the prevention of recurrent embolization in those patients with suprarenal lesions, as opposed to the morbidity and mortality associated with direct aortic replacement procedures.[3]

Penetrating Atherosclerotic Aortic Ulcers

In 1986 Stanson et al[14] described the penetrating atherosclerotic aortic ulcer as a distinct clinical and pathological entity in which aortic ulceration penetrated the internal elastic lamina into the media, resulting in a variable amount of intramural hematoma formation (Fig. 1). Additionally, penetrating aortic ulcers have been shown to be associated with intramural aortic hemorrhage, pseudoaneurysm formation, and aneurysmal dilatation.

The risk factors for patients with penetrating atherosclerotic aortic ulcers are similar to those patients presenting with systemic embolization from complicated aortic atheromas. The average age is 73 years

AORTIC ATHEROSCLEROTIC ULCERS

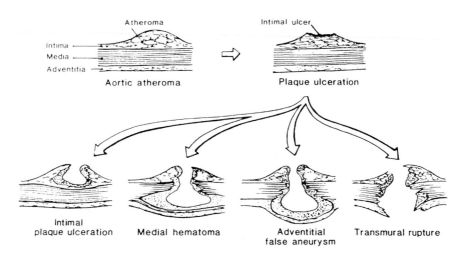

Figure 1. The spectrum of pathology of a penetrating atherosclerotic aortic ulcer. Reprinted from Reference 14, with permission.

with a high incidence of hypertension, coronary artery disease, smoking, hyperlipidemia, coexistent coronary artery disease, peripheral vascular disease, and cerebral vascular disease. Clinically, most patients present with symptoms of chest, epigastric, or back pain which may frequently be confused with acute aortic dissection. However, penetrating atherosclerotic aortic ulcer may be differentiated from acute aortic dissection by the absence of pulse deficits, the absence of aortic insufficiency, the absence of cerebrovascular insufficiency, and the absence of diminished blood flow in the visceral vessels.[15,18]

The imaging methods currently available for the diagnosis and follow-up of patients with penetrating atherosclerotic aortic ulcers include computed tomography, conventional aortography, and magnetic resonance imaging. Although the clinical presentation of penetrating aortic ulceration may be confused with acute aortic dissection, the imaging findings of penetrating aortic atherosclerotic ulcers differ from those of acute aortic dissection. The imaging studies of acute aortic dissection frequently demonstrate a false lumen, an intimal flap, and inward displacement of intimal calcifications. However, rather than a false lumen with intimal flap as seen in acute aortic dissection, a penetrating aortic ulcer may demonstrate an intramural hematoma with associated wall thickening on computed tomography (Fig. 2) and magnetic resonance imaging. Additionally, computed tomography may

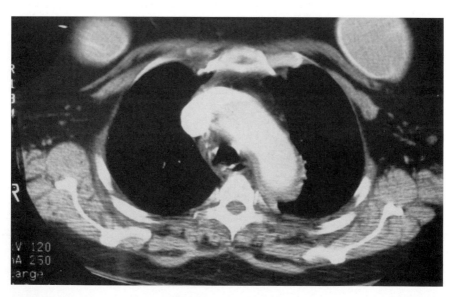

Figure 2. CT scan demonstrating an aortic intramural hematoma in the proximal descending thoracic aorta.

also demonstrate the sight of the penetrating ulcer. Computed tomography and magnetic resonance imaging may also demonstrate saccular aneurysms or pseudoaneurysms associated with an aortic ulceration.[14] Contrast-enhanced computed tomography has emerged as the primary imaging modality in this setting.[8]

The natural history of a penetrating atherosclerotic aortic ulcer may include intramural hematoma formation, limited aortic dissection, pseudoaneurysm formation, aortic rupture, and progressive aneurysmal dilatation. Stanson and associates[14] described the presence of intramural hematoma extending from an aortic ulcer in 10 of 14 patients undergoing surgical treatment. However, only one patient was described as having an extensive dissection. Harris et al[8] described only 1 of 18 patients with an aortic ulcer found to have a concomitant dissection originating from the atherosclerotic ulcer in a follow-up period of 1 to 7 years. Although some degree of intramural hematoma occurs in most ulcers, propagation of the dissection is probably prevented because of extensive fibrosis of the aortic wall from atherosclerosis.[8] Aortic pseudoaneurysm formation associated with penetrating atherosclerotic ulcer refers to a contained leakage of blood by overlying hematoma and aortic adventitia (Fig. 3). In the original report by Stanson et al,[14] 7 of 16 patients with penetrating aortic ulcers developed "contained" ruptures. Although uncommon, transmural rupture of an atherosclerotic ulcer has been reported. Nora and Hollier[16] reported one case of contained transmural rupture of the suprarenal aorta from a penetrating atherosclerotic aortic ulcer in a 56-year-old male presenting with complaints of low back pain. Computed tomography suggested a contained aortic perforation. This study was supplemented with an angiogram that demonstrated a penetrating ulcer with a contained rupture of the aorta at T-12 just above the level of the celiac axis origin. At operation a tube graft was placed from the distal thoracic aorta to the middle of the abdominal aorta, incorporating the celiac, superior mesenteric, and both renal arteries as a cuff in continuity with the distal anastomosis.[16] Additionally, Ma and Ang[17] reviewed 14 cases of spontaneous rupture of the aorta without associated aneurysm. In six patients the rupture was through an atheromatous plaque with the rupture site in the ascending aorta (1 case), transverse aortic arch (1 case), and descending aorta (4 cases).

Penetrating aortic ulcers may also progress to form saccular or fusiform aortic aneurysms. Harris et al[8] reported that 5 of 10 patients developed aneurysms from underlying atherosclerotic ulcers during a 1- to 7-year follow-up. Six penetrating ulcers with mean follow-up of 4.6 years progressed to aneurysms at an annual growth rate of 0.31 cm per year. Progressive enlargement of the ulcer with aneurysmal dilatation occurred in all cases once focal periaortic advential bulging developed. However, in an additional four patients there was no enlargement of the aortic ulcer in follow-up.

The treatment strategies for patients with penetrating aortic ulcers include medical therapy with control of blood pressure, close observation with serial follow-up imaging tests, and surgical resection of the aortic ulceration, pseudoaneurysm, or aneurysm in appropriately selected cases (Fig. 4).[15] Age and general health of the patient, location of the ulcer, the presence of a saccular or concentric dilatation, and the rate of growth should all be considered when deciding whether resection is appropriate.[8] Embolism, rupture, hemorrhage, recurrent

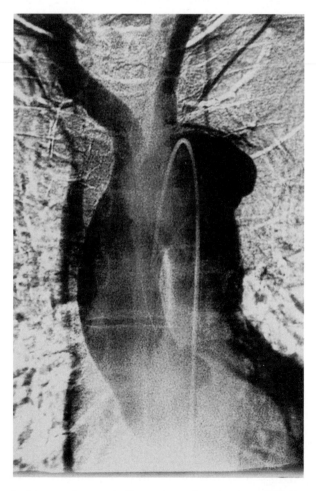

Figure 3. Aortogram demonstrating a pseudoaneurysm of the proximal descending thoracic aorta.

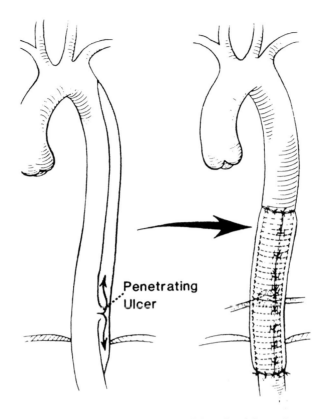

Figure 4. Penetrating athersclerotic ulcer of the distal thoracic aorta repaired by ulcer excision and segmental graft interposition. Reprinted from Reference 14, with permission.

chest or back pain, enlarging pseudoaneurysm, and progressive aneurysmal dilatation are considered indications for surgical therapy in this patient population.[8,15]

Summary

Complicated atherosclerotic aortic plaques are characterized by the presence of calcifications, ulceration, thrombosis, or hemorrhage. These complicated aortic plaques may be responsible for systemic embolization involving the cerebral, visceral, renal, or lower extremity circulations. The presence of proximal aortic atheromas has been demonstrated to be a statistically significant risk factor for cerebral ischemia independent of high-grade carotid artery stenosis. The most frequent locations of complicated aortic ulcerations include, in decreasing frequency, the distal descending thoracic aorta, infrarenal aorta, mid-descending thoracic aorta, proximal descending thoracic aorta, suprarenal aorta, and aortic arch. Aortography should be avoided in patients thought to be at risk for peripheral embolization from aortic sources. Spiral contrast-enhanced computed tomography has emerged as the diagnostic study of choice in this patient population. Axillo-bifemoral bypass with ligation of the external iliac arteries has emerged as the safest alternative for the prevention of recurrent embolization in patients with suprarenal aortic lesions responsible for peripheral embolization.

Penetrating atherosclerotic aortic ulcers may cause intramural hemorrhage, pseudoaneurysm formation, aortic rupture, and aneurysmal aorta dilatation. Symptomatic penetrating atherosclerotic aortic ulcers may be mistaken for acute aortic dissection. Physical examination and current imaging modalities may be used to differentiate primary aortic dissection from penetrating aortic ulceration. Embolism, rupture, hemorrhage, recurrent chest or back pain, enlarging psuedoaneurysm, and progressive aneurysm dilatation are all considered indications for surgical therapy in patients with penetrating atherosclerotic aortic ulceration.

References

1. Haust MD. Atherosclerosis–lesions and sequelae. In: Silver MD ed: *Cardiovascular Pathology*. New York: Churchill Livingstone; 1983:191–316.
2. Berliner JA, Navab M, Fogelman AM, et al. Atherosclerosis: Basic mechanisms oxidation, inflammation, and genetics. *Circulation* 1995;91:2488–2496.
3. Hollier LH, Kazmier FJ, Bowen JC, Procter CD. "Shaggy" aorta syndrome with atheromatous embolization to visceral vessels. *Ann Vasc Surg* 1991;5: 439–444.
4. Jones EF, Kalman JM, Calafiore P, et al. Proximal aortic atheroma: An independent risk factor for cerebral ischemia. *Stroke* 1995;26:218–224.
5. DiTullio MR, Sacco RL, Gersony D, et al. Aortic atheromas and acute ischemic stroke: A transesophageal echocardiographic study in an ethnically mixed population. *Neurology* 1996;46:1560–1566.
6. Khoury Z, Gottlieb S, Stern S, Keren A. Frequency and distribution of atherosclerotic plaques in the thoracic aorta as determined by transesophageal echocardiography in patients with coronary artery disease. *Am J Cardiol* 1997;79:23–27.
7. Amarenco P, Cohen A, Hommel M, et al. Atherosclerotic disease of the aortic arch as a risk factor for recurrent ischemic stroke. *New Engl J Med* 1996;334:1216–1221.
8. Harris JA, Bis KG, Glover JL, et al. Penetrating atherosclerotic ulcers of the aorta. *J Vasc Surg* 1994;19:90–99.
9. De Virgilio C, Hollier LH. Cerebral and spinal cord ischemia. In: White

RA, Hollier LH eds: *Vascular Surgery: Basic Science and Clinical Correlations.* Philadelphia: J.B. Lippincott Company; 1994:343–358.

10. Khatibzadeh M, Mitusch R, Stierle U, et al. Aortic atherosclerotic plaques as a source of systemic embolization. *J Am Coll Cardiol* 1996;27:664–669.

11. Keen RR, McCarthy WJ, Shireman PK, et al. Surgical management of atheroembolization. *J Vasc Surg* 1995;21:773–781.

12. Welch TJ, Stanson AW, Sheedy PF II, et al. Radiologic evaluation of penetrating aortic atherosclerotic ulcer. *Radiographics* 1990;10:675–685.

13. Webber JD, Foster E, Heidenreich P, et al. Three—dimensional transabdominal ultrasound identification of aortic plaque. *Am J Card Imaging* 1995; 9:245–249.

14. Stanson AW, Kazmier FJ, Hollier LH, et al. Penetrating atherosclerotic ulcers of the thoracic aorta: Natural history and clinicopathologic correlations. *Ann Vasc Surg* 1986;1:15–23.

15. Braverman AC. Penetrating atherosclerotic ulcers of the aorta. *Curr Opin Cardiol* 1994;9:591–597.

16. Nora JD, Hollier LH. Contained rupture of the suprarenal aorta. *J Vasc Surg* 1987;5:651–654.

17. Ma TKF, Ang LC. Spontaneous rupture of thoracic aorta through an atheromatous plaque: Case report and literature review. *Am J Forensic Med Pathol* 1996;17:38–42.

18. Kazmier FJ. Penetrating aortic ulcer. *Cardiovasc Clin* 1992,22:201–207.

Overview of Pathology:

The Vulnerable Plaque and Complications of Atherosclerosis

Dr. Fuster: We will have a discussion starting with our speakers, pathologists to the left and our imagers to the right. I start by asking a question to Dr. Falk and Dr. Bassiouny. From what I understand, the coronary lesion leading to rupture can be small, or can be large, but one thing, very important, is the size of the lipid pool. In the carotid system the plaques that lead to trouble are very stenotic and there is nothing to do with the size of the lipid pool, but basically with the distance between the lipid pool's microscopic area and the lumen. In the carotid system, flow is probably critical in leading to rupture or to erosion. The kinetic energy of blood during systole, hits where the lesion's body is very stenotic and the very soft surface can peel off. In the coronary arteries, it seems that most of the blood flow is doing diastole and the kinetic energy of blood is not high. The plaques have to be soft by principle in order to rupture. I'm asking whether you are in favor of this hypothesis or whether you are against it.

Dr. Falk: I don't know what to say because I don't believe much in sheer forces as a cause of plaque disruption. We know that wall stress here may peel away the stenotic area. But whether the wall force is of a magnitude that will also disrupt the plaque, I don't know. But if they are, then of course the mechanism you are describing could operate and maybe explain the difference. There's probably not so much data as on the coronary artery measuring the thickness of the fibrous cap. What has been measured is the width of the lipid pool, the core, and it's correlation with the plaque's vulnerability. But of course the distance from the core to the lumen and the thickness of the fibrous cap is also important. I believe that it must be even more important. If you have a huge lipid rich pool, but it is deep in the plaque and covered by a thick fibrous cap, then I don't think it's so dangerous.

Dr Fuster: I agree with what you said on the coronary arteries about the width of lipid pools. But the question in the carotid arteries is about flow kinetics, because you know you are really sending blood there at a very high kinetic energy with an 80 percent lesion that is a soft surface. For me to believe that flow doesn't play a role on that erosion, I have to be convinced because it just doesn't make sense.

Dr. Bassiouny: There's experimental evidence that in very fast stenoses, the sheer stress levels can go up to 400 to 600 dynes per cm squared and that can desquamate cells. But more interestingly, as in tomorrow's discussion on the flow and stenosis, that there is distal collapse of the vessel. Experimental evidence shows that with a very tight stenosis in the carotid bifurcation, the vessel collapses resulting in fatigue of the fibrous cap, and disruption. So I think that the hemodynamic factors do play a role in the disruption of the plaque. I think that reasons we don't see disruption in earlier degrees of stenosis in the carotid bifurcation may be related to the susceptibility of the carotid bifurcation itself, the nature of the lesions that develop there, and the extrinsic forces of angulation and bending and so forth that are not seen in the proximal and distal carotid arteries.

Dr. Fuster: Let me ask Dr. Fallon about comparing what we heard about the abdominal aorta and the peripheral vessels. What Dr. Hollier presented today is the relatively rare syndrome of the whole abdominal aorta ulcerated and generating showers of emboli and cholesterol. These don't appear in peripheral artery disease, why?

Dr. Fallon: I think what Dr. Hollier beautifully showed us this morning is a rather dramatic one end of the scale in which very large ulcerated and voluminous plaques of the aorta dump into the circulation where it goes principally into the kidneys, the visceral arteries, or the periphery. In contrast, in the smaller iliac and femoral arteries, the volume of the plaques that ulcerate and release their contents into the circulation is much, much smaller. Therefore, we don't see that type of embolic phenomenon occurring as a clinical event.

Dr. Fuster: But do you agree that the disease in the ileo-femoral region is probably similar to the disease that develops in the ascending aorta and in the thoracic aorta?

Dr. Fallon: Yes, it is also in the coronaries and in the carotid.

Dr. Fuster: The disease is the same but the manifestations and their impact are quite different. For example, the leg is a filter of emboli but the head is not. You will hear this afternoon that there is a very good indication that a large number of strokes and cerebral ischemic attacks are related to relatively small plaques in the aorta which are not severely stenotic, but are ulcerating.

Dr. Fallon: I certainly agree with that. Small emboli to the brain obviously can have very untoward and immediate clinical sequelae, whereas the same volume of material being embolized into the legs or even into the kidneys will not be seen clinically.

Dr. Fuster: Dr. Bassiouny, I want to go back to the question of hemodynamics. In the coronary arteries, Dr. Falk may contradict me, but the intracoronary hematoma leading to an acute coronary event is rare, so I think people miss the fissure. In the carotid artery, I don't think it's rare. I think you said that symptomatic and asymptomatic patients have hematomas but there is no fissuring. This will be presented this afternoon with magnetic resonance studies; there is like a dissection, and then the hematoma takes place.

Dr. Bassiouny: I tend to disagree with the concept that intraplaque hemorrhage is a primary event in carotid plaque disruption. That has not been our finding. It has been reported in earlier studies that intraplaque hemorrhage, in other words, disruption of the vasa vasorum within the plaque structure is the primary event leading to plaque disruption. In the 140 plaques that we have looked at, and Sy Glagov looked at each one, we could not find any evidence that plaque hemorrhage was the primary event. However, as you mentioned, there is intraplaque, intramural hematoma, and that is a consequence of plaque disruption more so than intraplaque hemorrhage arising from the disruption of the body of the plaque itself and leakage from the vasa vasorum.

Dr. Fuster: You think there is a fissure?

Dr. Bassiouny: Yes.

Dr. Fuster: What about inflammation?

Dr. Bassiouny: There is evidence for a concentration of macrophages at peak stress regions in carotid plaques. I think that there have been publications to that effect. However, I also feel that it's hard for us to really define which came first, the chicken or the egg? In other words, is the macrophage reaction in the fibrous cap a reaction to an element in the carotid core, or is there initial macrophage infiltration which in fact degrades the fibrous cap and makes it more thin, thus rendering the necrotic core closer to the lumen? I would say that based in mechanical studies, the regions of macrophage concentrations were regions of high stress gradient and regions of increased peak stress, so they tend to be areas that are more vulnerable to plaque destruction. This not from a standpoint of flow dynamic, but from structural fatigue in the plaque.

Dr. Falk: I think inflammation or anti-inflammations are markers of arterial disease and disease progression. There is very good data saying that, if for example, you give a rabbit cholesterol so it has hypercholesterolemia, it will be able to go into the vessel wall and the first thing that happens is the cell will express adhesion molecules, probably B-CAM. Monocytes will adhere to the vessel wall, they will go into the intima and become macrophages, and they will take up LDL probably after oxidation and become foam cells, the key cells of atherosclerosis. Thus you have development of the fatty streak. So, from the very beginning inflammation plays a very important part in the evolution of the early lesion. Also, in the advanced lesion you will have signs of inflammation. If after you have induced the advanced lesion experimentally, for example in a monkey, and you again lower the serum cholesterol, the first cell that disappears from the lesion is the macrophage. It is probably one of the mechanisms that is behind plaque stabilization. So the monocyte-macrophage activated in the endothelium is the first thing that appears when you induce a lesion, and it's the first thing that disappears when you try to induce regression. Hence, I think inflammation is very important in the progression of this disease.

Dr. Fuster: I'd like to make a point, if it is true, that the force driving the monocyte into the vessel wall in many circumstances is hyperlipidemia. It is quite interesting that epidemiological- pathological studies indicate that hyperlipidemia is an extreme risk factor for coronary disease, but it appears less convincingly for carotid disease. As it will be discussed, it can be important in the diseases of the aorta embolizing and causing strokes, but it's more questionable for carotid disease.

Discussant from the Audience: I have a comment. There is no strong correlation between high serum lipids, stroke, and modifications of lipids with statins.

Dr. Fuster: I disagree. You have to look at the Scandinavian Simvastatin Survival Study and the CARE Study just published. It's quite striking the relationship in these studies on patients who were control, versus patients who received simvastatin in terms of the incidence of stroke. They pointed out that in fact hyperlipidemia is an important risk factor for a stroke and treatment with statins is of sufficient benefit. The question is whether statins are preventing these very soft aortic lesions that might cause the stroke. In summary, the evidence is very strong in disease of the aorta. The evidence is not so strong in the carotid artery. We will discuss this later.

Dr. Guyton: My question relates to electron beam tomography and its relationship to the pathology of the plaques. We know that the calcification occurs within the lipid-rich core. Has any study looked at the correlation between the amount of calcium and the extent of core formation within atherosclerotic lesions? That could either be a pathologic study or it could be a study using IVUS.

Dr. Fallon: I have a comment. I think we see calcification in advanced healed plaques in the carotid territory. If you look at the necrotic core, it progresses from the gruelous material to hyalinization and then calcification. When we see regions of calcification in the plaque, they indicate stability. I'm not aware of any data from the coronary artery measuring the amount of calcium and trying to correlate it with the vulnerability of plaques.

Dr. Fuster: Right. But you may have calcium both in the lipid-rich core and also in the old sclerotic plaque component.

Dr. Taubman: My question is for Dr. Falk. You showed first that there were macrophages and inflammation occurring at the site of plaque rupture, and you said that the macrophages were activated. What markers have you looked at to show the macrophages are truly activated?

Dr. Falk: I have not looked for activation markers. I referred to a study by Van der Wal, but I would be happy if Peter Libby could answer the question because he knows much more about it.

Dr. Libby: The marker in the Van der Wal study from the Becker Group was a compatibility element which we had shown in the 1980s was inducible by gamma interferon, but was not expressed by smooth muscle cells. They found it in that study published in *Circulation*, I think at the end of '94, in both smooth muscle cells and macrophages.

Dr. Taubman: I have another question for Dr. Falk. Regarding your perfusion model, the histology slide showed the thrombus overlying the lipid-rich core with nothing on the sides which were rich in collagen. How do you know, or do you know, whether there was endothelium overlying the collagen-rich part of the vessel and not the lipid core? This might explain why the thrombus was located where it was?

Dr. Falk: Before we put this aortic specimen into the perfusion chamber, we scraped with a knife to remove the endothelium, we took the fibrous cap away, and we opened the core. We wanted to expose the interior of the plaque because that is what happens when plaque ruptures. So we removed the surface cells of the lesions.

Dr. Taubman: I have one more question for the pathologists. I don't know which speaker, but someone showed in a heart transplantation a regression of the lesions. What immunosuppressive therapy was that patient on?

Dr. Libby: We've been able to show that transplant coronary disease is two diseases. First, it's a disease that comes from the donor and has all the characteristics of conventional atherosclerosis. Second, it's a disease that occurs in the recipient due to immune mediated injury. They're completely different patterns of disease, and if you look at a transplant patient at any point in time, you are likely to see an overlap of both the acquired disease from the donor heart and the disease that came from transplant vasculopathy. So the answer to the question is, those lesions I showed are lesions that we know that came from the donor and were not coming from the recipient. And therefore, the immune mechanism is not relevant to their regression or progression. In fact, we've been able to show that immune mechanisms affect the acquired disease but not the disease that's transplanted.

Dr. Libby: I have a comment that was raised by Dr. Falk's wonderful exposition. I must say that by listening to people like Erling Falk and Michael Davies, I know what experiments to do next in my laboratory. But you raised very nicely the dichotomy between the importance of triggering and vulnerability. One study that's helped me to think about this is the study that was published in the *New England Journal* a few years ago that analyzed the incidents of acute coronary deaths in the Los Angeles earthquake. That study showed that with this very potent stimulus, the earthquake, there was a new peak in incidents of coronary deaths. But the most interesting part of that study, and the most unexpected, was then it was followed by a dip. What that means to me is that vulnerability is the key issue and the triggering merely determines exactly what micropoint in time an atheroma will erupt. The analogy was used earlier. So that was very helpful information for me in balancing between triggering, of which there's been a great deal of discussion, and the substrate, the underlying atheroma.

Dr. Fuster: Do you know the similar situation from Israel with the SCUD missiles? The increased numbers of admissions into the coronary care units was very significant, actually four times what it had been predicted the same time the year before. But was there a dip afterwards?

Dr. Libby: Yes. Because you harvest, you harvest a crop and it's going to be harvested sooner or later, but you do it sooner if there's a stimulus. I have one comment about Dr. Bassiouny's presentation, which I found very elegant and very helpful, and it's a small quarrel but it's one which I think may be very significant. You used the word "rate" of apoptosis to denote positive labeling cells. The word "rate" to me requires a duration in time—I do not believe that you can measure a rate of a process by looking at one point in time. I think this may be a key issue because of the number of labeling nuclei that you showed. So I think that we have to be very careful in thinking about the kinetics of this process and what it actually means. We can discuss that privately at length if you like. Thank you.

Discussant from the Audience: A question to Dr. Falk. Most people in the field, as far as I know, think that calcification is the result of a healing, possibly for previous microinfarcts. The concept is that there's some injury to the vessel wall and it heals with fibrosis and calcifies. The question is, if that happens all the time, why did it happen 20 to 30 times before without a heart attack or infarction, and then suddenly that particular event lead to a catastrophic syndrome? So something else is missing between all these other infarctions and one that led to the problem at this particular time. I wonder if anybody has any idea of why that may be?

Dr. Falk: Are you asking about calcification in the plaque?

Discussant from the Audience: I'm saying that we know the calcification relates to events, and we also know that calcifications probably is simply a marker for a previous mini event that did not lead to catastrophic heart attack. At least that's a concept.

Dr. Falk: I don't know whether calcification follows plaque disruption. I think you have calcifications in many plaques that have never ruptured. To me they don't look as if they have ruptured and there may be calcification in the lipid core, in the sclerotic plaque component. I have changed my way of looking at calcification in recent years. Just 5 or 10 years ago I thought calcification was a kind of dystrophic phenomena in the plaque, but it's not so. Later in the program we will hear that calcification in the plaque is an active process, that calcium is secreted with calcification proteins in the plaque so they lay the ground for calcification. It's not just a dystrophic phenomenon.

Discussant from the Audience: But you do not believe that it's a marker for previous injury?

Dr. Falk: No I don't think so, and I think they indicate that calcified plaques are not so prone to rupture as noncalcified lesions. I also think from the last presentation that calcification in the coronary artery or calcification score is just a marker of the plaque burden. There are data comparing culprit lesions with nonculprit lesions. In acute myocardial infarction, the nonculprit lesions were more calcified than culprit lesions.

Dr. Fuster: The spacial distribution of plaque components appears important. If you have calcification deep in the substance of the plaque, it doesn't make a difference. But if you have calcification that is in proximity to a soft region of the plaque, then you can foresee fatigue of the plaque and disruption occurring at that point.

Chapter 4

Coronary Angiography and the Vulnerable Plaque

David Waters, MD, FRCP(C), FACC

Introduction

Coronary arteriography has been widely used for 30 years to definitively diagnose coronary artery disease, to risk-stratify patients with disease, and to select the optimal mode of therapy. Coronary arteriography has also proved to be an important tool for clinical research. Although newer modalities, intracoronary ultrasound, and angioscopy, have already provided important insights into the pathological processes involved in coronary atherosclerosis, much of our fundamental clinical knowledge in this area has been gleaned from studies that use coronary arteriography.

Most coronary plaques are benign. Why some coronary plaques rupture or erode and precipitate coronary events is an important question that has been partially answered, mainly by autopsy evidence.[1-4] These studies have identified plaque composition and the functional integrity of the fibrous cap as key factors in the process. Studies that use coronary arteriography corroborate and extend the autopsy evidence, and are reviewed in this chapter.

Historical Perspective

For the first 20 years after its development, coronary arteriography was thought to be contraindicated during the acute phase of myocardial infarction. But in 1980, DeWood et al[5] reported the results of coronary arteriography performed within 24 hours of Q wave infarction in 322

From: Fuster, V (ed). *The Vulnerable Atherosclerotic Plaque: Understanding, Identification, and Modification*. Armonk, NY: Futura Publishing Company, Inc.; © 1999.

patients who were being evaluated for emergency surgery. A total occlusion of the infarct-related artery was demonstrated in 87% of patients studied within the first 4 hours after the onset of symptoms; this rate decreased to 65% in patients studied between 12 and 24 hours. The occlusion exhibited angiographic features consistent with acute thrombosis in 59 of the 79 patients who underwent surgery, and in most of them thrombotic material was retrieved by Fogarty catheter at the time of coronary bypass.

This report ended a controversy that had started in the 1940s, when autopsy studies began to question the conclusion that myocardial infarction was caused by coronary thrombosis, as James Herrick had first proposed in 1912.[6] Clinical trials of anticoagulant therapy for myocardial infarction in the 1940s and 1950s produced discordant results[7] and eroded enthusiasm for coronary thrombosis as an etiologic mechanism. By the 1970s, the consensus was that coronary thrombosis was probably a consequence, and not the cause, of myocardial infarction.[8,9] As a result of this errant conclusion, therapeutic efforts during this decade were concentrated on reducing myocardial infarct size, not by timely reperfusion, but by metabolic means or by manipulating the determinants of myocardial oxygen consumption.[10]

The demonstration with coronary arteriography that coronary occlusion was present early in most myocardial infarctions led to the rapid acceptance of thrombolytic therapy as rational treatment.[11] Thrombolytic therapy was initially administered by the intracoronary route. Consequently, the angiographic features of culprit lesions after thrombolysis were soon well appreciated, as discussed later in this chapter.

DeWood et al[12] also described the angiographic findings soon after non–Q-wave myocardial infarction. In contrast to Q wave infarction, total occlusion was infrequently observed in this condition. The occlusion rate in the infarct-related vessel increased from 26% in the first 24 hours to 37% from 24 to 72 hours, and to 42% after 72 hours. These observations provided a sound basis for developing different treatment for non–Q-wave than for Q wave infarctions.

Coronary arteriography was not as immediately helpful in furthering our understanding of the pathophysiology of unstable angina as it was for myocardial infarction. In the early 1980s, the angiographic pattern of coronary atherosclerosis was considered to be similar in unstable and stable angina, and coronary spasm was thought to be the most likely explanation for angina at rest.[13] Neither heparin nor aspirin were part of optimal management for unstable angina.[14] Coronary thrombus was initially described in a small proportion of patients with unstable angina, comprising only 16 of 3553 patients undergoing coronary arteriography at the Mayo Clinic over a 3-year period.[15] However, thrombus was increasingly recognized at angiography in reports of patients with unstable angina. Ambrose et al[16] demonstrated that asymmetric coronary lesions with narrow necks or irregular borders were much more common in unstable compared to stable angina patients. Confirmation that coronary thrombosis was important in the pathogenesis of unstable angina soon came from clinical trials showing that aspirin and heparin significantly reduced the early event rate.[17]

The Culprit Lesion After Thrombolytic Therapy

Studies of the culprit lesion after thrombolytic therapy for myocardial infarction have provided useful information about the process of thrombolysis and have also yielded clues as to the features of the plaque that is vulnerable to rupture. In one series of 119 consecutive myocardial infarction patients undergoing coronary arteriography within 48 hours after streptokinase, a residual diameter stenosis of at least 70% was found in 58% of cases, from 50% to 69% in 13% of cases, and less than 50% in only 4% of cases.[18] No culprit lesion greater than 60% diameter stenosis was found in 12.6% of 1636 patients undergoing coronary arteriography 18 to 48 hours after tissue plasminogen activator (rt-PA) in the Thrombolysis in Myocardial Infarction (TIMI) II Trial.[19] Similarly, in a report from the Thrombolysis and Angioplasty in Myocardial Infarction (TAMI) Trials, a stenosis of 50% or less was found in only 5.5% of 799 patients undergoing coronary angiography at 90 minutes after successful thrombolysis.[20] At restudy 7 to 10 days later, the culprit lesion had resolved to a stenosis of 50% or less in an additional 5.4% of the patients.

Patients with culprit lesions less than 50% comprised 21% of 198 patients in another series; they were younger and were more likely to have been smokers.[21] At the other end of the spectrum, antecedent angina was associated with a more severe residual culprit lesion, both in the TIMI II population[22] and in the report of Bergelson et al.[23]

The severity of the culprit lesion tends to decrease in the hours and days after thrombolysis, presumably due to further dissolution of thrombotic material and remodeling of the plaque. In a study where quantitative coronary angiography was performed on patent lesions at 1.5 to 4 hours after streptokinase treatment, and again at 18 to 48 hours, mean diameter stenosis decreased from 77.2% to 72.5% ($P<0.001$).[24] Between 24 hours and 4 weeks in another report, diameter stenosis by quantitative measurement decreased from $62 \pm 9\%$ to $55 \pm 13\%$ ($P<0.005$).[25] Spontaneous thrombolysis occurs in a substantial proportion of patients with myocardial infarction. As a result, stenosis severity late after the event may not differ between patients who received this form of therapy and those who did not. For example, van Lierde et al[26] reported that diameter stenosis at 10 to 14 days was 57% (range 36% to 75%) and 58% (range 44% to 71%) in treated and untreated patients, respectively.

Several investigators have studied the morphological features of culprit plaques after thrombolysis, as seen at angiography.[27-30] In a series of 308 patients studied 7 days after thrombolytic therapy for acute infarction, Gotsman et al[27] found that 78% of culprit arteries were patent, 34% exhibited a ruptured plaque, 7% an ulcerated plaque, and in 62% the lesion was eccentric. Coronary narrowings were most often located proximally and at bifurcations, similar locations to those seen in a series of patients with stable angina. Davies et al[28] also compared lesion characteristics between patients 1 to 8 days post-thrombolysis and patients with stable angina. Irregular, eccentric, ulcerated plaques with shoulders, globular or linear filling defects, and contrast staining were seen significantly more commonly in the postinfarction group. At follow-up angiography 2 to 10 days later, some of the filling defects, irregularities, and ulcerations had disappeared.

Brown et al[29] studied the sequence of changes to the culprit lesion during and after thrombolysis from magnified and traced angiographic images. They observed that the recanalized lumen formed along the interface between the thrombus and the vessel wall and progressively enlarged. In nine lesions restudied and found to be patent 5 weeks later, the lumen was larger and in seven, a thin film of contrast surrounding the thrombus faintly defined the boundaries of the original plaque. Mean diameter stenosis was $56 \pm 14\%$.

Nakagawa et al[30] also described the sequence of angiographic changes that occurs in the culprit lesion after thrombolysis, from a series of 43 consecutive patients who had angiography before, immediately after, and 1 month after intracoronary urokinase. Progressive removal of overlying thrombus often leads to a pooling of contrast within the lesion. The pool may be covered by single or paired radiolucencies. A cavity may develop within the lesion, followed by smoothing or rounding of the cavity edges. Figures 1 and 2 depict typical sequences of angiographic changes seen after thrombolysis.

In unstable angina and non–Q-wave infarction, thrombolytic therapy increases the short-term risk of infarction, as shown both by a series of small trials[31] and by the Thrombolysis in Myocardial Ischemia (TIMI) III Trial.[32] The culprit lesions for unstable angina have been measured before and after thrombolysis in more than a dozen trials.[33-39] In some studies, small degrees of improvement in stenosis severity were reported, while in others thrombolysis had no discernible effect. The results of the Thrombolysis in Myocardial Ischemia (TIMI) IIIA Trial[39] are representative. Substantial improve-

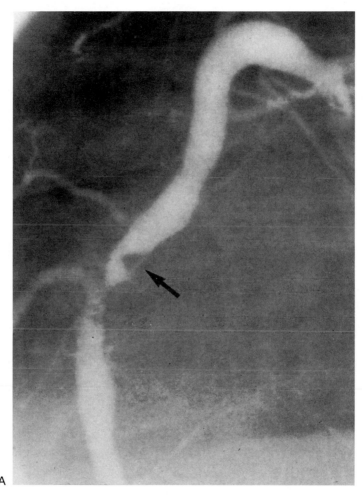

A

Figure 1. A. Right coronary angiogram 2 hours after the onset of acute inferior myocardial infarction, before initiation of thrombolytic therapy. A hazy, concentric 70;pc stenosis is seen enveloping a side branch. Proximal to this stenosis is a triangular-shaped intraluminal filling defect (arrow). A thin line of contrast can be seen between the defect and the vessel wall.

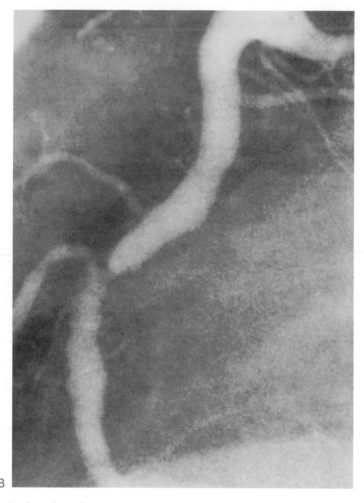

Figure 1. *(continued)*
B. Right coronary angiogram 6 days later, after thrombolysis. The filling defect has disappeared but the severity of the stenosis has not changed. *Continued.*

ment, defined as a reduction in stenosis severity of 20% or more, or of coronary flow by two TIMI grades or more, was seen in only 15% of culprit lesions in the t-PA group compared to 5% in controls. Angiographically apparent thrombus was present at baseline in one third of culprit lesions; patients with evident thrombus or non–Q-wave infarction were more likely to show angiographic improvement. However, the degree of angiographic improvement in unstable angina is much less impressive than it is in myocardial infarction. In unstable angina patients with obvious thrombus, the pattern of lysis is similar to that reported in myocardial infarction.[39]

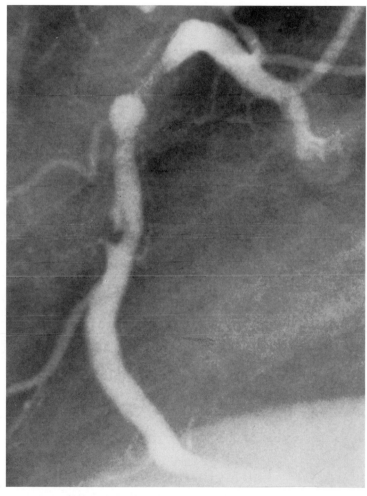

A

Figure 2. A. Right coronary angiogram 2 hours after the initiation of thrombo-lytic therapy in a patient with an acute inferior myocardial infarction. Two complex lesions are present: the proximal one has hazy, ill-defined margins characteristic of thrombus; the distal one is eccentric with a deep ulceration in its proximal portion, parallel to the vessel wall.

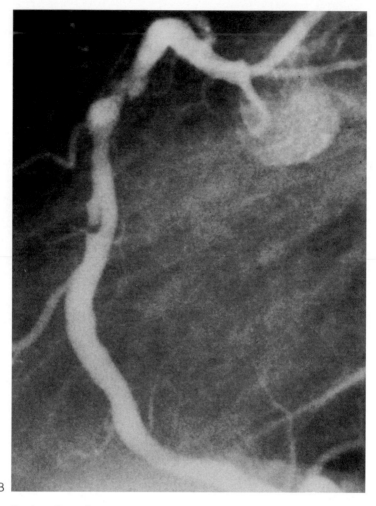

B

Figure 2. *(continued)*
B. Right coronary angiogram 6 days later, showing better definition of the margins of the proximal lesion and a well-defined ulceration. The distal lesion has not changed.

The Vulnerable Plaque
Before Myocardial Infarction

An alternate approach to the angiographic assessment of the culprit lesion after myocardial infarction, described above, is to study coronary lesions in patients before they develop myocardial infarction. This can be done either by scanning hospital and catheterization laboratory

Table 1

Severity of Culprit Lesions at Coronary Angiography Prior to Myocardial Infarction

First author	Number of patients	Months to MI (range)	Baseline stenosis <50%	Baseline stenosis 50% to 70%	Baseline stenosis >70%
Ambrose[40]	23	18 (1–84)	11 (48%)	7 (30%)	5 (22%)
Little[41]	29	24 (1–77)	19 (66%)	9 (31%)	1 (3%)
Nobuyoshi[42]	39	31 (1–120)	23 (59%)	6 (15%)	10 (26%)
Giroud[43]	92	26 (1–144)	72 (78%)	8 (9%)	12 (13%)
Total	183	–	125 (68%)	30 (16%)	28 (15%)

MI = myocardial infarction.

records to identify patients who underwent coronary angiography and later experienced myocardial infarction, or by examining a prospectively followed cohort of patients after their baseline angiogram. This approach has two main limitations. The first is selection bias; for example, patients with severe stenoses at baseline angiography are more likely to undergo revascularization and thus be excluded from the analysis. The second is the variable interval from angiography to infarction, when the severity and morphological features of the vulnerable plaque may be changing dramatically.

Table 1 lists four studies[40–43] in which coronary angiography was performed after myocardial infarction to define the culprit lesion in patients who had undergone an angiogram before their infarction, with no interval revascularization. The average interval between the first angiogram and the myocardial infarction was approximately 2 years. The severity of two thirds of the culprit lesions was less than 50% stenosis at the first angiogram, and only 15% were greater than 70%. This finding has important implications for the treatment of patients with coronary disease because it refutes the clinical myth that coronary revascularization reduces the risk of myocardial infarction. It also shifts attention from the minority of coronary lesions that are severe enough to cause myocardial ischemia to all of the epicardial coronary arteries, and thus to interventions that treat atherosclerosis globally. An example of a mild culprit lesion causing myocardial infarction is shown in Figure 3.

Although most myocardial infarctions develop at mild stenoses,

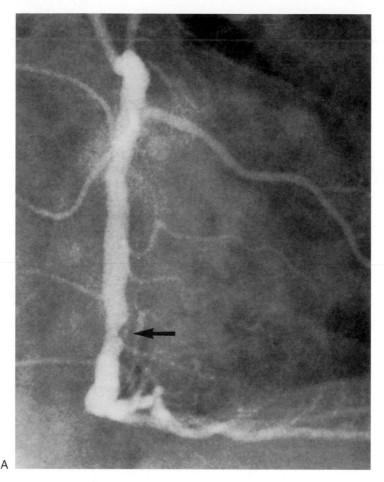

A

Figure 3. **A.** Right coronary angiogram from a patient with mild stable angina due to lesions in the left coronary system. Multiple minimal irregularities are present in the proximal part of the artery. A smooth, eccentric 40;pc stenosis (arrow) is seen in the mid-right coronary artery.

severe stenoses are more likely to progress to complete occlusion. Two factors account for this apparent paradox. First, mild lesions are much more numerous than severe lesions. For example, in a trial[44] where 335 patients had coronary angiography at baseline and at 2 years, with all lesions measured quantitatively, 1705 of 2092 lesions (82%) were less than 50% diameter stenosis at baseline.[45] The proportion of lesions that occluded during this trial increased from less than 1% for stenoses of less than 40% severity to 25% for stenoses of 70% or greater, as shown in Figure 4. The second factor is that severe stenoses are less likely than mild stenoses to produce a myocardial infarction when they occlude. In this series, only 1 of 15 occlusions in stenoses of 70% or greater resulted in a new infarction, compared to 12 of 59 occlusions of stenoses less than 70% (7% versus 20%, $P = $ NS). Ambrose et al[40] reported a mean

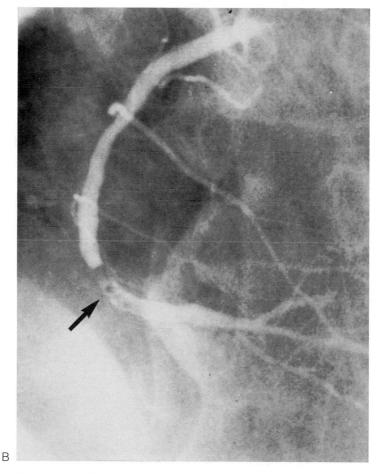

B

Figure 3. *(continued)*
B. Two months later, the patient developed an acute inferior myocardial infarction. Repeat angiography now reveals rapid progression of the previously mild lesion to a near total occlusion. A thrombus has produced a perpendicular surface at the lesion inflow and endoluminal filling defects (arrow) are visible distally.

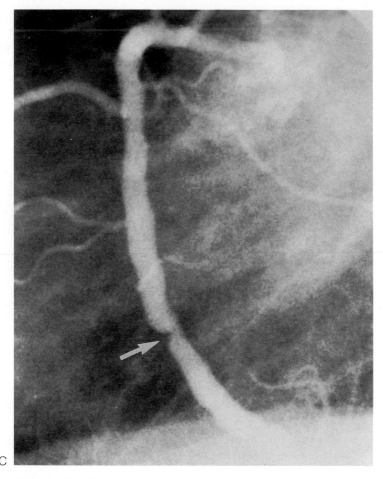

C

Figure 3. *(continued)*
C. Six days later, after thrombolytic therapy, the distal filling defects have completely disappeared and only a short, eccentric 50;pc stenosis (arrow) remains.

stenosis severity of 48% and of 73.5% in lesions that produced infarction when they occluded versus those that did not ($P<0.05$).

Other morphological features of coronary lesions, in addition to their severity, have been assessed as risk factors for infarction. Luminal roughness and lesion length were predictors in a study of left anterior descending coronary artery stenoses; by multivariate analysis, stenosis severity greater than 50%, lesion roughness, a concomitant circumflex stenosis, and smoking were predictive of anterior infarction.[46]

Taeymans et al[47] compared the qualitative and quantitative features of 38 coronary lesions that occluded within 3 years to cause an acute myocardial infarction to those of 64 control segments from the same patients that did not occlude. Compared with the control lesions, the lesions that occluded were more likely to have a division branch originating within the stenosis (76% versus 52%, $P<0.05$), were slightly more severe ($48\pm18\%$ versus $41\pm13\%$, $P<0.05$), and had significantly steeper inflow and outflow angles. A lesion with steep inflow and outflow angles is illustrated in Figure 5. Each of these lesion characteristics increases turbulence and thus would be expected to increase the risk of thrombosis if a thrombogenic surface developed. In this study stenosis length, eccentricity, and lesion irregularity were not predictive of occlusion.

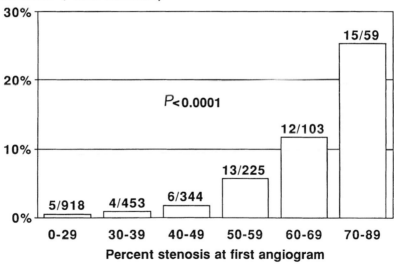

Figure 4. Proportion of coronary lesions progressing to occlusion during 2 years in a prospective trial with quantitative coronary angiography.[44] The fraction above each bar is the number of lesions occluding divided by the number of lesions in that category. Note that mild lesions are much more numerous than severe ones. The risk of developing occlusion is very low for mild lesions but increases incrementally as the baseline diameter stenosis becomes more severe. For stenoses of 70% or greater at baseline, the risk of occlusion is 25%.

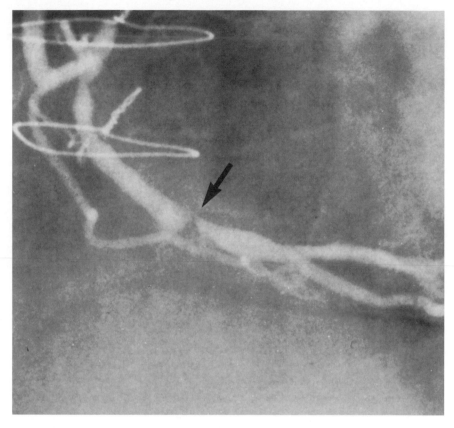

Figure 5. Distal right coronary artery lesion (arrow) with very steep inflow and outflow angles. The lesion is discrete, very eccentric, smooth, and measured 75% diameter stenosis. Factors increasing the risk of occlusion are the severity of the stenosis and the steep inflow and outflow angles. The lesion was totally occluded when coronary arteriography was repeated 1 week later.

The Vulnerable Plaque in Unstable Angina

The evolution of the vulnerable plaque in unstable angina has been defined from before, to during, to after the clinical event. In 1983, a series of 38 patients who had had an angiogram before and during an episode of unstable angina were compared to a series of 38 stable angina patients with two angiograms over a comparable time interval.[48] Progression had occurred in 76% of the unstable angina group and in 32% of controls ($P<0.0005$). The divergence between the two groups would probably have been even greater if the distinction between unstable and stable angina could be made more accurately from the patients' descriptions. One way to view unstable angina is as a clinical marker of underlying coronary disease progression.

What factors determine whether a plaque rupture leads to unstable angina, as opposed to myocardial infarction? We addressed this question by examining patients with identifiable culprit lesions who developed coronary events during two prospective coronary angiographic trials where baseline and 2-year follow-up angiograms were measured quantitatively.[49] The severity of the culprit lesion before the event was similar in the 23 unstable angina and 19 infraction patients, $52 \pm 22\%$ and $48 \pm 12\%$, respectively. However, after the event, the lesion was narrower in the infarction group, $92 \pm 11\%$ compared to $84 \pm 12\%$ in the unstable angina group ($P = 0.03$), and the degree of worsening was greater, $44 \pm 12\%$ versus $32 \pm 14\%$ ($P = 0.009$). The reference diameters of the segments containing the culprit lesions were identical in both groups, indicating that unstable angina was not due to plaque rupture and lesion progression occurring in a smaller sized vessel than in myocardial infarction.

Ambrose et al[16] developed a classification of coronary lesions and used it to compare lesions narrowed by 50% or greater in 47 patients with stable and 63 patients with unstable angina. Concentric lesions and multiple irregularities were more common in patients with stable angina. The type II eccentric lesion, defined as an asymmetric stenosis in the form of a convex intraluminal obstruction with a narrow neck or base, was seen in 54% of 92 lesions from unstable patients compared to 7% of 55 lesions from stable patients ($P < 0.001$). The authors postulated that this angiographic image represented ruptured atherosclerotic plaques, or partially occlusive thrombi, or both.

In a later study[50] the same authors compared the angiographic features of groups of patients with stable and unstable angina who had undergone a previous coronary angiogram. They observed that progression had occurred in three quarters of the unstable patients, usually from a lesion less than 50% at the earlier study. Most of the lesions that progressed to less than a complete occlusion in the unstable group were classified as type II eccentric. Other investigators have developed more complicated, quantitative parameters that also distinguish between the complex lesions of unstable angina and the simpler lesions of stable angina.[51]

Others have correlated the presence or absence of thrombus or angiographic morphology with either clinical outcome or clinical presentation. For example, Freeman et al[52] reported that the frequency of angiographic thrombus decreased within the first week after the onset of unstable angina, and that thrombus was strongly predictive of coronary events.[52] Bugiardini et al[53] found that the combination of complex lesion morphology and at least 60 minutes per 24 hours of ST segment depression on Holter monitoring defined a high-risk subgroup in unstable angina. In a more recent study,[54] complex lesions, intracoronary thrombus, and slow TIMI flow were associated with recent chest pain at rest, refractory unstable angina, or postinfarction unstable angina.

Investigators from St. George's Hospital Medical School in London have described the fate of the complex coronary lesion in a recent series of publications.[55-58] They studied 85 consecutive patients with unstable angina whose symptoms had been stabilized on medical therapy and who were put on waiting list for elective coronary angioplasty.[55] During a mean wait of 8 ± 4 months, one patient died and 25 others had nonfatal coronary events that were associated with culprit lesion progression. At repeat angiography, culprit stenoses were much more likely to progress than were other lesions, 25% versus 7% ($P = 0.001$). Complex stenoses were at higher risk for progression than were smooth lesions.[56] When this group of stabilized unstable angina patients was compared to a group of stable angina patients who also waited 8 ± 4 months for elective angioplasty, both complex lesion morphology ($P<0.001$) and unstable angina at initial presentation ($P<0.01$) were predictive factors for progression of the culprit lesion.[57]

Taken together, these studies describe, from an angiographic perspective, the entire lifetime of the vulnerable plaque responsible for unstable angina. A lesion that is usually mild or moderate undergoes plaque rupture and develops an overlying, eccentric thrombus that is usually not completely occlusive. This complex lesion causes unstable angina. Even when symptoms are subsequently controlled medically, the lesion often progresses rapidly within months to cause a recurrent coronary event.

Conclusion

Coronary angiographic studies have contributed immensely to our understanding of the vulnerable coronary plaque in acute coronary syndromes. The concepts derived from angiographic studies have led to the development of successful therapies for these conditions. Further studies, with use of newer tools, coronary angioscopy, and intracoronary ultrasound, hold the promise of further increasing our knowledge of the vulnerable plaque. Better identification of the high-risk plaque and better therapies to prevent plaque rupture will reduce the incidence of coronary events.

Acknowledgment   Angiographic images in Figures 1, 2, 3, and 5 courtesy of Dr. Jacques Lespérance, Montreal Heart Institute.

References

1. Falk E, Shah PK, Fuster V. Coronary plaque disruption. *Circulation* 1995; 92:657–671.
2. Farb A, Burke AP, Tang AL, et al. Coronary plaque erosion without rupture into a lipid core. A frequent cause of coronary thrombosis in sudden coronary death. *Circulation* 1996;93:1354–1363.
3. Davies MJ. Stability and instability: Two faces of coronary atherosclerosis. The Paul Dudley White Lecture 1995. *Circulation* 1996;94:2013–2020.
4. Burke AP, Farb A, Malcom GT, et al. Coronary risk factors and plaque morphology in men with coronary disease who died suddenly. *N Engl J Med* 1997;336:1276–1282.
5. DeWood MA, Spores J, Notske R, et al. Prevalence of total coronary occlusion during the early hours of transmural myocardial infarction. *N Engl J Med* 1980;303:897–902.
6. Forrester J. Intimal disruption and coronary thrombosis: Its role in the pathogenesis of human coronary disease. *Am J Cardiol* 1991;68:69B–77B.
7. Hilden T, Iversen K, Raaschow F, et al. Anticoagulants in acute myocardial infarction. *Lancet* 1961;2:327–331.
8. Roberts WC. Coronary thrombosis and fatal myocardial ischemia. *Circulation* 1974;49:1–3.
9. Chandler AB, Chapman I, Erhardt LR, et al. Coronary thrombosis in myocardial infarction. Report of a workshop on the role of coronary thrombosis in the pathogenesis of acute myocardial infarction. *Am J Cardiol* 1974:34: 823–832.
10. Rude RE, Muller JE, Braunwald E. Efforts to limit the size of myocardial infarcts. *Ann Intern Med* 1981;95:736–761.
11. Laffel GL, Braunwald E. Thrombolytic therapy. A new strategy for the treatment of acute myocardial infarction. *N Engl J Med* 1984;311: 710–717,770–776.
12. DeWood MA, Stifter WF, Simpson CS, et al. Coronary arteriographic findings soon after non-Q-wave myocardial infarction. *N Engl J Med* 1986;315: 417–423.
13. Scanlon PJ. The intermediate coronary syndrome. *Prog Cardiovasc Dis* 1981; 23:351–364.
14. Russell RO, Rackley CE, Kouchoukos NT. Unstable angina pectoris: Do we know the best management? *Am J Cardiol* 1981;48:590–591.
15. Holmes DR, Hartzler GO, Smith HC, et al. Coronary artery thrombosis in patients with unstable angina. *Br Heart J* 1981;45:411–416.
16. Ambrose JA, Winters SL, Stern A, et al. Angiographic morphology and the pathogenesis of unstable angina pectoris. *J Am Coll Cardiol* 1985;5:609–616.
17. Théroux P, Ouimet H, McCans J, et al. Aspirin, heparin, or both to treat acute unstable angina. *N Engl J Med* 1988;319:1105–1111.
18. Satler LF, Pallas RS, Bond OB, et al. Assessment of residual coronary arterial stenosis after thrombolytic therapy during acute myocardial infarction. *Am J Cardiol* 1987;59:1231–1233.
19. The TIMI Study Group. Comparison of invasive and conservative strategies after treatment with intravenous tissue plasminogen activator in acute myocardial infarction. Results of the Thrombolysis in Myocardial Infarction (TIMI) Phase II Trial. *N Engl J Med* 1989;320:618–627.
20. Kereiakes DJ, Topol EJ, George BS, et al. Myocardial infarction with mini-

mal coronary atherosclerosis in the era of thrombolytic reperfusion. *J Am Coll Cardiol* 1991;17:304–312.
21. Marshall JC, Waxman HL, Sauerwein A, et al. Frequency of low-grade residual coronary stenosis after thrombolysis during acute myocardial infarction. *Am J Cardiol* 1990;66:773–778.
22. Ruocco NA, Bergelson BA, Jacobs AK, et al. Invasive versus conservative strategy after thrombolytic therapy for acute myocardial infarction in patients with antecedent angina. A report from Thrombolysis in Myocardial Infarction Phase II (TIMI II). *J Am Coll Cardiol* 1992;20:1445–1451.
23. Bergelson BA, Ruocco NA, Ryan TJ, et al. Antecedent angina: A predictor of residual stenosis after thrombolytic therapy. *J Am Coll Cardiol* 1989;14:91–95.
24. Anderson JL, Sorensen SG, Moreno FL, et al. Multicenter patency trial of intravenous anistreplase compared with streptokinase in acute myocardial infarction. *Circulation* 1991;83:126–140.
25. Schröder R, Vöhringer H, Linderer T, et al. Follow-up after coronary arterial reperfusion with intravenous streptokinase in relation to residual myocardial infarct artery narrowings. *Am J Cardiol* 1985;55:313–317.
26. Van Lierde J, De Geest H, Verstraete M, et al. Angiographic assessment of the infarct-related residual coronary stenosis after spontaneous or therapeutic thrombolysis. *J Am Coll Cardiol* 1990;16:1545–1549.
27. Gotsman M, Rosenheck S, Nassar H, et al. Angiographic findings in the coronary arteries after thrombolysis in acute myocardial infarction. *Am J Cardiol* 1992;70:715–723.
28. Davies SW, Marchant B, Lyons JP, et al. Coronary lesion morphology in acute myocardial infarction: Demonstration of early remodeling after streptokinase treatment. *J Am Coll Cardiol* 1990;16:1079–1086.
29. Brown BG, Gallery CA, Badger RS, et al. Incomplete lysis of thrombus in the moderate underlying atherosclerotic lesion during intracoronary infusion of streptokinase for acute myocardial infarction: Quantitative angiographic observations. *Circulation* 1986;73:653–661.
30. Nakagawa S, Hanada Y, Koiwaya Y, et al. Angiographic features in the infarct-related artery after intracoronary urokinase followed by prolonged anticoagulation. Role of ruptured atheromatous plaque and adherent thrombus in acute myocardial infarction in vivo. *Circulation* 1988;78:1335–1344.
31. Waters D, Lam JYT. Is thrombolytic therapy striking out in unstable angina? *Circulation* 1992;86:1642–1644.
32. The TIMI IIIB Investigators. Effects of tissue plasminogen activator and a comparison of early invasive and conservative strategies in unstable angina and non-Q-wave myocardial infarction. Results of the TIMI IIIB Trial. *Circulation* 1994;89:1545–1556.
33. Ambrose JA, Alexopoulos D. Thrombolysis in unstable angina: Will the beneficial effects of thrombolytic therapy in myocardial infarction apply to patients with unstable angina? *J Am Coll Cardiol* 1989;13:1666–1671.
34. Williams DO, Topol EJ, Califf RM, et al. Intravenous recombinant tissue-type plasminogen activator in patients with unstable angina pectoris. Results of a placebo-controlled, randomized trial. *Circulation* 1990;82:376–383.
35. Ardissino D, Barberis P, De Servi S, et al. Recombinant tissue-type plasminogen activator followed by heparin compared with heparin alone for refractory unstable angina pectoris. *Am J Cardiol* 1990;66:910–914.
36. Sansa M, Cernigliaro C, Campi A, et al. Effects of urokinase and heparin

on minimal cross- sectional area of the culprit narrowing in unstable angina pectoris. *Am J Cardiol* 1991;68:451–456.

37. Bär FW, Verheugt FW, Col J, et al. Thrombolysis in patients with unstable angina improves the angiographic but not the clinical outcome. Results of UNASEM, a multicenter, randomized, placebo- controlled, clinical trial with anistreplase. *Circulation* 1992;86:131–137.

38. Freeman MR, Langer A, Wilson RF, et al. Thrombolysis in unstable angina. Randomized double-blind trial of t-PA and placebo. *Circulation* 1992;85: 150–157.

39. The TIMI IIIA Investigators. Early effects of tissue-type plasminogen activator added to conventional therapy on the culprit coronary lesion in patients presenting with ischemic cardiac pain at rest. Results of the Thrombolysis in Myocardial Ischemia (TIMI IIIA) Trial. *Circulation* 1993;87:38–52.

40. Ambrose JA, Tannenbaum MA, Alexopoulos D, et al. Angiographic progression of coronary artery disease and the development of myocardial infarction. *J Am Coll Cardiol* 1988;12:56–62.

41. Little WC, Constantinescu M, Applegate RJ, et al. Can coronary angiography predict the site of a subsequent myocardial infarction in patients with mild-to-moderate coronary artery disease? *Circulation* 1988;78:1157–1166.

42. Nobuyoshi M, Tanaka M, Nosaka H, et al. Progression of coronary atherosclerosis: Is coronary spasm related to progression? *J Am Coll Cardiol* 1991; 18:904–910.

43. Giroud D, Li JM, Urban P, et al. Relation of the site of acute myocardial infarction to the most severe coronary arterial stenosis at prior angiography. *Am J Cardiol* 1992;69:729–732.

44. Waters D, Lespérance J, Francetich M, et al. A controlled clinical trial to assess the effect of a calcium channel blocker on the progression of coronary atherosclerosis. *Circulation* 1990;82:1940–1953.

45. Waters D, Lespérance J, Hudon G. Progression of coronary atherosclerosis: A prospective, quantitative angiographic study. *Circulation* 1990;82(suppl III):III-251. Abstract.

46. Ellis S, Alderman E, Cain K, et al. Morphology of left anterior descending coronary territory lesions as a predictor of anterior myocardial infarction: A CASS Registry Study. *J Am Coll Cardiol* 1989;13:1481–1491.

47. Taeymans Y, Théroux P, Lespérance J, et al. Quantitative angiographic morphology of the coronary artery lesions at risk of thrombotic occlusion. *Circulation* 1992;85:78–85.

48. Moise A, Théroux P, Taeymans Y, et al. Unstable angina and progression of coronary atherosclerosis. *N Engl J Med* 1983;309:685–689.

49. Mercho N, Waters D, Craven T, et al. Quantitative coronary arteriographic comparison of the culprit lesions of unstable angina and myocardial infarction in a prospectively defined population. *Circulation* 1995;92(suppl I):I-719. Abstract.

50. Ambrose JA, Winters SL, Arora RR, et al. Angiographic evolution of coronary artery morphology in unstable angina. *J Am Coll Cardiol* 1986;7: 472–478.

51. Kalbfleisch SJ, McGillem MJ, Simon SB, et al. Automated quantitation of indexes of coronary lesion complexity. Comparison between patients with stable and unstable angina. *Circulation* 1990;82:439–447.

52. Freeman MR, Williams AE, Chisolm RJ, et al. Intracoronary thrombus and complex morphology in unstable angina. Relation to timing of angiography and in-hospital cardiac events. *Circulation* 1989;80:17–23.

53. Bugiardini R, Pozzati A, Borghi A, et al. Angiographic morphology in unstable angina and its relation to transient myocardial ischemia and hospital outcome. *Am J Cardiol* 1991;67:460–464.
54. Dangas G, Mehran R, Wallenstein S, et al. Correlation of angiographic morphology and clinical presentation in unstable angina. *J Am Coll Cardiol* 1997;29:519–525.
55. Chen L, Chester MR, Redwood S, et al. Angiographic stenosis progression and coronary events in patients with 'stabilized' unstable angina. *Circulation* 1995;91:2319–2324.
56. Kaski JC, Chester MR, Chen L, et al. Rapid angiographic progression of coronary artery disease in patients with angina pectoris. The role of complex stenosis morphology. *Circulation* 1995;92:2058–2065.
57. Chen L, Chester MR, Crook R, et al. Differential progression of complex culprit stenoses in patients with stable and unstable angina pectoris. *J Am Coll Cardiol* 1996;28:597–603.
58. Chester MR, Chen L, Tousoulis D, et al. Differential progression of complex and smooth stenoses within the same coronary tree in men with stable coronary artery disease. *J Am Coll Cardiol* 1995;25:837–842.

Chapter 5

Detection of Atherosclerosis and Identification of Vulnerable Plaque: Potential Role of Intravascular Ultrasound

Steven E. Nissen, MD, Khalid Ziada, MD, and E. Murat Tuzcu, MD

Introduction

Until recently, atherosclerotic coronary lesions could not be visualized in vivo by any imaging modality. Accordingly, detection of coronary atherosclerotic disease has traditionally relied on indirect methods that either depict the vessel lumen (angiography) or unmask the ischemic effect of coronary obstructions (functional testing). However, both methods are insensitive to the early, minimally obstructive disease associated with the most lethal consequences of atherosclerosis—acute coronary syndromes. Recent technical advances have enabled intraluminal coronary interrogation using small catheter-delivered intravascular ultrasound probes.[1-7] For intravascular imaging, high frequencies of ultrasound are used, which range from approximately 20 MHz to 50 MHz, and enable very high spatial resolution.

Intravascular ultrasound represents a radically different approach to imaging of vessel wall anatomy, providing important insights into diverse phenomena, which range from the pathophysiology of coronary syndromes to the mechanical effects of interventional devices.[8] Whereas angiography depicts the complex cross-sectional anatomy of a human coronary as a planar silhouette, ultrasound *directly* examines the anatomy within the vessel wall. This capability

From: Fuster, V (ed). *The Vulnerable Atherosclerotic Plaque: Understanding, Identification, and Modification.* Armonk, NY: Futura Publishing Company, Inc.; © 1999.

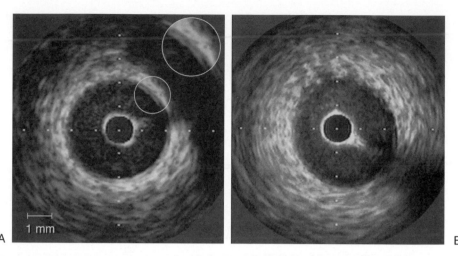

Figure 1. Normal anatomy by coronary intravascular ultrasound. **A.** A trilaminar arterial structure is evident within the magnified inset in the upper right hand corner. **B.** The artery is monolayered. Both images represent variants of normal anatomy by intravascular ultrasound.

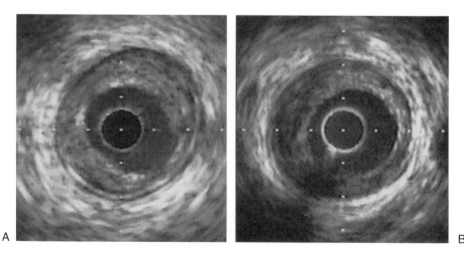

Figure 2. "Soft" sonolucent atheroma. Both panels show examples of plaque with relatively low echogenicity. Atheromas with this appearance have been shown to contain a high lipid content.

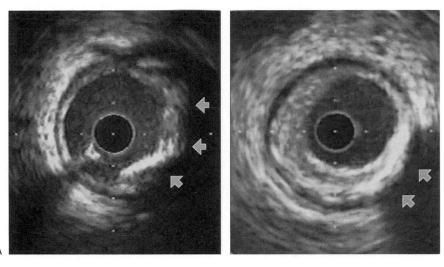

Figure 3. Fibrocalcific coronary atheromata. Both panels show atheromata with relatively high echogenicity consistent with fibrous and/or fibrocalcific plaque. The areas identified by the gray arrows exhibit "acoustic shadowing," marked attenuation of ultrasound transmission, consistent with calcification.

allows the operator to precisely measure atheroma size, distribution, and composition (Figs. 1—3). The incremental value of coronary ultrasound originates principally from two key features: its cross-sectional, tomographic perspective, and the ability to directly image atheromata. Accordingly, miniaturized intravascular devices are increasingly used in both clinical practice and research to confirm, refute, or supplement angiographic data.

Rationale for Ultrasound

Limitations of Angiography

Coronary angiography depicts the vessel anatomy as a simple two-dimensional projection of the vascular lumen. Clinical, histologic, and animal investigations have revealed many deficiencies inherent in this method for evaluation of coronary artery disease.[9–17] Necropsy studies demonstrate that the vessel wall in atherosclerotic coronaries is complex with highly variable luminal shapes and sizes. Accordingly, the

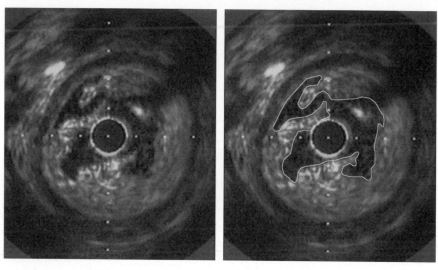

Figure 4. Complex coronary luminal shape. **A.** An atheroma following treatment with balloon angioplasty. The lumen is highly eccentric with many flaps and crevices. **B.** The blood—atheroma border is outlined in white. The angiographic appearance of a complex plaque such as the one shown here will predictably overestimate lumen size.

silhouette or "luminogram" of the artery is a relatively poor representation of coronary anatomy and a limited standard on which to base diagnostic or therapeutic decisions (Fig. 4).

Visual interpretation of angiograms exhibits significant observer variability with observer differences in the visual estimation of stenosis severity approaching 50%.[13,14] Comparisons of angiography to postmortem histology have documented major discrepancies between the apparent angiographic severity of lesions and postmortem histologic examination.[10–12] Nearly all necropsy studies demonstrate that angiography significantly underestimates the extent of atherosclerosis.

Angiography provides no direct information on the hemodynamic effects of coronary stenoses. This limitation is particularly important when evaluating intermediate lesions, generally in the range of 40% to 75% narrowing, which often fall on the borderline between a recommendation for medical therapy or revascularization. With use of functional testing, investigators have demonstrated a striking discordance between angiographic lesion severity and measurements of the physiological effects of the stenosis.[15] Accordingly, most ischemic disease patients require one or more functional tests, in addition to angiography, to enable appropriate clinical decision making.

Percentage Stenosis

The traditional method for characterization of angiographic lesion severity depends on visual or computer measurements of the percentage stenosis. This approach compares the luminal diameter within the lesion to the caliber of an adjacent, uninvolved "normal" reference segment. However, necropsy examinations have demonstrated that coronary atherosclerosis is often diffuse, involving long segments of the diseased vessel. Therefore, in many patients, no truly normal segment exists; this precludes accurate calculation of the percentage diameter reduction. In the presence of diffuse disease, calculation of percentage stenosis will always underestimate disease severity. In the most dramatic circumstances, diffuse, concentric, and symmetrical coronary disease can affect the entire length of the vessel, resulting in an angiographic appearance of a small artery with minimal luminal irregularities (Fig. 5).[18]

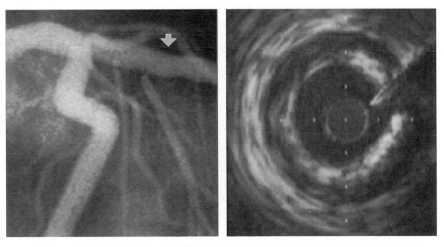

A   B

Figure 5. Diffuse coronary disease. **A.** An angiogram showing trivial luminal narrowing. **B.** Ultrasound from the site marked by the gray arrow illustrates a well—formed fibrous cap with diffuse atherosclerosis. Because the entire vessel was diseased, the angiogram is false-negative.

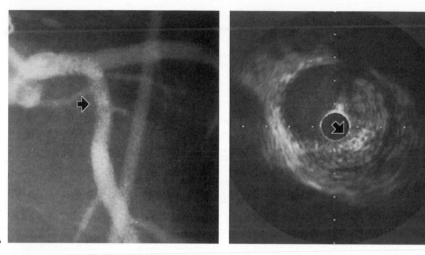

A   B

Figure 6. Coronary remodeling. **A.** A coronary angiogram shows no discrete luminal narrowing. Ultrasound obtained from the site marked by the black arrow shows a large crescentic atheroma. The adventitia overlining this atheroma is expanded outward, thus preventing luminal encroachment. This process is known as coronary remodeling (Glagov phenomenon).

Coronary Remodeling

Angiography is particularly confounded by the phenomenon of coronary "remodeling," first described in 1987 by Glagov et al[19] The remodeling process is observed histologically as the outward displacement of the external vessel wall in vascular segments with significant atherosclerosis. In the early stages of coronary disease, this adventitial enlargement prevents the atheroma from encroaching on the lumen, thereby concealing the presence, on angiography, of a lesion (Fig. 6). Necropsy studies demonstrate that lumen reduction does not occur until the plaque occupies more than 40% of the total vessel cross-sectional area. Although remodeled lesions do not restrict blood flow, observational studies demonstrate that minimal, nonobstructive angiographic lesions represent an important substrate for acute coronary syndromes.[20] Other studies demonstrate that angiographically unrecognized disease virtually always underlies an ergonovine-positive response in symptomatic patients with "normal" coronary angiograms.[21]

Ultrasound Advantages

Several characteristics of intravascular ultrasound have potential value in the precise detection and quantitation of atherosclerotic coronary disease.[5–8,22—26] The tomographic orientation of ultrasound enables visualization of the full 360° circumference of the vessel wall, rather than a 2-dimensional projection of the lumen. The cross-sectional perspective of ultrasound enables characterization of disease in vessels that are difficult to assess by conventional angiographic techniques, including diffusely diseased segments, bifurcation or ostial lesions, and eccentric plaques. Measurement of lumen area can employ direct planimetry performed on a cross-sectional image, which unlike angiography, is not dependent on the projection angle. The constant velocity of sound in soft tissue permits ultrasound scanners to overlay a highly accurate, electronically generated distance scale within the image. This capability obviates the need to correct for radiographic magnification, a troublesome requisite of angiographic methods.

Ultrasound Limitations

Normal first-order epicardial coronaries range from 1.0 to 5.0 mm, while atherosclerotic lumina frequently reach 0.1 to 0.5 mm. Accordingly, the physical size of ultrasound catheters (currently about 1.0 mm) constitutes an important limitation in certain clinical applications. Although the operator may be able to interrogate most critical stenoses with a 1.0-mm device, lesional morphology or quantitative measurements will be distorted by the distending effect of the catheter.

Evaluation of small coronaries or second-order branches requires imaging close to the transducer surface. However, ring-down artifact, a defect that appears in virtually all medical ultrasound devices, impairs the ability to image close to the transducer surface. Ring-down artifacts are produced by acoustic oscillations in the piezoelectric transducer material that results in high-amplitude ultrasound signals that obscure near-field imaging. Inability to image structures immediately adjacent to the transducer results in an "acoustic" catheter size slightly larger than its physical size. Recent designs use carefully chosen transducer materials, ultrasound-absorbent backings, specialized coatings, and electronic filtering to suppress ring-down artifacts.

All tomographic imaging techniques are vulnerable to distortion produced by imaging in oblique planes not perpendicular to the long axis of the vessel. Noncoaxial alignment of the transducer within the artery results in an elliptical rather than circular cross-sectional imaging plane.[27] This artifact can represent a significant confounding variable in application of intravascular ultrasound for quantitative plaque and lumen measurements. Mechanical transducers also exhibit cyclical oscillations in rotational speed, resulting in an artifact known as nonuniform rotational distortion (NURD). Nonuniform rotational speed variation produces a readily visible type of distortion recognized as circumferential stretching of a portion of the image with compression of the contralateral vessel wall.

Intravascular Ultrasound

Catheter Designs

Intracoronary ultrasound equipment consists of two major components, a catheter incorporating a miniaturized transducer, and a console containing the electronics necessary to reconstruct the image. Two very different approaches to ultrasound catheter design are currently employed—mechanically rotated devices, and multi-element electronic arrays. Multi-element designs usually result in catheters with greater mechanical flexibility, while actively rotated probes typically offer superior image quality. Currently available ultrasound catheters for intracoronary applications have an outer diameter between 2.6 and 3.5 French (diameter of 0.87 to 1.17 mm). For most mechanical ultrasound systems, a rotation rate of 1800 rpm is used, which corresponds to 30 full revolutions per second, yielding 30 images per second.

Since the transducer is placed in close proximity to the vessel wall, high ultrasound frequencies are typically employed for intravascular imaging, centered at 20 MHz to 50 MHz for coronary imaging. The use of high frequencies provides excellent theoretical resolution because the ultrasound wavelength, which determines the theoretical maximum resolution, is inversely proportional to the frequency. At 30 MHz, the wavelength is approximately 50 μm (0.05 mm), which permits axial resolution approaching 100 μm. Determinants of lateral resolution are more complicated and are dependent on imaging depth and beam shape. Lateral resolution for a 30-MHz device averages approximately 250 μm at the typical distances most prevalent in coronary imaging. In the electronic systems, an annular array of multiple piezoelectric transducer elements (currently up to 64) are activated sequentially to generate a tomographic image. The electronic signals are processed and multiplexed by several ultraminiaturized integrated circuits near the catheter tip.

Examination Technique

Standard interventional techniques for intracoronary catheter delivery are used for intraluminal ultrasound examination. Intravenous heparin (5000 to 10,000 units) and intracoronary nitroglycerin (100 to

300 μg) are routinely administered prior to imaging. Most practitioners employ a 7- or 8-French guiding catheter, and subselectively cannulate the vessel using a steerable a 0.0140-inch angioplasty guidewire. A stable guiding catheter position with good support is desirable, since current ultrasound catheters have less trackability and a larger profile than modern balloon angioplasty catheters. The operator careful advances or retracts the imaging catheter over the wire to examine the vessel in real time, recording images on videotape for subsequent quantitative or qualitative analysis.

Some centers use a motorized pullback device to withdraw the catheter at a constant speed (between 0.25 and 1 mm/s, most frequently 0.5 mm/s). However, it must be emphasized that a single pullback, even when controlled by a precise motor, may be insufficient for a complete diagnostic ultrasound examination. Accordingly, motorized pullback should only be used as a means to "survey" the coronary prior to more prolonged and thorough examination of sites of interest. The principal advantage of motorized pullback is the ability to perform serial studies in which the analyzed segments are carefully matched to determine the long-term effect of a disease process or intervention. For mechanical systems, some catheter designs that allow the withdrawal of the imaging cable within an external sheath minimize the risk of catheter rotation or uneven velocity during pullback. Side-branches, visualized with both angiography and ultrasound, are extremely useful as landmarks to facilitate interpretation and comparisons of sequential examinations.

Safety of Intravascular Ultrasound

Intravascular ultrasound has been performed safely in a wide variety of clinical situations with few serious untoward effects.[28] Focal coronary spasm occurs occasionally (5% to 10% of patients), but is usually transient and responds rapidly to intracoronary administration of nitroglycerin (100 to 300 μg). Additional care is required when imaging small distal vessels or tight stenoses, because the imaging transducer can partially or totally occlude blood flow. However, most patients do not experience chest pain if the catheter is promptly withdrawn. Most centers experienced in ultrasound examination do not routinely image coronaries with an estimated normal diameter that is too small to safely accommodate the device (usually less than 1.3 to 1.5 mm). Although the safety of intracoronary ultrasound is well documented, any device placed subselectively in the coronaries carries the potential risk of vessel injury.

Image Interpretation

Normal Anatomy

A series of investigations has characterized the appearance of normal coronary anatomy by intravascular ultrasound.[6,29-34] At the high frequencies typically used for coronary imaging (25 MHz and above), the vessel lumen is characterized by faint, finely textured, specular echoes that move and swirl with blood flow. The echogenicity within the lumen arises from the reflection of acoustic energy by circulating blood elements. In many situations, blood "speckle" assists image interpretation by providing a means to confirm the communication between tissue planes and the lumen. The pattern of blood speckle is dependent upon the velocity of flow, exhibiting increased intensity and a coarser texture when flow is reduced. In some cases, fresh (nonorganized) thrombus can be recognized as a region of reduced blood flow echogenicity.

Investigations performed either in vivo or with use of excised, pressure distended vessels have characterized the appearance of normal and abnormal coronaries by intravascular ultrasound. Important determinants of the vessel wall appearance include both the normal arterial structure and the inherent properties of ultrasound. An abrupt change in acoustic impedance between adjacent tissue layers is the most important factor responsible for the ultrasound appearance of the vessel wall. The leading edge of the intima (at the interface between the blood-filled lumen and the endothelium) and the outer border of the media (at the junction of media and external elastic membrane) are two particularly strong acoustic interfaces. As a result, both boundaries are typically well visualized by ultrasound in human coronaries.

The two classic interfaces are not well visualized in all normal subjects (Fig.1).[32] The magnitude of the acoustic impedance shift at the blood-tissue interface is highly dependent on patient-related factors, particularly the composition of the intima. In normals, the intima is thin and consists principally of a superficial layer of endothelial cells and connective tissue, resulting in a relatively small impedance difference between blood and intima. Accordingly, in young subjects, ultrasound imaging frequently cannot distinguish intima from the deeper wall layers. This finding has led some observers to propose that a trilaminar wall morphology represents evidence of early coronary atherosclerosis.[32] Others have studied young subjects and report a range of normal values for the intimal thickness, typically about 0.15 ± 0.07 mm.[6] Most investigators use 0.25 to 0.30 mm as an upper limit of normal (2 standard deviations greater than normal).

In older subjects, progressive intimal thickening or the development of pathological intimal changes results in an ultrasound pattern
consisting of two distinct echogenic layers sandwiching a sonolucent
intermediate layer (three-layered appearance). A clear delineation of
the inner border of the media (internal elastic membrane) is frequently
difficult or impossible, so that only two layers are normally distinguished with ultrasound. The inner-wall layer, often described as intima or intimal plaque, should be more correctly described as "intima-
media complex." Whether the artery is trilaminar or monolayered, the
deepest layers, representing the adventitia and peri-adventitial tissues,
exhibit a characteristic "onion skin" pattern. The outer border of the
vessel is usually indistinct, primarily because there are no acoustic differences between the adventitia and other encasing tissues. Accordingly, total wall thickness cannot be measured with use of ultrasound,
except in vessels with a distinct outer border such as aortocoronary
saphenous vein grafts.

Atherosclerotic Wall Morphology

Atherosclerotic arteries exhibit a diversity of features that reflect
the distribution and composition of the atheromata. (Figs. 2,3, and 7).
The subtle changes, such as fatty streaks, observed by histology early
in the development of coronary atherosclerosis are not visible with use
of current 30-MHz ultrasound devices. Sites with unequivocal atherosclerosis exhibit generalized or focal thickening of the intimal leading
edge, while advanced lesions appear as large echogenic masses within
the lumen. Most classification schemes differentiate coronary atheromata into one of three categories (soft, fibrous, or calcified) according
to plaque echogenicity. However, the echogenicity of plaque components is also not dependent on the acquisition settings (gain, compression, etc.) of the ultrasound system. Accordingly, most classification
schemes compare the echointensity of the plaque to the surrounding
adventitia to correct for differences in technique.

Plaques are termed *soft* if they are less echogenic than the adventitia. These echolucent lesions represent either highly cellular fibromuscular proliferation (eg, restenosis) or diffuse lipid infiltration, both of
which exhibit low echogenicity. Plaques with an echodensity similar
to the adventitia are described as *fibrous* or *hard*. In vitro studies that
compare ultrasound appearance with histology confirm that echogenic
lesions have a high fibrous tissue content. "Calcified" lesions are recognized as highly echogenic plaques that attenuate transmission of the
ultrasound signal, thereby obscuring deeper layers, a phenomenon
known as *acoustic shadowing*. Obstruction of ultrasound transmission,

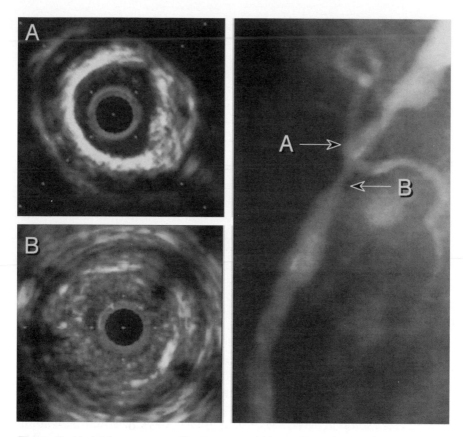

Figure 7. Variable coronary atheroma morphology. Two sites labeled **A** and **B** in the angiogram have very different atheroma morphologies. In **A** the lesion is heavily calcified, whereas in **B** the lesion is soft and sonolucent.

not merely a high degree of echogenicity, is a requisite for identification of calcium. With the exception of multiple scattered microcalcification, ultrasound can be considered highly specific and sensitive for the detection of calcified plaque.

The traditional approach to identification of calcification uses cinefluoroscopy to visualize moving opacities in proximity to the vessel silhouette. However, this approach is limited by many factors, including the moderate spatial and contrast resolution of angiography and the confounding effects produced by the overlap of other calcium-containing structures. Studies which compare ultrasound and angiography studies demonstrate poor sensitivity for angiography in detection of coronary calcification.[35,36] Of 1155 coronary lesions, Mintz et al[35] detected calcium in 73% by ultrasound and only 38% by angiography.

At interventional target lesions, Tuzcu et al[36] reported that angiography identified less than half (45%) of patients with calcification by ultrasound. Even in the presence of more extensive calcification, the sensitivity of angiography remains poor, correctly identifying only 52% of patients with calcium subtending more than 90° of vessel circumference and only 63% of lesions with greater than 180° of involvement.

Appropriate caution must be exercised in interpretation of intravascular ultrasound images. Although ultrasound devices produce remarkably detailed views of the vessel wall, interpretation usually employs visual inspection of acoustic reflections to determine plaque morphology. Validated methods do not yet exist for objective or automated classification of atheromatous lesions. The echogenicity and texture of different histologic features may exhibit comparable acoustic properties, appearing quite similar by intravascular ultrasound. For example, a sonolucent plaque may represent intracoronary thrombus, while a nearly identical appearance may result from an atheroma with a high lipid content. Thus, intravascular ultrasound can delineate the thickness and echogenicity of vessel wall structures, but does not provide actual histology.

Clinical and Research Applications

Angiographically Unrecognized Disease

Normal angiograms are present in 10% to 15% of patients undergoing coronary angiography for suspected coronary artery disease. In patients with symptoms of coronary disease, intravascular ultrasound commonly detects atherosclerosis at angiographically normal sites.[6] Erbel et al[37] observed atherosclerotic abnormalities in 21 of 44 patients (48%) with suspected coronary artery disease and normal coronary angiograms. Other studies demonstrate that, if any luminal irregularity is present by angiography, ultrasound will usually reveal disease at nearly all other examined sites.[6] The prevalence of disease at angiographically normal sites confirms the finding, previously reported from necropsy studies, that coronary disease is more extensive than what is apparent by angiography.[9,10]

There are multiple mechanisms by which angiography may underestimate the extent of atherosclerosis. As previously noted, in order to detect disease, angiography relies on comparison of the diseased segment of the vessel to a normal reference site. However, atherosclerosis is typically a diffuse process, and a diffusely diseased vessel may be reduced in caliber along its entire length, containing no truly normal segment for comparison. In the absence of a focal stenosis, the angiographer could erroneously conclude that the vessel is simply "small in caliber." There are physical limitations that prevent an angiographer from obtaining optimal radiographic projections in some patients. For example, at certain angles, overlapping structures, such as adjacent vessels, can obscure some segments of the coronary. Accordingly, an eccentric lesion may not be visualized by angiography. Vessel foreshortening can conceal short "napkin-ring" lesions (usually less than 1 to 2 mm in length) from angiographic detection.

The phenomenon of coronary remodeling, originally described by Glagov[19] from necropsy examinations, represents another important mechanism underlying false-negative angiography (Fig. 6).[18,38,39] As previously discussed, compensatory enlargement (remodeling) of the vessel wall overlying the plaque preserves lumen diameter, resulting in an angiographic diameter similar to those of adjacent, uninvolved coronary segments.

Despite the high sensitivity of ultrasound in detecting atherosclerosis, the tomographic orientation of intravascular ultrasound can represent a problem in quantifying disease severity. Since each image contains information from only a single tomographic slice of the vessel, quantification of atheroma burden requires integration of multiple cross sections. In this application, motorized pullback devices are increasing used to facilitate measurements. Since motor speed is kept constant, the operator can obtain a series of evenly spaced cross sections, which are individually measured and summated to approximate total atheroma burden. A second approach to atheroma quantitation employs three-dimensional (3-D) reconstruction of the vessel from the ultrasound images. Unfortunately 3-D methods are exceedingly complex, have many unresolved confounding variables, and remain largely unvalidated.

Ambiguous Lesions

Despite thorough examination with use of multiple angiographic projections, ambiguous lesions remain a common diagnostic problem. Difficult lesions include ostial lesions, bifurcation lesions, and moderate stenoses (angiographic severity ranging from 40% to 75%) in patients whose symptomatic status is difficult to evaluate. Such lesions are particularly problematic in patients who are unable to tolerate functional testing or whose symptomatic status is difficult to evaluate. For patients with ambiguous lesions, ultrasound provides precise tomographic measurements, enabling quantitation of the stenosis independent of the radiographic projection.

Cardiac Allograft Vasculopathy

Transplant coronary vasculopathy is the leading cause of death beyond the first year after cardiac transplantation. Because cardiac allografts are functionally denervated, major clinical events such as myocardial infarction, congestive heart failure, and sudden death may occur without prodromal angina. Although most transplant centers perform coronary arteriograms annually for screening, these surveillance studies often fail to detect atherosclerosis prior to a clinical event.[40-43] Angiography systematically underestimates coronary atherosclerosis in transplant recipients, primarily because these patients frequently have diffuse disease that, for reasons already enumerated, conceals atherosclerosis from angiography. Increasingly, transplant centers routinely perform intravascular ultrasound annually in cardiac transplant recipients.[44]

Intracoronary ultrasound is an effective and reproducible method of measuring intimal proliferation in cardiac transplant recipients. Studies which employ ultrasound to detect transplant vasculopathy report a very high incidence of this disease. Tuzcu et al[45] demonstrated abnormal intimal thickening in 80% of patients at 1 year and more than 92% of patients studied 4 or more years after transplantation. Intracoronary ultrasound has been shown to have prognostic value after heart transplant, as the presence of a mean intimal thickness greater or equal to 0.3 mm is an independent predictor of overall and cardiac survival and of freedom from repeat transplantation.[46]

The studies performed in patients early after transplantation have helped to define the normal appearance of young healthy arteries, but have also shown that advanced atherosclerotic changes can be present in apparently normal donor hearts.[45-47] Recent studies have revealed two distinctive pathways to transplant—associated atherosclerosis.[44] Some patients receive atherosclerotic plaques transmitted via the donor heart, while others develop an immune-mediated vasculopathy. Available data indicate that the ultrasound disease pattern is related to the origins of the vasculopathy. Traditional atherosclerosis (usually donor-transmitted) has an eccentric plaque distribution with patchy longitudinal involvement, whereas immune-mediated (acquired) disease is more circumferential and diffuse.

"Unstable" Atherosclerotic Lesions

Little et al[20] have clearly demonstrated that plaques of minimal to moderate angiographic severity are the most likely to rupture and cause acute myocardial infarction. The ability of intravascular ultrasound to differentiate predominantly fibrous or calcified plaques from atheromata with a high lipid content offers the potential to determine which plaques are most susceptible to progression to acute coronary syndromes. When intracoronary ultrasound is used to interrogate lesions associated with acute coronary syndromes, the plaques frequently contain relatively echolucent material, consistent with a high lipid content. Some plaques contain a zone of reduced echogenicity within the main body of the atheroma. In individual cases, one cannot determine whether these represent areas of lipid deposition and necrotic degeneration, both of which can appear as zones of low density. It some cases, the echolucent zone is covered by a distinct "cap" that exhibits greater echogenicity and presumably represents the classic fibrous cap described by histology.

The appearance of unstable or degenerating atheromata by ultrasound remains incompletely characterized.[48,49] Spontaneous plaque degeneration or fissuring within low-grade lesions is sometimes evident during ultrasound examination of the culprit lesions in patients with unstable coronary ischemic syndrome, hours to days following the event (Fig. 8). This phenomenon commonly has the appearance of multiple channels within the plaque that communicate with the lumen. However, at the 30-MHz imaging frequency most often used in coro-

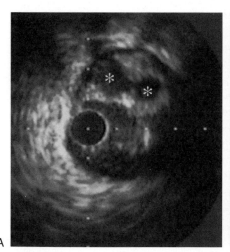
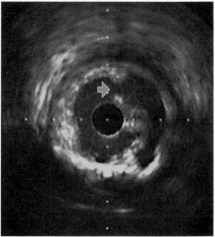

A   B

Figure 8. Intravascular ultrasound in an unstable coronary lesion. These are images from two different patients. In **A** there is a complex flow channel deep within the plaque, marked by the asterisks. In **B** a fibrous cap remnant is seen following rupture of an atheroma at the site indicated by the gray arrow. Both of these appearances are common in intravascular ultrasound imaging following recovery from an acute coronary syndrome.

nary ultrasound, organizing thrombus may appear visually indistinguishable from other types of plaques. The presence of mobile or pedunculated intraluminal masses suggests the presence of thrombi, but definitive conclusions are often not possible.

Intravascular Ultrasound and Restenosis

Angiographic parameters, including quantitative angiographic measurements, are poor predictors of the long-term results following balloon angioplasty. Accordingly, an important evolving application of intravascular ultrasound is the detection of lesions that are at high risk for development of restenosis at the time of the initial procedure. Theoretically, this would allow the operator to perform further interventions to improve the long-term outcome. Despite this promise, preliminary studies have shown conflicting data concerning the factors predictive of restenosis after balloon angioplasty.[50,51] A more complete understanding of restenosis has evolved from serial ultrasound measurements of plaque and lumen areas at follow-up studies after balloon angioplasty and directional atherectomy.[51]

In some studies, repeated ultrasound examinations have shown that a late reduction in total vessel area (chronic negative remodeling) is an important mechanism of restenosis after many nonstent interventional procedures.[51] These observations suggest that mechanical interventions (such as stenting) to prevent chronic recoil may be more important in the prevention of restenosis than pharmacological treatment to prevent intimal hyperplasia. If further validated, this concept would explain the lower restenosis rate observed in randomized multicenter studies that compare balloon angioplasty and stent implantation.[52,53] Although some strong evidence of "negative remodeling" exists, this concept remains incompletely developed and should still be considered speculative. In particular, the proportion of lumen loss produced by vessel shrinkage after intervention versus neointimal proliferation remains poorly defined.

Other phenomena observed by ultrasound may also play a role in determining the outcome following coronary interventions. The relatively poor correlation between angiographic and ultrasonic dimensions following angioplasty raises a provocative issue. In certain patients, does "restenosis" represent a failure in adequate augmentation of the luminal area, rather than the subsequent loss of luminal gain? Can ultrasound assessment of the residual lumen predict short-term post-interventional complications or identify patients with a high likelihood of poor long-term results? Several multicenter clinical trials, currently underway or recently completed (but unpublished), are examining whether ultrasound can reliably predict restenosis following various types of intervention.

Future Directions

Technological advances in intravascular imaging, including further reductions in the size of imaging catheters to guidewire dimensions (<0.025 inches), are anticipated during the next several years. A guidewire-sized ultrasound probe would improve the ease and safety of the examination and might enable simultaneous transluminal imaging during the revascularization procedure. Smaller devices would also enable imaging of nearly all coronary stenoses prior to treatment.

Analysis of backscattered ultrasound signals has been used by several investigators to perform "tissue characterization" of coronary plaques. Intrinsic characteristics of the backscattered ultrasound signals, including the amplitude distribution, frequency response, and power spectrum of the signal, convey specific information about tissue types.[53-56] Soft plaque consists of an amorphous collection of lipid substances, fibrosis, cholesterol clefts, and a variable amount of collagen and elastin. Thrombus, on the other hand, consists of a fairly organized layering of fibrous strands packed with a dense collection of red blood cells. Preliminary studies have shown that computer-based analysis of the unprocessed radiofrequency backscatter from the vessel wall can differentiate the histologic layers of the normal vessel wall and distinguish the cellular infrastructure of noncalcific plaque and thrombus, based on first-order moments of the probability distribution function.

Higher frequency ultrasound catheters are also in the advanced stages of development and will likely yield significantly improved spatial resolution, although the incremental clinical benefit remains to be demonstrated (Fig. 9). There may exist significant trade-offs in moving beyond the current 30-MHz frequency. For example, although high-frequency probes enable better axial and lateral resolution, penetration is likely to be impaired in comparison to more conventional devices. In addition, greater backscatter from blood cells at high frequencies may interfere with discrimination of the interface between lumen and vessel wall. However, as the demand for catheter miniaturization becomes more intense, a shorter wavelength becomes more important in preserving near-field image quality. Use of a center frequency of 40 MHz to 50 MHz, for example, would allow discrimination of small fatty deposits or zones of fibrous tissue separated by as little as three to four times the size of a red blood cell. It remains apparent that the physical limits of intravascular imaging technology have not been reached. Accordingly, further improvements in the performance of these devices are anticipated.

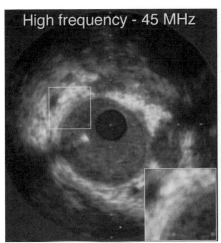 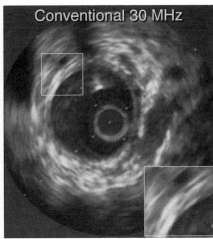

A   B

Figure 9. The advantages of high frequency imaging. Both images were obtained in a porcine animal model. **A.** A 45-MHz intravascular ultrasound image is shown with magnification of a portion of the vessel wall in the inset image. **B.** A conventional 30-MHz image in the same vessel. The high frequency image exhibits much improved lateral resolution and increased image detail.

Three-dimensional reconstruction of intravascular ultrasound has been proposed as a means to facilitate understanding of the spatial relationship between the structures within different tomographic cross sections.[57,58] A prerequisite for 3-D reconstruction is the use of a motorized pullback, which allows the acquisition of successive cross sections separated by known distance. In some 3-D approaches, an image segmentation algorithm is used to process the ultrasound images and distinguish between blood pool and structures of the vessel wall for automatic measurements of lumen area. Despite the promise of these methods, many unresolved problems remain. The algorithms applied for 3-D reconstruction do not allow for the presence of curvatures of the vessel, and assume that the catheter passes in a straight line through the center of consecutive cross sections. The systolic expansion of the coronary vessel and the movements of the catheter within the vessel during the cardiac cycle also generate characteristic artifacts. Accordingly, the reconstructed images should not be considered faithful representations of the vessel and should not be used for volumetric plaque determination. Simultaneous digitization of biplane fluoroscopic tracking of the radiopaque transducer and catheter tip has the potential to overcome some of these limitations, but at present is practical only for small-scale research purposes.

Summary

Coronary intravascular ultrasound continues to undergo rapid development. This imaging modality remains the only readily available means to examine coronary atherosclerotic plaque morphology in vivo. Accordingly, intravascular ultrasound is increasingly used in atherosclerosis research. This new imaging modality has the potential to provide valuable insights into the process by which stable coronary disease undergoes transition to unstable coronary syndromes. If such investigations provide valuable prognostic information, intravascular ultrasound may enable early identification of patients at risk for coronary events. Conceivably, this approach would enable triage of at-risk patients to more aggressive therapy designed to improve clinical outcome.

References

1. Bom N, Lancee CT, Van Egmond FC. An ultrasonic intracardiac scanner. *Ultrasonics* 1972;10:72–76.
2. Yock PG, Johnson EL, Linker DT. Intravascular ultrasound: Development and clinical potential. *Am J Card Imaging* 1988;2:185–193.
3. Roelandt JR, Bom NY, Serruys PW. Intravascular high-resolution real-time, two-dimensional echocardiography. *Int J Card Imaging* 1989;4:63–67.
4. Hodgson JM, Graham SP, Savakus AD, et al. Clinical percutaneous imaging of coronary anatomy using an over-the-wire ultrasound catheter system. *Int J Cardiac Imaging* 1989;4:187–193.
5. Nissen SE, Grines CL, Gurley JC, et al. Application of a new phased-array ultrasound imaging catheter in the assessment of vascular dimensions: In vivo comparison to cineangiography. *Circulation* 1990;81:660–666.
6. Nissen SE, Gurley JC, Grines CL, et al. Intravascular ultrasound assesment of lumen size and wall morphology in normal subjects and patients with coronary artery disease. *Circulation* 1991;84:1087–1099.
7. Tobis JM, Mallery J, Mahon D, et al. Intravascular ultrasound imaging of human coronary arteries in vivo. Analysis of tissue characterization with comparison to in vitro histological specimens. *Circulation* 1991;83:913–926.
8. Nissen SE, Tuzcu EM, De Franco AC. Coronary intravascular ultrasound: Diagnostic and interventional applications. In: Topol EJ ed: *Update to Textbook of Interventional Cardiology*. Philadelphia: W. B. Saunders; 1994:207–222.
9. Arnett EN, Isner JM, Redwood CR, et al. Coronary artery narrowing in coronary heart disease: Comparison of cineangiographic and necropsy findings. *Ann Intern Med* 1979;91:350–356.
10. Grodin CM, Dydra I, Pastgernac A, et al. Discrepancies between cineangiographic and post-mortem findings in patients with coronary artery disease and recent myocardial revascularization. *Circulation* 1974;49:703–709.
11. Isner JM, Kishel J, Kent KM. Accuracy of angiographic determination of left main coronary arterial narrowing. *Circulation* 1981;63:1056–1061.
12. Vlodaver Z, Frech R, van Tassel RA, Edwards JE. Correlation of the antemortem coronary angiogram and the postmortem specimen. *Circulation* 1973;47:162–168.

13. Zir LM, Miller SW, Dinsmore RE, et al. Interobserver variability in coronary angiography. *Circulation* 1976;53:627–632.
14. Galbraith JE, Murphy ML, Desoyza N. Coronary angiogram interpretation: Interobserver variability. *JAMA* 1981;240:2053–2059.
15. White CW, Wright CB, Doty DB, et al. Does visual interpretation of the coronary arteriogram predict the physiologic importance of a coronary stenosis? *N Engl J Med* 1984;310:819–824.
16. Waller BF, Orr CM, Slack JD, et al. Anatomy, histology, and pathology of coronary arteries: A review relevant to new interventional and imaging techniques. Part III. *Clin Cardiol* 1992;15(8):607–615.
17. Roberts WC, Jones AA. Quantitation of coronary arterial narrowing at necropsy in sudden coronary death. *Am J Cardiol* 1979;44:39–44.
18. Topol EJ, Nissen SE. Our preoccupation with coronary luminology. The dissociation between clinical and angiographic findings in ischemic heart disease. *Circulation* 1995;92:2333–2342.
19. Glagov S, Weisenberg E, Zarins CK, et al. Compensatory enlargement of human atherosclerotic coronary arteries. *N Engl J Med* 1986;316:1371–1375.
20. Little WC, Constantinescu M, Applegate RJ, et al. Can arteriography predict the site of a subsequent myocardial infarction in patients with mild-to-moderate coronary artery disease? *Circulation* 1988;78:1157–1166.
21. Yamagishi M, Miyatake K, Tamai J, et al. Detection of atherosclerosis at the site of focal vasospasm in angiographically normal or minimally narrowed coronary segments by intravascular ultrasound. *J Am Coll Cardiol* 1994;23: 352–357.
22. Nissen SE, Gurley JC. Application of intravascular ultrasound to detection and quantitation of coronary atherosclerosis. *Int J Card Imaging* 1991;6: 165–177.
23. Nissen SE, Gurley JC. Quantitative assessment of coronary dimensions, lumen shape and wall morphology by intravascular ultrasound. In: Tobis P, Yock P eds: *Intravascular Ultrasound*. New York, New York: Churchill Livingstone, Inc.; 1992:71–83.
24. Nissen SE, Gurley JC, DeMaria AN. Assessment of vascular disease by intravascular ultrasound. *Cardiology* 1990;77(5):398–410.
25. Nissen SE, DeFranco A, Tuzcu EM. Detection and quantification of atherosclerosis: The emerging role for intravascular ultrasound. In: Fuster V ed: *Syndromes of Atherosclerosis: Correlations of Clinical Imaging and Pathology.* Armonk, NY: Futura Publishing Company, Inc.; 1996:291–312.
26. Nissen SE, Gurley JC, DeMaria AN. Intravascular ultrasound of the coronaries: Current applications and future directions. *Am J Cardiol* 1992;69: 18H–29H.
27. Di Mario C, Madretsma S, Linker D, et al. The angle of incidence of the ultrasonic beam: A critical factor for the image quality in intravascular ultrasonography. *Am Heart J* 1993;126:76–85.
28. Hausmann D, Erbel R, Alibelli-Chemarin MJ, et al. The safety of intracoronary ultrasound. A multicenter survey of 2207 examinations. *Circulation* 1995;91(3):623–630.
29. Gussenhoven EJ, Essed CE, Lancee CT, et al. Arterial wall characteristics determined by intravascular ultrasound imaging: An in vitro study. *J Am Coll Cardiol* 1989;4:947–952.
30. Potkin BN, Bartorelli AL, Gessert JM, et al. Coronary artery imaging with intravascular high-frequency ultrasound. *Circulation* 1990;81:1575–1585.
31. Nishimura RA, Edwards WD, Warnes CA, et al. Intravascular ultrasound

imaging: In vitro validation and pathologic correlation. *J Am Coll Cardiol* 1990;16:145–154.

32. Fitzgerald PJ, St. Goar FG, Connolly AJ, et al. Intravascular ultrasound imaging of coronary arteries: Is three layers the norm? *Circulation* 1992;86: 154–158.

33. St. Goar FG, Pinto FJ, Alderman EL, et al. Intravascular ultrasound imaging of angiographically normal coronary arteries: An in vivo comparison with quantitative angiography. *J Am Coll Cardiol* 1991;18:952–958.

34. Di Mario C, The SHK, Madretsma S, et al. Detection and characterization of vascular lesions by intravascular ultrasound: An in vitro study correlated with histology. *J Am Soc Echocardiogr* 1992;5:135–146.

35. Mintz GS, Popma JJ, Pichard AD, et al. Patterns of calcification in coronary artery disease. A statistical analysis of intravascular ultrasound and coronary angiography in 1,155 lesions. *Circulation* 1995;91:1959–1965.

36. Tuzcu EM, Berkalp B, DeFranco AC, et al. The dilemma of diagnosing coronary calcification: Angiography versus intravascular ultrasound. *J Am Coll Cardiol* 1996;27:832–838.

37. Erbel R, Ge J, Kearney P, et al. Value of intracoronary ultrasound and Doppler in the differentation of angiographically normal coronary arteries: A prospective study in patients with angina pectoris. *Eur Heart J* 1996;17: 880–889.

38. Hermiller JB, Tenaglia AN, Kisslo KB, et al. In vivo validation of compensatory enlargement of atherosclerotic coronary arteries. *Am J Cardiol* 1993;71: 665–668.

39. Ge J, Erbel R, Zamorano J, et al. Coronary artery remodeling in atherosclerotic disease: An intravascular ultrasonic study in vivo. *Coron Artery Dis* 1993;4:981–986.

40. Uretsky BF, Kormos RL, Zerbe TR, et al. Cardiac events after heart transplantation: Incidence and predictive value of coronary arteriography. *J Heart Transplant* 1992;11:S45–S50.

41. O'Neill BJ, Pflugfelder PW, Single NR, et al. Frequency of angiographic detection and quantitative assessment of coronary arterial disease one and three years after cardiac transplantation. *Am J Cardiol* 1989;63:1221–1226.

42. Dressler FA, Miller LW. Necropsy versus angiography: How accurate is angiography? *J Heart Lung Transplant* 1992;11(part 2):S56–S59.

43. Johnson DE, Alderman EL, Schroeder JS, et al. Transplant coronary artery diease: Histopathological correlations with angiographic morphology. *J Am Coll Cardiol* 1991;17:449–457.

44. Tuzcu EM, DeFranco AC, Goormastic M, et al. Dichotomous pattern of coronary atherosclerosis 1 to 9 years after transplantation: Insights from systematic intravascular ultrasound imaging. *J Am Coll Cardiol* 1996;27: 839–846.

45. Tuzcu EM, Hobbs H, Rincon G, et al. Occult and frequent transmission of atherosclerosis coronary disease with cardiac transplantation. *Circulation* 1995;91:1706–1713.

46. Rickenbacher PR, Pinto FJ, Lewis NP, et al. Prognostic importance of intimal thickness measured by intracoronary ultrasound after cardiac transplantation. *Circulation* 1995;92:3445–3452.

47. St.Goar FG, Pinto FJ, Alderman EL, et al. Detection of coronary atherosclerosis in young adult hearts using intravascular ultrasound. *Circulation* 1992; 86:756–763.

48. de Feyter PJ, Ozaki Y, Baptista J, et al. Ischemia-related lesion characteristics

in patients with stable or unstable angina. A study with intracoronary angioscopy and ultrasound. *Circulation* 1995;92:1408–1413.

49. Alibelli-Chemarin MJC, Pieraggi MT, Elbaz M, et al. Identification of coronary thrombus after myocardial infarction by intracoronary ultrasound compared with histology of tissues sampled by atherectomy. *Am J Cardiol* 1996;77:344–349.

50. The GUIDE Trial Investigators. IVUS-determined predictors of restenosis in PTCA and DCA: An interim report from the GUIDE Trial, Phase II *Circulation* 1994;90;4;2:I–23(113). Abstract.

51. Mintz GS, Popma JJ, Pichard AD, et al. Arterial remodeling after coronary angioplasty. A serial intravascular ultrasound study. *Circulation* 1996;94: 35–43.

52. Serruys PW, de Jaegere P, Kiemeneij, et al, on behalf of the Benestent Study Group. A comparison of balloon-expandable-stent implantation with balloon angioplasty in patients with coronary artery disease. *N Engl J Med* 1994;331:489–495.

53. Fischman DL, Leon MB, Baim DS, et al. A randomized comparison of coronary-stent placement and balloon angioplasty in the treatment of coronary artery disease. *N Engl J Med* 1994;331:496–501.

54. Barzilai B, Saffitz JE, Miller JG, et al. Quantitative ultrasonic characterization of the nature of atherosclerotic plaques in human aorta. *Circ Res* 1987; 60:459–463.

55. Wickline SA, Barzilai B, Thomas LJ, et al. Quantification of intimal and medial thickness of human coronary arteries by acoustic microscopy. *Coron Artery Dis* 1990;1:333–340.

56. Fitzgerald PJ, Connolly AJ, Watkins RD, et al. Distinction between soft plaque and thrombus by intravascular tissue characterization. *J Am Coll Cardiol* 1991;17:11A.

57. Roelandt JRTC, Di Mario C, Pandian NG, et al. Three-dimensional reconstruction of intracoronary ultrasound images: Rationale, approaches, problems and directions. *Circulation* 1994;90:1044–1055.

58. Di Mario C, von Birgelen C, Prati F, et al. Three dimensional reconstruction of two-dimensional intracoronary ultrasound: Clinical or research tool? *Br Heart J* 1995;73:26–32.

Chapter 6

Angioscopic Detection of Vulnerable Plaques and Prediction of Acute Coronary Syndromes

Yasumi Uchida, MD

Introduction

Unstable angina and acute myocardial infarction are called acute coronary syndromes because their underlying mechanisms are essentially the same. Usually, the syndromes occur suddenly and unexpectedly. It still cannot be predicted in whom these syndromes occur, and when. If we succeed in predicting and preventing occurrence of these fatal syndromes, one of the great burdens of humankind may be minimized. To attain this purpose, we must know more precisely about the detailed characteristics of coronary atherosclerotic plaques, the mechanisms of their disruption, and thrombus formation.

Natural History of Coronary Plaques

Figure 1 shows a possible natural history of coronary plaques and the differences between unstable angina and acute myocardial infarction. Unstable angina and acute myocardial infarction can be differentiated based upon whether persistent occlusion with thrombi and resultant irreversible myocardial damages occurs. This is why they are classified into one entity and called *acute coronary syndromes*.

From: Fuster, V (ed). *The Vulnerable Atherosclerotic Plaque: Understanding, Identification, and Modification*. Armonk, NY: Futura Publishing Company, Inc.; © 1999.

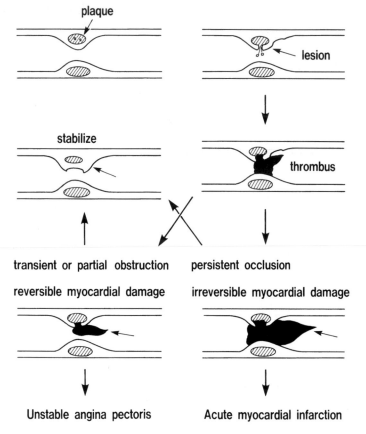

Figure 1. Mechanisms of acute coronary syndromes and differences in mechanisms between unstable angina and acute myocardial infarction.

Mechanisms of Plaque Disruption

There are organic and functional mechanisms for plaque disruption and thrombus formation. Organic mechanisms include: (1)mismatch between atheroma growth and fibrous cap growth; (2) mismatch between plaque growth and remodeling of media and adventitia; and (3) fragile fibrous cap formation due to inflammatory or other processes, or thinning of the cap by certain substances (Fig. 2).

Functional mechanisms of plaque disruption include: (1) overstretching of the plaques due to hypertension and resultant disruption; (2) vasospasm-induced deformation and rupture; and (3) prestenotic thrombosis due to rheological mechanisms and embolization of the stenotic portion with the detached thrombi (Fig. 3).

a) Mismatch between cholesterol deposition and
fibrous cap growth → thinning of the cap → rupture

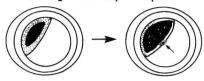

b) Mismatch between plaque growth and remodeling of media
and adventitia → protrusion of plaque → rupture

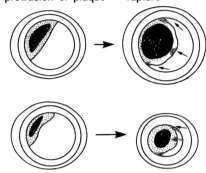

c) Regression of and cell infiltration
into fibrous cap → fragile and thinning → rupture

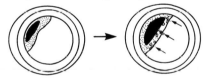

Figure 2. Three possible major organic mechanisms of acute coronary syndromes.

Angioscopy Systems Used In Our Laboratory

Coronary angioscopy has greatly contributed to the understanding of acute coronary syndromes. This method is now routinely used for plaque characterization and evaluation of interventional and surgical therapies in our laboratory.[1–4] Figures 4 and 5 show angioscopy systems used in our laboratory. We select the one of these five systems that is most feasible for target plaque. One system is composed of a 5-F balloon-guiding catheter, a fiberscope 0.5 mm in diameter, and a 0.014-inch guidewire. The fiberscope is steerable in this system and the

a) Hypertension

luminal pressure rise → overstretching →
rupture → thrombus formation

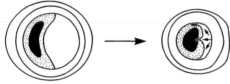

b) Spasm

shear stress → rupture → thrombus formation

c) blood turburence and

hypercoagulability →

pre-, post-stenotic thrombus formation → embolization

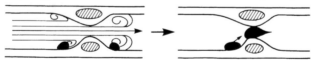

Figure 3. Three possible major functional mechanisms of acute coronary syndromes.

system is used for observation of middle to distal segments. The second system is composed of an 8- or 9-F balloon-guiding catheter and a fiberscope 1.4 mm in diameter. The fiberscope is steerable and this system is usually used for observation of proximal coronary segments (Fig. 4). The other three systems are simpler and now most frequently used (Fig. 5).

Angioscopic Classification of Coronary Plaques

Coronary plaques are angioscopically classified into regular and complex plaques. Based on coloration of the plaques, the former is

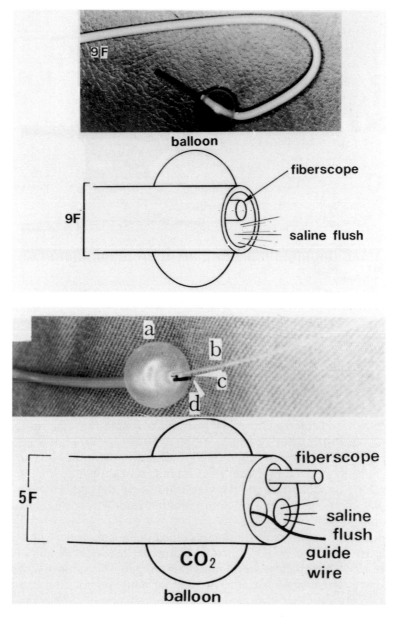

Figure 4. Angioscopy systems. **A.** Nine-F guiding balloon catheter with one channel and a steerable fiberscope 1.4 mm in diameter. **B.** Five-F balloon-guiding catheter with three channels and a steerable fiberscope 0.5 mm in diameter. a = balloon; b = guide wire; c = fiberscope; d = flush channel.

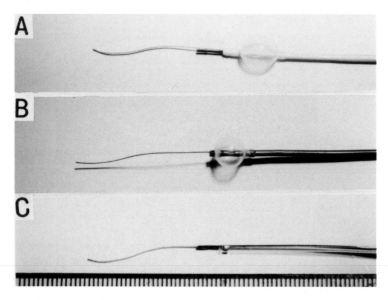

Figure 5. Angioscopy systems. **A.** Five-F guiding balloon catheter with one channel and with a steerable fiberscope 0.5 mm in diameter. **B.** Five-F guiding balloon catheter with a fixed fiberscope. **C.** Transparent guiding catheter without balloon and a steerable fiberscope 0.5 mm to 0.8 mm in diameter.

further classified into white, nonglistening yellow, and glistening yellow plaques (Table 1). Our ex vivo study[5] revealed that plaque coloration is determined by thickness of the fibrous cap. When the fibrous cap is thin, the plaque becomes yellow due to atheroma beneath the cap. Reflection of illumination in a certain group of yellow plaques is probably due, in addition to the very thinness of the cap, to abundant cholesterol crystals, small calcium particles, and/or rearrangement of endothelial cells.[5]

Luminal surfaces of the angiographically intact coronary artery in adult patients are angioscopically white or yellow and are either smooth or have shallow spiral folds (Fig. 6, panel A). Figure 6, panel B shows a representative example of regular white plaque, and Figure 7 shows representative examples of regular nonglistening yellow plaque, regular glistening yellow plaque, and complex plaques.

We examined the relationship between plaque appearance and clinical classification of ischemic heart disease. Complex plaques were frequently observed in unstable angina, acute myocardial infarction, and in old myocardial infarction, while regular plaques were more

Table 1

Classification of Coronary Plaques

	Color	Histologic changes
A. Regular plaques		
	White	Thick fibrous cap
	Nonglistening yellow	Relatively thin fibrous cap
	Glistening yellow	Thin fibrous cap (rich cholesterol cristals, Ca particles, rearranged endothelium)
B. Complex plaques		
	White, yellow, mosaic	Disruption of plaque with or without thrombi (bleeding, dissection, red or white thrombi, etc)
C. Regular plaque with just proximal thrombus		

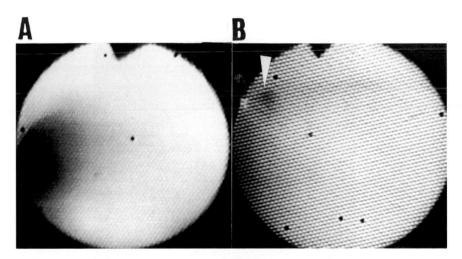

Figure 6. **A.** Normal coronary artery (LMT). **B.** Regular white plaque observed in LMT. Arrow = pin—point residual lumen.

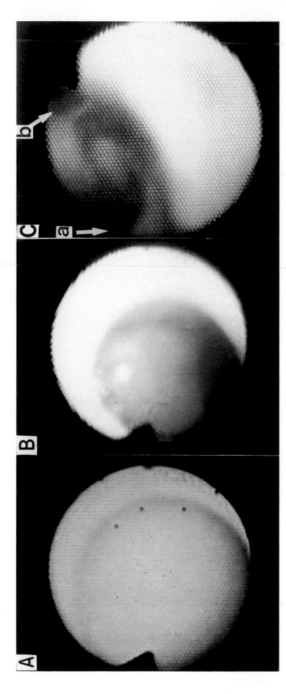

Figure 7. **A.** Regular nonglistening yellow plaque. **B.** Regular glistening yellow plaque. **C.** Complex plaque. a = residual lumen; b = mural thrombus.

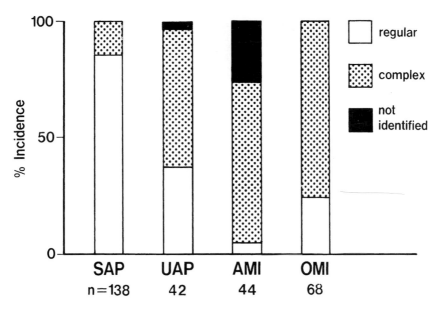

Figure 8. Relationship between angioscopic appearance of coronary plaques and clinical manifestations. SAP = stable angina pectoris; UAP = unstable angina pectoris; AMI = acute myocardial infarction; OMI = old myocardial infarction.

commonly observed in stable angina (Fig. 8). Complex plaques were mostly yellow, while regular plaques were mostly white. Those white and yellow plaques, in mosaic fashion, were more frequently observed in old myocardial infarction (Fig. 9).

Postinfarction Angina

We examined the relationship between plaque appearance and presence or absence of angina in patients with old myocardial infarction.[5] In this study, the patients were examined 1 month after the attack of acute myocardial infarction. At least three types of plaques were observed: (1) irregular and yellow plaque, abundant residual atheroma inside (Fig. 10, panel A); (2) yellow plaque with a crater at the top, covered with or not covered with thrombi (Fig. 10, panel B), probably with abundant atheroma inside and exposed thrombogenic tissues resembling an active volcano; and (3) a large crater covered with white fibrous tissue, with yellow and irregular tissues surrounding the crater (Fig. 10, panel C), probably due to almost complete loss of atheroma at the time of disruption. The former two types were frequently observed in patients with postinfarction angina (Fig. 11).

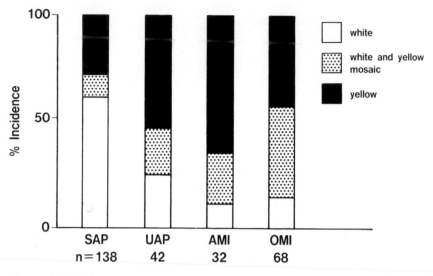

Figure 9. Relationship between coloration of plaques and clinical manifestations.

As summarized in Figure 12, it seems that the magnitude of loss of atheroma at the time of disruption determines postinfarction events.

Angioscopic Classification of Thrombi

Thrombus formation is considered to be essential for development of acute coronary syndromes. Fresh thrombi are classified into red (Table 2, Fig. 13, panel A), white (Fig. 13, panel B), and red and white in mosaic fashion. In a rare occasion, a doughnut-like thrombus was observed just proximal to the regular plaque (Fig. 14). It seems that the color of thrombi is determined by the presence or absence of blood flow and by age (Table 2).

We examined the relationship between thrombus appearance and clinical manifestations. Thrombi were observed in the majority of patients with acute coronary syndromes. White thrombi were more frequently observed in patients with unstable angina, probably due to flow existence and resultant washout of red blood cells (Fig. 15).

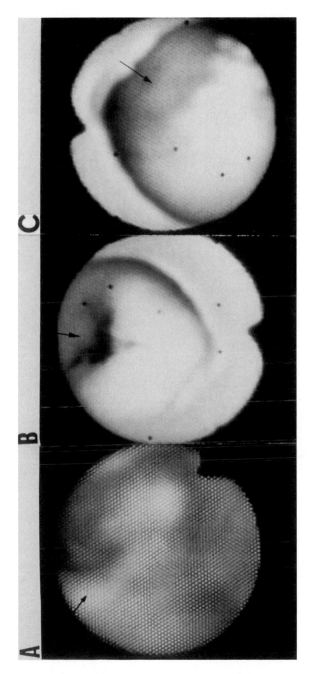

Figure 10. Three different types of complex plaques observed in patients with old myocardial infarction. **A.** Irregular yellow plaque. **B.** Smooth-surfaced yellow plaque with a crater and thrombus at the top (arrow). **C.** A large crater (arrow) surrounded by residual yellow tissues.

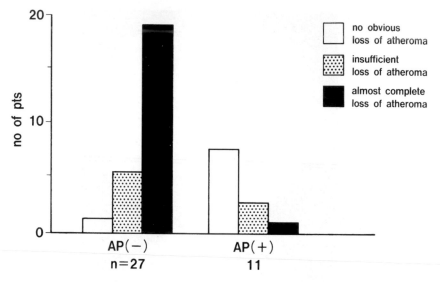

Figure 11. Relationship between the magnitude of atheroma loss at the time of disruption and presence or absence of postinfarction angina.

Angioscopic Prediction
of Acute Coronary Syndromes

Based on plaque and thrombus characterization, we carried out an angioscopic prospective follow-up study on prediction of acute coronary syndromes. A total of 157 patients, in whom only regular plaques were detected, were successfully followed up for 12 months.

The patients were classified into "white plaque" and "yellow plaque" groups. The latter was further classified into "glistening yellow" and "nonglistening yellow" groups. Besides cholesterol, there were no differences in background (Table 3). Figures 16 and 17 show angiographic and angioscopic changes of the right coronary artery in a patient with stable angina. The initial coronary arteriography (CAG) revealed an insignificant stenosis in the proximal segment of the right coronary artery. Six weeks later, acute myocardial infarction occurred in this patient. Repeated CAG revealed obstruction of the segment with a mass suggesting a globular thrombus. Angioscopy at the initial CAG revealed a glistening yellow plaque. Angioscopy immediately after the attack revealed disrupted identical plaque and growth of a globular red thrombus from the plaque.

Figure 18 shows angioscopic changes of the left circumflex coro-

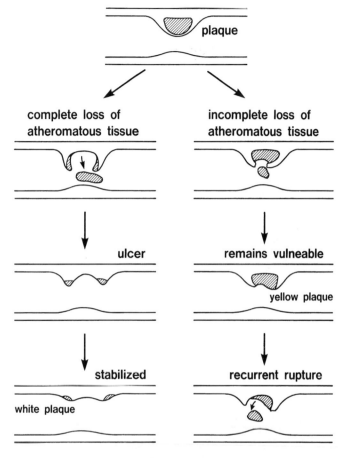

Figure 12. Possible fate of ruptured plaques.

Table 2

Classification of Thrombi

Color	Age	Blood flow	Histologic changes
Red	Fresh	Usually absent	RBC rich
White or pink	Fresh	Usually present	Fibrin, platelet rich
Mixed	Fresh	Absent or present	
Dark red	Relatively old	Absent or present	Rich in RBC
Yellow	Old	Absent or present	Organized

RBC = red blood cell.

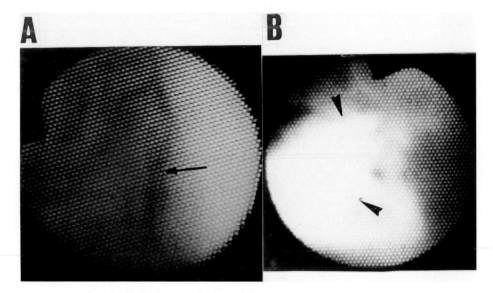

Figure 13. Coronary thrombi. **A.** Red thrombus (arrow). **B.** White thrombus.

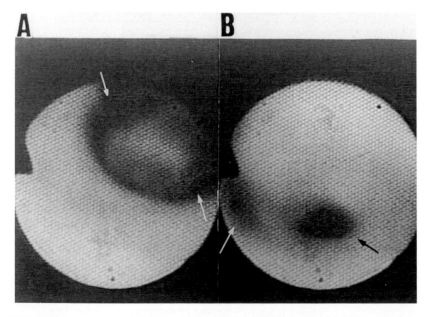

Figure 14. A doughnut-like mural thrombus (white arrows in **A**) located just proximal to a regular white plaque (black arrow in **B**).

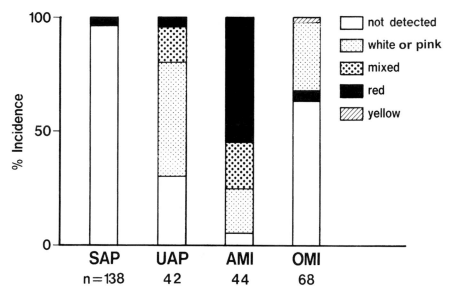

Figure 15. Relationship between angioscopic appearance of coronary thrombi and clinical manifestations.

Table 3

Patient Characteristics

Plaque	White	Yellow	P value	Yellow nonglistening	Glistening	P value
No. of patients	118	39		26	13	
Age (range in yrs)	41–77	38–76	NS	51–76	38–72	NS
Mean + SE	59.7 ± 4.1	61.5 ± 5.3		62.0 ± 4.8	60.2 ± 5.8	
Sex (F/M)	26/92	8/21	NS	6/19	2/12	NS
Blood pressure (mm Hg)						
Systolic	140.9 ± 18	139.5 ± 20	NS	145.3 ± 22	135.0 ± 27	NS
Diastolic	83.9 ± 9	80.1 ± 11	NS	81.8 ± 13	79.5 ± 16	NS
Serum cholesterol (mg/dL)	216.1 ± 36	238.4 ± 48	0.03	230.2 ± 43	240.6 ± 46	0.04
Body-mass index	26.2 ± 3.4	24.6 ± 4.0	NS	23.8 ± 4.3	25.3 ± 4.7	NS
History of diabetes mellitus	11	4	NS	2	2	NS
Smoking	28	10	NS	6	4	NS
Antiplatelet agents	0	0	NS	0	0	NS

Student's *t* test or Fisher's exact probability test. SE = standard error; NS = not significant.

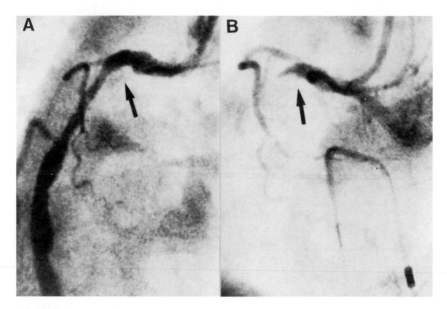

Figure 16. Angiographic changes in the right coronary artery (RCA) before (**A**) and immediately after (**B**) the occurrence of acute myocardial infarction in a 72-year—old female. Arrow in **A** = a nonsignificant stenosis; arrow in **B** = a globular thrombus. From Reference 5.

nary artery (LCX), before and immediately after occurrence of acute myocardial infarction in a patient with vasospastic angina. Angioscopy before the attack revealed a white plaque in LCX. Immediately after the attack, angioscopy revealed exposed atheroma and thrombus formation on it.

During 12 months' months follow-up, acute coronary syndromes occurred more frequently in the yellow plaque group. Furthermore, the syndromes occurred in about 70% of patients with glistening yellow plaques (Table 4). In addition, the syndromes occurred within 3 months, and in 1.9 months in average, in this group of patients (Fig. 19).

Discussion

Our prospective angioscopic study indicated that regular but glistening yellow plaques are prone to disrupt within 3 months. Therefore, this category of plaques can be called vulnerable, fragile, or malignant

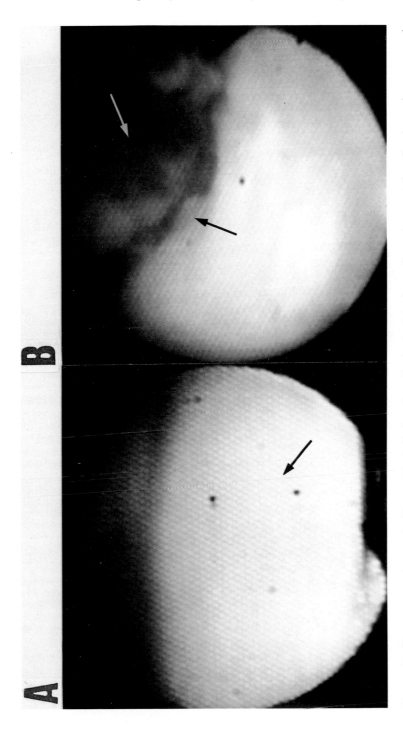

Figure 17. The same patient as in Figure 16. **A.** Before the attack. A glistening yellow plaque at the site shown by an arrow in Figure 15, panel **A**. **B.** Disrupted identical plaque (black arrow) and thrombus formation (white arrow). From Reference 5.

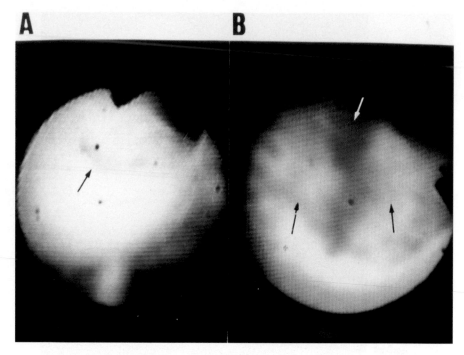

Figure 18. White plaque before (**A**) and protrusion of atheromatous tissues from the disrupted identical plaque immediately after (**B**) the occurrence of acute myocardial infarction observed in a 60-year-old male. From Reference 5.

Table 4

Relation Between Angioscopic Appearance of the Plaque and the Clinical Outcome

Plaque	No. of patients	No. of plaques	Stenosis (%)	Eccentricity index	Acute coronary syndrome			Incidence of acute coronary syndrome (%)		Cardiac death
					UA	AMI	Total	Patient	Plaque	
White	118	182	48.6 ± 3.2	0.31 ± 0.08	1	3‡	4	3.3	2.1	1
Yellow	39	48	51.0 ± 5.2*	0.34 ± 0.10*	2	7	11	28.2§	22.8¶	5††
Yellow										
Nonglistening	26	34	49.0 ± 5.8	0.32 ± 0.11	0	2**	2	7.6	5.9	2
Glistening	13	14	52.3 ± 7.3†	0.35 ± 0.12†	2	7	9	68.4‖	64.2#	31‡‡

UA = Unstable angina pectoris; AMI = acute myocardial infarction; * Not significant vs white plaque; † Not significant vs nonglistening yellow plaque; ‡ With endothelial exfoliation; § With mural thrombus proximal to the plaque; ‖ P = 0.00021 vs white plaque; ¶ P = 0.00026 vs non-glistening yellow plaque; # P = 0.00048 vs white plaque; **P = 0.00003 vs nonglistening yellow plaque; †† P = 0.001 vs white plaque; ‡‡ P = 0.091 vs nonglistening yellow plaque; P = 0.009 vs white plaque. Student's t test or Fisher's exact probability test.

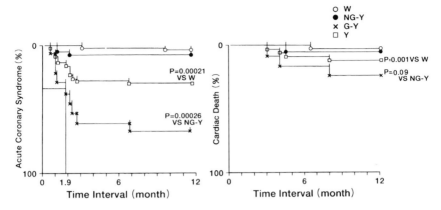

Figure 19. **A.** Relationship between occurrence of acute coronary syndromes and time duration from the initial angioscopy. **B.** Relationship between cardiac death and time duration from the initial angioscopy. From Reference 5.

plaques. Further angioscopic mass study is required to confirm our results. Follow-up studies on complex plaques are also necessary in order to clarify the relationship between the fate of disrupted plaques and clinical manifestations.

In the near future, prophylactic removal of, regression therapy of, and inhibitory therapy of birth of vulnerable plaques may be established and acute coronary syndrome, a great burden on human beings, may be minimized.

References

1. Uchida Y, Tomaru T, Nakamura F, et al. Percutaneous coronary angioscopy in patients with ischemic heart disease. *Am Heart J* 1987;114:1216–1222.
2. Uchida Y, Hasegawa K, Kawamur K, Shibuya I. Angioscopic observation of coronary luminal changes induced by percutaneous transluminal coronary angioplasty. *Am Heart J* 1989;117:769–776.
3. Uchida Y. Percutaneous cardiovascular angioscopy. In: Kulwer AG ed: *Lasers in Cardiovascular Medicine and Surgery*. Boston: Academic Publishers; 1989.
4. Uchida Y. Percutaneous coronary angioscopy. *Jpn Heart J* 1992;33:271–294.
5. Uchida Y, Nakamura F, Tomaru T, et al. Prediction of acute coronary syndromes by percutaneous coronary angioscopy in patients with stable angina. *Am Heart J* 1995;130:195–203.

Chapter 7

Ultrafast Computed Tomography in Coronary Heart Disease

Alan D. Guerci, MD

The Pathological Basis of Coronary Calcification

In 1959, Blankenhorn[1] reported an association between coronary calcification and coronary atherosclerosis. Based on examination of 3500 serial sections from 76 hearts, Blankenhorn later noted that coronary calcification was, in all cases, confined to the intima and associated with atherosclerotic plaque.[2] More importantly, the amount of calcium was related to the amount of plaque. These observations were subsequently confirmed by five other autopsy studies involving more than 2500 hearts.[3–7] Atherosclerosis was the sole cause of coronary calcification in these studies, and all investigators commented on the strength of the relationship between the amount of calcium and the severity of underlying atherosclerosis. One of these studies[5] lends itself to statistical analysis, and the correlation coefficient between the calcium content and severity of underlying coronary disease is 0.75.

An accumulating body of evidence indicates that lipid-rich, "soft" atherosclerotic plaques are most vulnerable to fissuring or rupture.[8] This raises a question as to whether coronary calcification, which is associated with more advanced and perhaps more stable atherosclerotic lesions, is an appropriate target for noninvasive screening. The autopsy literature suggests an answer: the calcium content of the coronary arteries in persons dying of coronary disease is two to five times

Supported by the St. Francis Hospital Foundation

From: Fuster, V (ed). *The Vulnerable Atherosclerotic Plaque: Understanding, Identification, and Modification.* Armonk, NY: Futura Publishing Company, Inc.; © 1999.

greater than the calcium content of the coronary arteries of persons dying of other causes.[4]

Ultrafast Computed Tomographic (CT) Scanning: Methods, Accuracy and Reproducibility

The results of ultrafast or electron beam CT scanning of the coronary arteries are usually reported as a "calcium score." The CT technician designates suspected coronary calcium deposits as regions of interest, and proprietary software then calculates the number of pixels with attenuation coefficients greater than 130 Hounsfield units (130 Hounsfield units is two standard deviations above the mean attenuation coefficient of blood). The number of pixels with attenuation coefficient greater than 130 is then multiplied by an integer representing maximal attenuation for that lesion: one for attenuation coefficients 130 to 199, two for attenuation coefficients 200 to 299, three for attenuation coefficients 300 to 399, and four for attenuation coefficients greater than or equal to 400.

The electron beam CT coronary calcium score correlates closely ($r = 0.93$) with actual calcium phosphate (hydroxyapatite) content[9] and with histochemical estimates of coronary calcification ($r = 0.96$).[10]

The electron beam CT coronary calcium score is also highly reproducible ($r = 0.96$ to 0.99).[11–13] Reproducibility is lower among subjects with lower scores (eg, ≤ 20), but the importance of this observation is uncertain. Coronary calcium scores below 20 generally indicate minimal amounts of coronary atherosclerosis and minimal risk (vide infra).

Diagnostic Significance

Three studies indicate that electron beam CT estimates of coronary calcium content correlate closely with the severity of coronary atherosclerosis in persons without symptoms of coronary disease. Rumberger et al[15] scanned 13 autopsied hearts and then dissected out the coronary arteries and repeated the scan. Because scan thickness was 3 mm, the coronary arteries were sliced into 3-mm-thick sections. Within each section, the volume of atherosclerotic plaque was determined by planimetry. The correlation between the volume of atherosclerotic plaque and the electron beam CT calcium area (which, in turn, correlates with the calcium score with a coefficient of 0.99)[14] was 0.84 per coronary artery and 0.93 per heart.[15]

Chou et al[16] performed electron beam CT and intravascular ultrasound examinations on the left main coronary artery and proximal left anterior descending (LAD) artery in 20 asymptomatic men and women with hyperlipidemia. The correlation of the coronary calcium score and plaque volume was 0.90 for the left main and 0.75 for the LAD.[16]

In a third study, Guerci et al[17] reported the results of coronary arteriography in 18 apparently healthy, asymptomatic middle-aged men and women with high coronary calcium scores. In order to extend the range of observation to subjects with low calcium scores, angiographic and electron beam CT data were analyzed for 18 men and women with valvular heart disease and low coronary calcium scores or exertional dyspnea of unknown etiology and low calcium scores. Coronary arteriograms were analyzed by use of computer-assisted quantitative coronary arteriography at a remote site by observers blinded to the coronary calcium score. The 18 subjects with high coronary calcium scores had a mean age of 55 ± 7 years, a mean calcium score of 573 ± 504, and a mean worst stenosis of 45%. For all 36 subjects, the worst stenosis in any major coronary arterial segment was given by the following equation: worst stenosis (%) = 1.78 (calcium score)$^{1/2}$ + 3, with a regression coefficient of 0.85, SEE = 0.19, and $P<0.0001$ (Fig. 1).[17]

Without exception, correlative studies comparing angiographic and electron beam CT findings in (a total of more than 2300) patients undergoing coronary arteriography for clinical indications have reported a relationship between the coronary calcium score and the severity of underlying coronary disease.[14,18–24] Because the prevalence of the three disease states of interest (normal coronary arteries, nonobstructive disease, and obstructive disease) is unknown, these data cannot be used to predict the severity of atherosclerosis in asymptomatic persons. Nevertheless, they are consistent with evidence which indicates that coronary calcium content is related to the severity of underlying coronary atherosclerosis. Table 1 provides an example of the distribution of coronary calcium scores in a symptomatic population.[24]

Prognostic Significance

Clearly, the electron beam CT coronary calcium score is related to the severity and extent of coronary disease. On the other hand, the atherosclerotic plaques responsible for most myocardial infarctions and sudden coronary deaths are not calcified.[8] Proponents of electron beam CT coronary screening argue that only 10% to 20% of atherosclerotic plaque is calcified,[15,25] and the close correlation between coronary calcium score and the severity of underlying atherosclerosis can be accounted for only if the calcium score is related to other atheromatous lesions. Opponents of electron beam CT coronary screening argue that

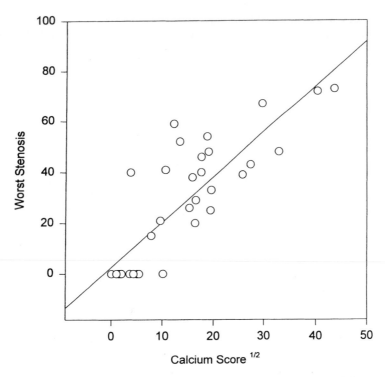

Figure 1. Relationship of worst stenosis in any major coronary arterial segment (percent reduction in lumenal diameter) to the coronary calcium score in 36 subjects without symptoms of coronary disease. r = 0.85.

Table 1

Distribution of Coronary Calcium Scores in 715 Symptomatic Patients by Category of Coronary Disease

Category	n	Percentile		
		25th	50th	75th
Normal	222	0	2	34
Nonobstructive	172	16	107	376
Obstructive	321	143	462	1137

the calcified plaque is not the plaque of interest. The two positions are not irreconcilable.

Arad et al[26] recently reported 19 months of follow-up (range 14 to 22 months) on 1173 asymptomatic men and women. As might be expected, the coronary event rate (death, nonfatal myocardial infarction, or need for revascularization) at 19 months in this population of apparently healthy men and women (mean age 53 years) was low, only 1.5 percent. However, the mean calcium score differed widely between those with and those without events (mean $\pm$ SD), 935 ± 1070 versus 144 ± 446, respectively ($P<0.0001$). A calcium score threshold of 160, which maximized overall test accuracy, was associated with a sensitivity of 0.89, specificity of 0.82, positive predictive value of 0.07, negative predictive value of 0.998, and an odds ratio of 35.4. The area under the receiver operator characteristics (ROC) curve was 0.91. The latter two figures are unprecedented for any screening test for coronary disease.

Two other reports of short-term follow-up (1 to 2 years) and one report of intermediate follow-up (3 to 6 years) also indicate that coronary calcification is a significant risk factor for future coronary events. Wong et al[27] followed 206 men and women for 1 to 2 years after electron beam CT scanning and analyzed the results according to the presence or absence of coronary calcification. Subjects with coronary calcification had a sixfold increase in the risk of cardiac death or nonfatal myocardial infarction. In a series of 862 men and women followed for 1 to 2 years, Balogh et al[28] reported that all 10 patients undergoing coronary revascularization had coronary calcium scores above the 70th percentile. There were no myocardial infarctions or cardiac deaths in this series.

Agatston et al[29] recently reported 3 to 6 years of follow-up on 367 asymptomatic men and women. Mean age at the time of the electron beam CT scan was 52 years. Twenty-six patients (7.0%) sustained coronary events. The mean coronary calcium scores for subjects with and subjects without events were 399 ± 424 and 76 ± 207, respectively ($P<0.0001$). The odds ratio for myocardial infarction and death associated with a coronary calcium score greater than 26 (roughly the 67th percentile of the population) was 21.2 (95% CI 2.8 to 172, $P<0.0001$).

Together, these studies of more than 2600 asymptomatic middle-aged men and women followed for 1 to 6 years after electron beam CT scanning indicate that coronary calcification is a significant risk factor for future cardiac events. However, one study stands in contrast to this otherwise consistent pattern. Secci et al[30] recently reported that the coronary calcium score was highly predictive of future revascularization procedures, but failed to predict myocardial infarction or sudden death in the South Bay Heart Watch.

Why did coronary calcification fail to predict nonfatal myocardial infarction and cardiac death in the South Bay Heart Watch? In fact, it really did not. The South Bay Heart Watch began as a study of the predictive accuracy of cardiac fluoroscopy in 1459 asymptomatic high-risk adults. These 1459 subjects underwent fluoroscopy between 1990 and 1992; 1289 asymptomatic survivors underwent electron beam CT scanning from 1992 to 1994. In the original cohort, 28% had fluoroscopically evident calcification of two or three coronary arteries. Compared to subjects with zero or one calcified coronary artery, those with multivessel coronary calcification had an odds ratio for death of 3.1 at an average follow-up of 50 ± 10 months ($P = 0.004$).[31] For the 1289 asymptomatic survivors who underwent electron beam CT scanning between 1992 and 1994, the coronary calcium score has not been a significant predictor of nonfatal myocardial infarction and coronary death.[30] The explanation probably has more to do with study design than with any inherent advantage of number of calcified vessels by fluoroscopy over the electron beam CT coronary calcium score. The South Bay Heart Watch was a study of *high-risk* adults. To qualify, individuals must have been at or above the 70th percentile for coronary risk according to Framingham criteria. Excluding age, subjects had a mean ($\pm$SD) of 2.6 (1.0) risk factors for coronary artery disease. Thus, the high prevalence of coronary artery disease in this population increased the likelihood that a low coronary calcium score was a false-negative. In addition, hypertensive subjects with electrocardiographic evidence of left ventricular hypertrophy, including a "strain" pattern, were included in the South Bay Heart Watch. Such persons are at risk for noncoronary sudden cardiac death.

Table 2, section A contains the data for myocardial infarction and cardiac death in the three studies[26,29,30] that have reported myocardial infarction and cardiac death as a function of the coronary calcium score. Section B is an update that was added after this chapter was completed. The South Bay Heart Watch experience notwithstanding, the data indicate that the coronary calcium score is a highly significant predictor of nonfatal myocardial infarction and coronary death in asymptomatic persons. This observation is in keeping with two abundantly documented relationships, the first between coronary calcium content and the severity of underlying coronary atherosclerosis,[1–7,14–23] the second between the severity of coronary atherosclerosis and the risk of death.[32] Although not the lesion of interest, the calcified plaque is a marker for the presence of the lesion of interest.

Incremental Value

In 1995 at the annual meeting of the American College of Cardiology, Kennedy et al[33] reported the results of a multivariate risk factor

Table 2

A. Prediction of Myocardial Infarction and Sudden Death in Asymptomatic Persons by Electron Beam CT Scanning

Study	n	#MIs/SDs	In top third	OR	P
Arad et al[26]	1173	8	7	14	<0.0001
Agatston et al[29]	367	11	10	22	<0.0001
Secci et al[30]	326	14	6 to 9	–	–
Total	1866	33	23 to 26	4.7 to 7.7	≤0.0001

In Reference 30 data were reported by quartile. Three events occurred among patients in the third quartile, but their position within the overall population (ie, the top third versus the bottom two thirds) was not reported. Therefore, best case (all three events fell within the top third) versus worst case (all three events fell between the 50th and 67th percentiles) analyses were performed. In either case, the coronary calcium score was highly predictive of nonfatal MI.

B. Prediction of Nonfatal Myocardial Infarction and Cardiovascular Death by Electron Beam CT Scanning: Highest Tercile Versus Two Lowest Terciles

Study	n	f/u (yrs)	MI/Death (%)	OR (95% CI)	P
St. Francis[41]	1171	3.6	3.33 vs 0.26	13.4 (3.0–59.5)	<0.001
Mt. Sinai[29]	367	4.5	8.20 vs 0.41	21.8 (2.8–170)	0.004
Subtotal	1534	3.8	4.49 vs 0.29	16.1 (6.5–39.7)	<0.0001
South Bay[42]	1196	2.8	5.26 vs 2.01	2.7 (1.4–5.3)	0.003
Total	2730	3.4	4.83 vs 1.04	4.8 (2.9–7.9)	<0.0001

The South Bay Heart Watch is a study of high-risk subjects (see text). The limited range of coronary risk associated with the relative homogeneity of the study population probably accounts for the low observed odds ratios. CT = computed tomography; MI = myocardial infarction; SD = sudden death.

analysis of 263 patients who had undergone coronary arteriography for clinical indications and electron beam CT scanning. In multiple logistic regression, the coronary calcium score emerged as the most accurate predictor of obstructive coronary disease. Age, male gender, and hypercholesterolemia were also significant predictors of the presence of obstructive coronary disease.

In 1996 at the annual meeting of the American College of Cardiology, Spadaro et al reported the results of a comparison of electron beam CT scanning and conventional risk factor assessment for the prediction of coronary artery disease in 290 symptomatic adults.[34] This study differed from the aforementioned study by Kennedy et al in that the ratio of total cholesterol to high-density lipoprotein (HDL) cholesterol (ie, not just total cholesterol) was included in the multiple logistic regression model. In addition to analyses of the association of coronary calcium score and conventional risk factors with obstructive disease, the relationship between coronary calcium score and conventional risk factors in the identification of subjects with any coronary disease (ie, nonobstructive as well as obstructive disease) was also examined. After adjustment for serum lipid values and nonlipid risk factors, the coronary calcium score remained highly predictive of the presence and severity of coronary disease ($P<0.0001$). The coronary calcium score added significantly to the ability of conventional risk factors to predict the presence or severity of coronary disease over a range of zero to six risk factors (Figs. 2 and 3). Patients who met the National Cholesterol Education Program (NCEP) guidelines for treatment with lipid-lowering medications had an average worst stenosis of 47 ± 40 percent compared to an average worst stenosis of 36 ± 37 percent for patients who did not meet treatment criteria ($P=0.02$). Patients meeting NCEP treatment criteria also had more extensive disease as judged by a score of 2.5 ± 1 versus 2.2 ± 1 ($P=0.04$) on an ordinal scale in which a score of 1 was assigned for normal coronary arteries, a score of 2 was assigned

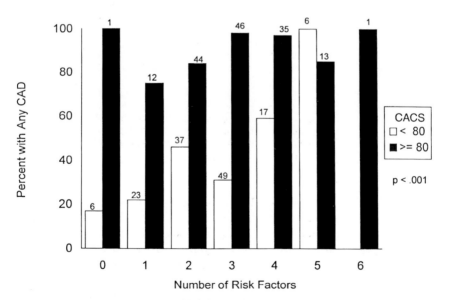

Figure 2. Percentage of patients with any coronary disease as a function of the number of risk factors and the coronary calcium score. Solid bars refer to patients with calcium scores <80; open bars refer to patients with calcium scores <80. Numbers at the top of each bar refer to the number of patients in each group. CACS = coronary artery calcium score.

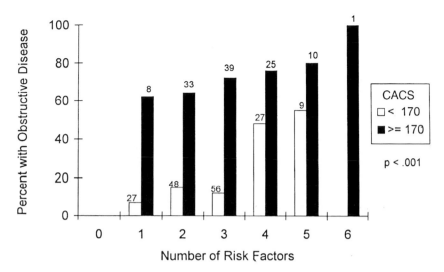

Figure 3. Percentage of patients with obstructive coronary disease as a function of the number of risk factors and the coronary calcium score. Solid bars refer to patients with calcium scores ≥170; open bars refer to patients with calcium scores <170. Numbers at the top of each bar refer to the number of patients in each group. No patient with obstructive disease had no risk factors. CACS = coronary artery calcium score.

for nonobstructive coronary disease, a score of 3 was assigned for obstructive single-vessel coronary disease, a score of 4 was assigned for obstructive double-vessel coronary disease, and a score of 5 was assigned for obstructive triple-vessel coronary disease. In contrast, a coronary calcium score greater than or equal to 170 was associated with an average worst stenosis of 61 ± 34 percent, compared to an average worst stenosis of 17 ± 29 percent for patients with calcium scores less than 170 ($P<0.001$). Patients with calcium scores greater than or equal to 170 had a score of 3.0 ± 1.2 on the ordinal scale for extent of disease, compared to 1.5 ± 0.8 for patients with calcium scores less than 170 ($P<0.001$). Thus, not only did the coronary calcium score identify subjects with more severe coronary stenoses and greater number of diseased vessels more accurately than the NCEP guidelines, but patients identified as being at high risk by the coronary calcium score had more severe disease and more extensive disease than patients so identified by the NCEP guidelines. Conversely, patients identified as being at lesser risk by the coronary calcium score had less severe and less extensive disease than those deemed not in need of treatment by the NCEP guidelines.

These findings are in keeping with a report of 1 to 2 years of follow-up of 1461 apparently healthy asymptomatic men and women who underwent cardiac cinefluoroscopy.[35] The presence of coronary calcification was a significant independent risk factor for coronary death, nonfatal myocardial infarction, and coronary revascularization. Despite the fact that there was no opportunity to relate event rates to the amount of calcium in the coronary arteries (ie, cinefluoroscopy cannot quantify coronary calcium content and the analysis was therefore restricted to the presence or absence of coronary calcification), the presence of coronary calcium negated total cholesterol and the ratio of total cholesterol to HDL cholesterol as risk factors for coronary events.

Application to Asymptomatic Populations

In the absence of direct evidence that the coronary calcium score can be used to reduce cardiovascular morbidity and mortality in a cost-effective manner, what, if any, are the indications for electron beam CT scanning of the coronary arteries? The answers to this question must be prefaced by a general statement about how the coronary calcium score might be used.

The diagnostic and prognostic meanings of the coronary calcium score expose the arbitrariness of traditional distinctions between primary prevention and secondary prevention of coronary disease. The former is based on risk factors, the latter on clinical events. In fact, the focus should be on risk for coronary events (low, intermediate, high . . .), which, in turn, is dependent on the severity and extent of coronary atherosclerosis. It is in this sense, as the only noninvasive test that can quantify with reasonable accuracy the severity and extent of coronary disease in middle-aged populations, that electron beam CT scanning can make a unique contribution to coronary risk stratification.

Although a powerful and independent predictor of the presence and severity of coronary artery disease, the coronary calcium score has not consistently nullified the predictive power of other risk factors. Therefore, the coronary calcium score must be interpreted in the context of the number and severity of other coronary risk factors. We would propose that the coronary calcium score be incorporated into the NCEP guidelines for the treatment of hypercholesterolemia. Very high coronary calcium scores ($\geq$95th percentile for age and gender) might be considered the equivalent of clinical coronary disease because these calcium scores are frequently associated with obstructive coronary disease.[17] Other elevated coronary calcium scores might be regarded as equivalent to one or two additional risk factors. Thus, a coronary calcium score at the 85th or 90th percentile in a middle-aged man or woman with a low-density lipoprotein (LDL) cholesterol of 170 mg/dL and no other risk factors might be sufficient to trigger therapy with a cholesterol-lowering drug. At the other extreme, in a fashion analogous to the influence of elevated HDL on the treatment algorithm, very low calcium scores might cancel one or two conventional risk factors. This approach is unproven, but it is consistent with a substantial body of evidence relating coronary calcification to coronary atherosclerosis and coronary atherosclerosis to coronary events.

Empirically defined cost-effectiveness data are not yet available, but mathematical modeling suggests that electron-beam-CT–based primary prevention is highly cost effective. For primary prevention in men aged 40 to 65, Lieberman et al[37] reported a net cost of just $70 per patient over 5 years. Although this estimate is debatable, to the extent that electron beam CT scanning can reduce the use of hepatic hydroxymethyl glutaryl coenzyme A (HMG CoA) reductase inhibitors, it is on secure footing. At $1000 per year to reduce LDL cholesterol with HMG CoA reductase inhibitors, $375 per scan, and a 5-year interscan interval, reduction in the use of HMG CoA reductase inhibition by just 7.5% (in absolute terms) would pay for all the electron beam CT scans. To put this figure in perspective, about 40% of hypercholesterolemic middle-aged men and women have calcium scores of zero.[38]

Who, then, should be scanned? The most defensible answer is middle-aged men and women with an intermediate number (eg, one to three) of risk factors for coronary artery disease. Modification of treatment of such persons on the basis of electron beam CT scan results seems reasonable. Scanning of individuals with four or more risk factors is probably ill-advised, because currently available data indicate at least an intermediate prevalence of coronary disease[34] and at least an intermediate risk of coronary events.[30] Finally, despite the fact that as many as 30% of patients with clinical coronary disease have no risk factor other than age, there are insufficient data to endorse routine screening of persons with no risk factors.

Electron Beam Computed Tomography for the Diagnosis of Obstructive Coronary Disease in Symptomatic Patients

In symptomatic men over age 40 and symptomatic women over age 50, electron beam CT scanning of the heart identifies obstructive coronary disease with sensitivities and specificities of approximately 77% and areas under the ROC curve of ranging from .80 to .90 (Table

Table 3

Sensitivity, Specificity, Overall Accuracy, and Area Under The Receiver Operating Characteristics Curve (ROC) of Electron Beam CT Scanning for the Diagnosis of Obstructive Coronary Disease

Reference	n	Sensitivity	Specificity	Accuracy	ROC Area
Kaufmann[14]	160	.86	.81	.83	.90
Rumberger[21]	139	–	–	–	.88 (M)
					.82 (F)
Kajinami[22]	251	.77	.86	.81	–
Budoff[23]	710	–	–	–	.82
Guerci[24]	715	.74	.75	.75	.81 (M)
Subtotal	1126	.76	.78	.77	–
Subtotal	1684	–	–	–	.80–.90

M = men; F = women.

3).[14,18–23] These figures are superior to published data on the sensitivity and specificity of conventional exercise testing[36] and, although inferior to figures for sensitivity published from leading laboratories for single photon emmission computed tomography (SPECT) thallium scintigraphy, are probably similar to the overall accuracy of thallium scintigraphy in most community hospitals or private laboratories. Kajinami et al[22] have reported equivalence of electron beam CT scanning and SPECT thallium scintigraphy in 256 patients undergoing cardiac catheterization for clinical indications, and Spadaro et al[34] have reported the superiority of electron beam CT scanning of the heart when compared to thallium stress testing performed in a community hospital/private laboratory setting in 196 men and women with chest pain or shortness of breath.

These data suggest two applications of electron beam CT scanning, both consistent with the previously described relationship between coronary calcification and the severity of underlying coronary atherosclerosis. The first of these would simply be electron beam CT scanning of the heart as a standard diagnostic test for the evaluation of patients with chest pain or exertional dyspnea thought to be due to obstructive coronary disease. At approximately $400 per scan, compared to about $250 for a conventional stress test and more than $1000 for a thallium stress test, electron beam CT scanning would appear to offer excellent value. This would particularly appear to be the case in women, in whom the specificity of conventional stress testing and thallium scintig-

Table 4

Cost of Different Testing Pathways for Diagnosis of Obstructive CAD

	Cath alone		TM + Cath		TH + Cath		EC + Cath		EBCT + Cath	
P	$C	%ND	$C	%ND	$C	%ND	$C	%ND	$C	%ND
0.2	2.7	0	1.1	30	2.0	15	1.8	20	1.2	15
0.7	2.7	0	1.7	31	2.9	16	2.6	18	2.1	16
1.0	2.7	0	2.1	32	3.4	15	3.1	18	2.6	16

In this analysis, catheterization was used as a first test for all patients with chest pain (cath alone) or a second test in patients with abnormal conventional stress test (TM), thallium stress test (TH), stress echocardiogram (EC) or electron beam CT. Cost ($C) data are expressed in thousands. %ND is the percentage of patients with obstructive disease who are not diagnosed (ie, only those with abnormal first tests go on to catheterization). Costs are actually charges in Rochester, MN. At different pretest probabilities of disease (P), electron beam CT scanning is as accurate and less expensive than thallium stress testing and stress echo, more accurate and more expensive than conventional stress testing. CAD = coronary artery disease Table adapted from Reference 40.

raphy are relatively low. Indeed, Rumberger et al[39] have calculated that electron beam CT scanning is less expensive and as accurate as thallium stress testing and stress echocardiography across all probabilities of obstructive coronary disease. Conventional stress testing is less expensive, but also significantly less accurate, than electron beam CT (Table 4).

A second, more radical application of electron beam CT scanning would require its use prior to coronary angiography in certain subgroups of patients with suspected coronary disease. In particular, this strategy could be applied in women with atypical chest pain, in whom the prevalence of obstructive coronary disease tends to be rather low.

In its recent statement on coronary artery calcification, the American Heart Association endorsed the use of electron beam CT scanning as a diagnostic test in patients with suspected coronary artery disease:

> *There are sufficient data to suggest that coronary calcium evaluation, especially with electron beam CT, is ready for clinical application in the de novo patient with chest pain, particularly with an "atypical" chest pain presentation, and that this anatomic evaluation may be useful by itself or in addition to exercise testing.*[40]

Summary

Electron beam CT scanning of the heart is a noninvasive test that can be used to exploit the relationship between coronary calcification and the severity of underlying coronary atherosclerosis. Electron beam CT scans of the heart measure coronary calcification accurately and with a high degree of reproducibility. The resulting coronary calcium score is closely related to the severity of coronary disease in symptomatic and asymptomatic populations. The coronary calcium score is also predictive of future cardiac events in symptomatic and asymptomatic populations. In the latter, unprecedented levels of prognostic accuracy have been achieved. Electron beam CT scanning adds significantly to the predictive accuracy of conventional risk factor assessment in symptomatic populations, and coronary calcification is a significant independent risk factor for future cardiac events in all of the unselected asymptomatic populations studied to date. Electron beam CT scanning of the coronary arteries is also known to be almost as accurate or as accurate as thallium scintigraphy for the diagnosis of obstructive coronary disease in symptomatic populations. These data indicate that electron beam CT scanning can be used as a diagnostic test in patients with chest pain or shortness of breath and that its use as a screening test, although unproven in terms of cost-effectiveness, is both logical and reasonable.

References

1. Blankenhorn DH, Stern D. Calcification of the coronary arteries. *Am J Roentgenol* 1959;81:772–777.
2. Blankenhorn DH. Coronary artery calcification. A review. *Am J Med Sci* 1961;242:41–49.
3. Beadenkopf WG, Daoud AS, Love BM. Calcification in the coronary arteries and its relation to atherosclerosis and myocardial infarction. *Am J Roentgenol* 1964;92:865–871.
4. Eggen DA, Strong JP, McGill HC. Coronary calcification: Relationship to clinically significant coronary lesions and race, sex and topographic distribution. *Circulation* 1965;32:948–955.
5. Warburton RK, Tampas JP, Soule AB, et al. Coronary artery calcification: Its relationship to coronary artery stenosis and myocardial infarction. *Radiology* 1968;91:109–115.
6. Frink RJ, Achor RWP, Brown AL, et al. Significance of calcification of the coronary arteries. *Am J Cardiol* 1970;26:241–247.
7. McCarthy JH, Palmer FJ. Incidence and significance of coronary artery calcification. *Br Heart J* 1974;36:499–506.
8. Davies MJ. A macro and micro view of coronary vascular insult in ischemic heart disease. *Circulation* 1990;82(suppl II):II-38–II-46.
9. Detrano R, Tang W, Kang X, et al. Accurate coronary calcium phosphate mass measurements from electron beam computed tomograms. *Am J Card Imaging* 1995;9(3):167–173.
10. Mautner GC, Mautner SL, Froelich J, et al. Coronary artery calcification: Assessment with electron beam CT and histomorphometric correlation. *Radiology* 1994;192:619–623.

11. Kajinami K, Seki H, Takekoshi N, et al. Quantification of coronary artery calcification using ultrafast computed tomography: Reproducibility of measurements. *Coron Artery Dis* 1993;4(12):1103–1108.
12. Bielak LF, Kaufmann RB, Moll PP, et al. Small lesions identified by electron beam computed tomographic exams of the heart: Calcification or noise? *Radiology* 1994;192:631–636.
13. Shields JP, Mielke CH, Rockwood TH, et al. Reliability of electron beam CT to detect coronary artery calcification. *Am J Card Imaging* 1995;9(2): 62–66.
14. Kaufmann RB, Peyser PA, Sheedy PF, et al. Quantification of coronary artery calcium by electron beam computed tomography for determination of angiographic coronary disease severity in younger patients. *J Am Coll Cardiol* 1995;25:626–632.
15. Rumberger JA, Simons DB, Fitzpatrick LA, et al. Coronary artery calcium area by electron beam computed tomography and coronary atherosclerotic plaque area: A histopathologic correlative study. *Circulation* 1995;92: 2157–2162.
16. Chou TM, Redberg RF, Ko E, et al. Screening for coronary atherosclerosis by detection of calcium on electron beam computed tomography: Correlation with intravascular ultrasound in asymptomatic patients with primary hyperlipidemia. *Circulation* 1996;94:I–360. Abstract.
17. Guerci AD, Spadaro LA, Popma JJ, et al. Relation of coronary calcium score by electron beam computed tomography to arteriographic findings in asymptomatic and symptomatic adults. *Am J Cardiol* 1997;79:128–133.
18. Breen JF, Sheedy PF, Schwartz RS, et al. Coronary artery calcification detected with ultrafast CT as an indication of coronary artery disease. *Radiology* 1992;185(2):435–439.
19. Agatston AS, Janowitz WR, Kaplan G, et al. Ultrafast computed tomography-detected coronary calcium reflects the angiographic extent of coronary arterial atherosclerosis. *Am J Cardiol* 1994;74:1272–1274.
20. Devries S, Wolfkiel C, Fusman B, et al. Influence of age and gender on the presence of coronary calcium detected by ultrafast computed tomography. *J Am Coll Cardiol* 1995;25:76–82.
21. Rumberger JA, Sheedy PF, Breen JR, et al. Coronary calcium as determined by electron beam computed tomography, and coronary disease on arteriogram: Effect of patient's sex on diagnosis. *Circulation* 1995;91:1363–1367.
22. Kajinami K, Seki H, Takekoshi N, et al. Noninvasive prediction of coronary atherosclerosis by quantification of coronary artery calcification using electron beam computed tomography: Comparison with electrocardiographic and thallium exercise stress test results. *J Am Coll Cardiol* 1995;26:1209–1221.
23. Budoff MJ, Georgiou D, Brody A, et al. Ultrafast computed tomography as a diagnostic modality in the detection of coronary artery disease: A multicenter study. *Circulation* 1996;93:898–904.
24. Guerci AD, Spadaro LA, Sherman SJ, et al. Accuracy of electron beam CT in the diagnosis of coronary artery disease. *Am J Cardiac Imaging* 1996; 10(suppl 1)5. Abstract.
25. Mautner SL, Lin F, Mautner GC, et al. Comparison in women versus men of composition of atherosclerotic plaques in native coronary arteries and in saphenous veins used as aortocoronary conduits. *J Am Coll Cardiol* 1993; 21:1312–1318.
26. Arad Y, Spadaro LA, Goodman K, et al. Predictive value of electron beam CT of the coronary arteries: 19 month follow-up of 1173 asymptomatic subjects. *Circulation* 1996;93:1951–1953.

27. Wong N, Vu A, Abrahamson D, et al. Prediction of coronary events from noninvasive calcium screening by ultrafast CT. *Circulation* 1993;88:(suppl I):I–15. Abstract.
28. Balogh T, Hoff J, Rich S, et al. Development of coronary artery disease in asymptomatic subjects undergoing coronary artery calcification screening by electron beam tomograph. *Circulation* 1995;92(suppl I):I-650. Abstract.
29. Agatston AS, Janowitz WR, Kaplan GS, et al. Electron beam CT predicts future coronary events. *Circulation* 1996;94(suppl I):I-360. Abstract.
30. Secci A, Wang S, Wong N, et al. Both thin and thick slice electron beam tomographic coronary calcium predict future coronary endpoints in high risk adults. *Am J Card Imaging* 1996;10(suppl I):I-6. Abstract.
31. Detrano R, Schwendener C, Doherty T, et al. Coronary calcium results predict coronary heart disease deaths in high risk asymptomatic adults. *J Am Coll Cardiol* 1997;29:128A.
32. Emond M, Mock MB, Davis KB, et al. Long term survival of medically treated patients in the Coronary Artery Surgery Study (CASS) Registry. *Circulation* 1994;90:2645–2657.
33. Kennedy JM, Budoff MJ, Georgiou D, et al. Coronary calcification by ultrafast computed tomography is an independent predictor of obstructive coronary artery disease: A multivariate risk factor analysis. *J Am Coll Cardiol* 1995;25:387A. Abstract.
34. Guerci AD, Spadaro LA, Goodman KJ, et al. Comparison of electron beam CT scanning and conventional risk factor assessment for the prediction of coronary artery disease in symptomatic adults. *J Am Coll Cardiol* 1998. In press.
35. Detrano RC, Wong ND, Tang W, et al. Prognostic significance of cardiac cinefluoroscopy for coronary calcific deposits in asymptomatic high risk subjects. *J Am Coll Cardiol* 1994;24:354–358.
36. Detrano R, Froelicher VF. Exercise testing: Uses and limitations considering recent studies. *Prog Cardiovasc Dis* 1988;31:173–204.
37. Lieberman SM, Wolfkiel CJ, Freels S, et al. Use of electron beam tomography (UFCT) to develop cost effective treatments for primary prevention of coronary disease. *Circulation* 1995;92:I-512.
38. Wong ND, Kouwabunpat D, Vo AN, et al. Coronary calcification and atherosclerosis by ultrafast computed tomography in asymptomatic men and women: Relation to age and risk factors. *Am Heart J* 1994;127:422–430.
39. Rumberger JA, Behrenbeck T, Breen JF, et al. Electron beam computed tomography for diagnosis of coronary artery disease: A cost analysis of various diagnostic testing pathways. *Circulation* 1995;92:I-650. Abstract.
40. Wexler L, Brundage B, Crouse J, et al. Coronary artery calcification: Pathophysiology, epidemiology, imaging methods, and clinical implications. A statement for health professionals from the American Heart Association. *Circulation* 1996;94:1175–1192.
41. Arad Y, Spadaro LA, Goodman K, et al. 3.6 years follow-up of 1136 asymptomatic adults undergoing electron beam CT (EBCT) of the coronary arteries. *J Am Coll Cardiol* 1998;31:210A. Abstract.
42. Detrano RC, Wong N, Tang W, Doherty TM. Determining coronary event risk in asymptomatic high risk subjects: Risk factor versus an anatomic approach. *Circulation* 1997;96:I-104. Abstract.

Overview of Imaging:

Characterization of the Vulnerable Plaque with Emphasis on Coronary Atherosclerosis

Discussant from the Audience: This is a question to Dr. Nissen and it relates to the tissue characterization with the IVUS technique and the interpretation we can make in terms of describing the atherosclerotic plaque. You said first that a normal vessel didn't have any differentiation, whereas in the atherosclerotic arteries we get some thick echolucent regions which are really different. Why is that?

Dr. Nissen: First of all, what you're seeing is that the sonalucent zone is not the media per se. One of the problems with ultrasound, one of its limitations, is that when you get a reflection, you get a reflection because there's a change in acoustic impedance at a tissue boundary. The leading edge of all structures is located precisely where you see that reflection. The trailing edge, on the other hand, is very much a function of beam properties, ultrasound frequency, and so on. Hence, you can't measure accurately the thickness of the media in an ultravascular image. And so it may appear to be a thick media, but you really can't be certain what the actual thickness of the media is. In normal arteries, you see two patterns. You see a pattern where it's monolayered and where there is no trilamellar structure. The reason for that is when we're born, we have a single layer of endothelial cells. Even with 30 MHz you can't resolve that thin a layer. As you get into the twentieth and thirtieth years of age, most "normals" will have a trilamellar pattern. What you're seeing is the fact that they really aren't quite normal anymore. So we think that a real normal, and we've done this in children, is a monolayered artery because the intima's just too thin to resolve.

Discussant from the Audience: My second question is how the lipid infiltrations you showed are also echolucent. How do you make the difference between those regions and the region of lipid infiltration? Is there a way to make a difference for the core?

Dr. Nissen: There's not. You know one of the limitations of intravascular ultrasound is that we must infer plaque characteristics from the echogenicity and texture of the image. If you have two principally sonar lucent structures, they're not likely to look any different. Now, fortunately, what we've found is that as you push the frequency up, which we're about to do, as you get to about 50 MHz, even more subtle differentiation is possible. I think you're going to see a whole wave of new observations in the coronary with a high-frequency ultrasound. It's going to be a very, very successful approach.

Discussant from the Audience: In terms of detecting and measuring regression, especially in the bifurcation, how do you deal with core registration between 6 months apart in terms of location and catheter emulation?

Dr. Nissen: There's no question that we have to work very hard to come back to the same site every time. We've been doing this now for a number of years in our transplant patients where we bring them back every year for repeat imaging. Generally there are points that you can find. There are perivascular structures that are easily identified and you can come back to those points time and time again. We've been able to show actually very, very good reproducibility in doing so, but like any imaging technique, be it angiography or IVUS, you have to work hard to be able to come back to the same points. There is one way to get around that problem almost entirely and it's one that we're now using more and more. This is to put the catheter at a distal point and then do a precise motorized pullback of the transducer so that one millimeter or a half of a millimeter is one second's pullback. So if you know where you're starting from, then you can line up all of those slices and actually get a summated volume of atherosclerosis that's very reproducible, very precise, and very easy to do in repeated studies.

Dr. Rosenfeld: I'd like to make a comment and pose a question perhaps to both panels. The comment has to do with the point about the size of the atheroma's core, the lipid core, and the problem with the carotid and coronary plaques. The comment is that the key is not the size of the lipid core but the composition of that lipid. The published case reports say cholesterol emboli are very proinflammatory. There is something about the nature of the lipid that is both attracting the inflammatory cells and killing the inflammatory cells. Perhaps the difference in the carotid and the coronaries is actually the composition of the lipid. My question is whether it's possible with the imaging modalities to detect differences in the composition of the lipid? Perhaps Dr. Witztum's talk tomorrow will address imaging of oxidation products within the plaque. I think the key is the degree of oxidation because if you look at the antioxidant data in the animal models, what disappears with antioxidant treatment are the macrophage foam cell components. So I wonder if you might want to address the question of whether it's possible, using imaging modalities, and whether using an approach from a pathologist point of view, to look at differences in composition, not just size and thinning of the cap.

Dr. Fuster: This is going to be discussed tomorrow, but maybe you have a comment, Dr. Nissen.

Dr. Nissen: I think it's an interesting concept, I don't know if anybody's really looked at the chemical composition of the necrotic core in the various arterial territories. I don't know if imaging can discriminate. There's an instrument that is going to be entering human trials shortly that I think is going to be very useful for research. It consists of a directional atherectomy device with an ultrasound transducer built into the blade. We've done a lot of animal work with this and we're just about ready to begin human studies. You see out the window of the cutting device. You see the plaque that you're going to cut, and then you can take a sample of it, like a shaving off of it. And so we're going to be able to supply to our pathology colleagues samples taken from different points in the plaque and know, because of the ultrasound, exactly where we took the sample. Was it at the shoulder? Was it at the center? And then as you cut deeper, you'll begin to cut into the deeper material. I'm very eager, once we get this FDA approved, to do some studies where we really do look at the composition of those plaques and correlate that with their ultrasound appearance. Interestingly, this device, we've now mounted a 50 MHz transducer, not only can you sample the plaque, you can also image it at a very high frequency. So I think this is going to be very useful for research.

Discussant from the Audience: I want to comment. I think Peter Libby made a very interesting comment about the earthquakes and the MIs. Dr. Fuster, you mentioned the SCUD missile. I often present that SCUD missile study showing that there's an increase in MIs in Israel. However, it does decrease. The highest peak was at the very, very first attack and I've always assumed that the subsequent decrease, which does trail off, was due to the Israeli's becoming accustomed to the missile attacks. Might not be. The MIs have been harvested. Peter Libby, you may be right.

My question deals with something that I've never been sure of as whether it's a sampling problem or whether it varies from patient to patient. So I guess I'm looking to the pathologists, but maybe also to the imagers. We know that plaque composition varies over the length of the plaque, there are lipid-rich areas, and there are fibrous regions. Does anybody have a feeling whether there are subsets of patients who are more prone to develop the fibrous lesions and who don't get the lipid lesions. I mean I've been always looking in the literature to see if we could do an epidemiological study of patients who develop keloids or hyperplastic scars, to see if they develop more fibrous lesions.

Does anybody have comments?

I don't know. I don't think there are many data telling you how the risk factors for clinical coronary artery disease operate at the plaque level. In fact, in the May 1st, 1997 issue of *New England Journal of Medicine*, Dr. Virmani's group reported on sudden death that serum lipids were very closely associated with vulnerable lesions, while smoking was not. It was associated with thrombotic complications to the lesions, so there may be something here.

Dr. Fuster: Dr. William Roberts has looked at autopsy data according to risk factors. There are major differences in plaque morphology in patients according to whether their major risk factor is hypertension, hyperlipidemia, smoking, or family history. We don't understand these yet, but I assume that there are classes of patients who have different plaques from others. However, the disease is so heterogenous. When you look at the coronary artery of any patient with any risk factor, you see all the lesions there. And to begin to quantify if the patient is "more fibrotic" than "lipid core" prone is very difficult because you're dealing there with many, many lesions. The question's a very important one, but I'm not sure if there is a clear answer.

Panel Member: Well my answer is that younger people who have acute myocardial infarctions appear to have more lipid-laden plaques within their coronaries. Older patients, and I stress the age differences here, tend to have very severely stenotic plaques, which tend to have fibro- proliferative plaques and less lipid in them. But the real difference comes in the transplant population, where the plaques are very fibrous and have very little lipid. But you certainly get severe stenosis. It's a different mechanism.

Discussant from the Audience: My question is directed to Professor Uchida. He's been the first one to make a presentation today in which he was able to predict the vulnerable plaque. This was because within the few months he followed the patients, there were events with the yellow glistening lesions. My question is, have you had the opportunity to check the pathology of any of those lesions against the morphology by angioscopy?

Dr. Uchida: No I did not examine the pathology.

Discussant from the Audience: It would be highly attractive. Of course that requires the death of the patient, but if by chance it occurred, even a few cases would be very helpful in order to correlate your angioscopy images with the pathology. Then we'd have a better definition of what the vulnerable lesion is.

Discussant from the Audience: This morning several speakers referred to the plaque's shoulder region as the most vulnerable region. However, this is a two dimensional. You will note that atherosclerotic plaques are three dimensional. I wonder if there is any information about how the plaque's progress along the longitudinal axis, proximal, distal, or from the central part of the plaque.

Dr. Fuster: You have a sense of morphology and geometry. I would have thought that was a pathological question in the sense that it's related to the pathology. The way a thrombus propagates appears to be independent of where the initial fracture occurs. How a plaque propagates may be a different story.

Dr. Badimon: Several years ago we did three-dimensional pathological reconstructions. In a small subset of those reconstructured areas, we found in the proximal plaque area a fracture at the shoulder region, and then in the distal area there would also be a fracture. The plaque could fracture almost anywhere, but more often that not, the fracture was in the middle of the fibrous cap. Interestingly enough, in the proximal area, it appeared that there was blood or hematoma within the plaque, and in the distal area often was this volcano type of pathology, with the cholesterol going out into the lumen of the coronary artery. I think a couple of the images that we were shown on the video this morning actually showed the combination of a proximal tear and distal rupture. The situation is complicated more in the carotid territory. The plaques don't just occur at the outer wall of the bifurcation, they tend to have a helical distribution as you go up, so they're lateral and then they become posterior. A three-dimensional reconstruction becomes very important.

Dr. Fuster: I have a number of questions for the imaging people. Dr. Guerci, did you have a fast electron beam CT for calcium yourself?

Dr. Guerci: Your question is actually very important. We've had our scanner in operation for about $3\frac{1}{2}$ years now. I'm 47 years old. My total cholesterol is 180, my HDL is 76 to 80, my blood pressure is 110/70. Both paternal grandparents died in their late 80s, age 87 and 88, of prostate cancer. One maternal grandmother died of complications of a fractured hip and one did die of atherosclerosis. She had a stroke at the age of 99. We have discouraged people without risk factors from undergoing ultrafast scanning, but I carry in my mind the impression that about 30 percent of patients with acute myocardial infarction have no known risk factors for coronary disease. Im referring to the standard five: diabetes, smoking, hypercholesterolemia, hypertension, and family history. Very clearly we know today that there are other things that play a risk role, measurable humoral factors, as homocystine for example. These likely account for some of that unexplained 30 percent. But basically we discourage people who don't have risk factors from undergoing scanning.

Well I think the concept of the degree of distribution and calcification is a significant advance compared to 3 or 4 years ago when it was graded presence or absence of calcification. The severity of calcification is a marker of extension of the disease, the plaque burden.

Dr. Fuster: Dr. Nissen, I have a pressing question about intravascular ultrasound. What is the sensitivity and the specificity of what you see? I cannot see well what is in the pictures and the literature and I am sure the best are selected. If somebody in the audience here wants to get into the predictability of plaques, would you tell them to get into intravascular ultrasound?

Dr. Nissen: Absolutely. Now first of all, it's important to understand that this is a very new technology and that if you go back just a few years, the images were not as good. Let me say unequivocally, that the pictures I showed today are typical, they're not exceptional. I showed them because the cases were interesting, not necessarily because the pictures were extraordinary. One can obtain very good quality images, reliably every time, 98 percent of the time let's say in patients with coronary disease. We've only been able to make pictures of that quality for just a very short few years. Second, I think that the science of how to use that information is certainly lagging. I don't think that this is solved yet, and I think that the next leap, with the use of a little higher frequency, will take us to the point where we can really show details of the pathology of the plaque that are very, very useful. I'm looking forward to being able to sample those plaques with an atherectomy device so we can correlate what we see with the precise pathology of the tissue. I guess my answer is, you ought to expect to get good pictures every time, and anybody, when properly trained, can interpret these pictures now.

Dr. Fuster: Will you try to get into the peripheral vasculature or even the carotid arteries?

Dr. Nissen: Absolutely. We've made pictures in the peripheral arteries. It's a little different problem. Actually it's a little easier because the limitation here is the size of the transducer. The bigger the transducer, the better the picture. We're working with a 1-millimeter catheter. In the periphery you can actually work with a 2- or 3-millimeter catheter and make just exquisite pictures. It hasn't been used very much there for reasons I can't necessarily answer, but it's a very effective technique for looking at peripheral disease. Perhaps the reason it hasn't been used more is you can look at carotid disease from the surface, and so everybody takes the noninvasive route to look.

Dr. Fuster: However, surface ultrasound cannot discriminate the components well, as the frequency and resolution are much lower.

Dr. Nissen: We have been imaging all the patients, getting carotid stents. We don't have a big enough number of patients to determine any difference between the coronary lesions and the carotid lesions. Ultimately, we should be able to address that. I want to make a few points. First of all, one of the things that I think is very striking in the intravascular ultrasound follow-up study we did and the people that we're now studying as a part of an intervention study, is that a significant proportion of patients have absolutely no risk factors, and yet have very high calcium scores. It's quite impressive. We know that people have disease. In a few cases where we find extremely high calcium scores, and completely asymptomatic people with no risk factors, when for other reasons they end up with an angiogram, invariably, they have severe disease.

Discussant from the Audience: While the National Cholesterol Education Program guidelines include age as a risk factor, let's forget about that for the purpose of this discussion. About 10 percent of subjects have no known risk factors for coronary disease, but have coronary calcium scores that are at or above roughly the 80th percentile for age and gender.

Dr. Guerci: I think what's more important than the actual score is where an individual is in the distribution of coronary calcium scores for persons of his age and gender.

Dr. Fuster: The point is very important to the community. What you are saying is in the population without risk factors, you see a significant number with high calcium scores. My question is in a population of 100 people, how many, without risk factors, will have a score of 160 and above?

Dr. Guerci: Fifteen percent.

Discussant from the Audience: I'd like to make two other comments. The first comment is the inverse of what was just said. For people with high risk factors, no matter what they are, an extremely low calcium score basically rules out disease. The clinical value of this was not emphasized. My last point is that calcium score is really a procedure from the past. Currently intravenous electron beam CT coronary angiography simultaneously gives coronary imaging, coronary perfusion, and wall motion abnormalities. The calcium score was the first use of this machine. It's been progressing from then on.

Dr. Nissen: I'm a little troubled by the assertion that a negative fast CT in a patient with risk factors rules out disease because we see by intravascular ultrasound a large population with extensive coronary atherosclerosis and not one speck of calcium anywhere in the coronary.

Dr. Guerci: The coronary calcium score rules out obstructive coronary disease with a likelihood of 98 percent. So there's a 2 percent chance that middle-aged men and women with a calcium score of zero have obstructive disease, symptomatic or not.

Dr. Fuster: The point is that with a calcium score below a certain threshold, the likelihood of some amount of coronary disease remains a function of the number of risk factors. For the patient with one or two risk factors, a calcium score of zero is a very good sign. With four, five, or six risk factors for coronary disease and a calcium score of zero, the patient may still have a problem with obstructive disease.

Discussant from the Audience: I'm not an expert in this area. A recently published study reported fast electron beam CT of a 400- to 500-person population that they had followed for risk factors and outcome since childhood. Thirty-one percent have a positive CT. Of those 31 percent, who were calcium positive at average age 30, all had three positive risk factors. Women had obesity, hypertension, and low HDL. Men had these three risk factors plus high LDL. They are very highly correlated, which would go along with calcium, indicating it to be a marker for the same process.

Dr. Fuster: We can close the discussion this morning and touch into the world of imaging. As a summary, coronary arteriography has become a standard. We have learned a lot about coronary arteriography and we are continuing to learn. Intravascular ultrasound is moving forward. Dr. Nissen is very excited about its future and we should follow the developments. I am very impressed about Professor Uchida's angioscopic data as a predictor of coronary events. Regarding fast electron beam CT, I think it's coming along. We are beginning to learn what this tool can do in terms of predicting coronary disease and I think it may have its use in the future in specific populations. We are all dealing with the same disease, but the manifestations are a little bit different depending upon how the trigger acts in the different arterial regions. Furthermore, the brain doesn't have much leeway, as any little anatomical event is usually, but not necessarily always, noticeable. In the legs it seems we don't notice much. We will reconvene at 2:00. Thank you all!

Chapter 8

Magnetic Resonance Imaging of the Vessel Wall in Carotids and Coronaries

Meir Shinnar, MD, PhD, Zahi A. Fayad, PhD, John T. Fallon, MD, PhD, and Valentin Fuster, MD, PhD

Introduction

Coronary artery disease and its complications remain the major cause of morbidity and mortality in the United States. Current diagnostic techniques for evaluating the coronary arteries, such as exercise testing and angiography, focus on the reduction of flow by either measuring the pathophysiological consequences of a decreased lumen diameter or by imaging the lumen diameter invasively. It is now known that many acute coronary syndromes, including unstable angina, myocardial infarction, and sudden death, are the consequence of a ruptured atherosclerotic plaque in a coronary artery that had a minimal obstruction to flow when imaged in the year prior to the infarct.[1] It is thought that many of these infarctions are secondary to the instability of a non-occlusive American Heart Asssociation type IV atherosclerotic lesion, leading to plaque rupture and thrombosis.[2,3] Thus, simply measuring coronary stenosis is inadequate to assess the risk.

There is, therefore, a need for a technique that can discriminate between different types of plaque. In particular, it should discriminate between lesions with a thick fibrous cap and lesions with a lipid core

This work was supported in part by NIH HL54469 and funds from The Cardiovascular Institute at Mount Sinai Medical Center.

From: Fuster, V (ed). *The Vulnerable Atherosclerotic Plaque: Understanding, Identification, and Modification.* Armonk, NY: Futura Publishing Company, Inc.; © 1999.

and a thin fibrous cap. Furthermore, for more universal applicability, it should be relatively noninvasive.

Magnetic resonance imaging (MRI) has emerged as a leading candidate for such a technique. Studies have shown that MRI can discriminate different tissue types.[4,5] Furthermore, recent studies show that it can be done in vivo.[6–8]

This chapter summarizes current research into imaging the vessel wall in carotids and coronaries. It aims to achieve the following objectives: (1) explain the MRI characteristics of different plaque components; (2) explain some of the methodological problems in extending the in vitro work to in vivo work in coronary and carotid lesions; and (3) explain the problems and current status of imaging coronary artery lesions in vivo. Data are presented which show that characterizing such lesions is feasible.

Magnetic Resonance Imaging

One of the major advantages of MRI over other imaging technologies is the range of contrast mechanisms available. In x-ray techniques, ranging from ultrafast CT to fluoroscopy, image contrast is solely dependent on the tissue's absorbance of x-rays or Hounsfield units. Ultrasound only measures the scattering of sound by tissue or, by use of Doppler, its velocity.

In MRI multiple contrast mechanisms are available. These include the proton density; T1 relaxation and T2 relaxation, which relate to the physical state of the water; the motion of the tissue; and the diffusion coefficient of water. As we shall see, several different contrast mechanisms are needed to fully characterize plaque.

Early work on the application of magnetic resonance techniques to the characterization of plaque focused on spectroscopy.[9,10] Magnetic resonance spectroscopy allows for the determination of the different biochemical components of plaque, and has therefore been very valuable. This research has provided much valuable information about the nature of the plaque.

Unfortunately, the concentration of these chemicals in the plaque is very low in comparison with that of water. Therefore, it has been difficult to extend these techniques to an in vivo setting. Most in vivo applications of spectroscopy use large pixels to compensate for the low signal—pixels larger than even a big plaque.

Other groups tried to image the lipids within the plaque.[11,12] This work was interesting, but the signal to noise was still low.

Recent studies[4–8] have shown that standard MRI techniques can distinguish plaque components. These techniques image the water and

Table 1

Magnetic Resonance Imaging Characteristics of Plaque Components

Plaque component	MRI Characteristic
Fibrocellular	Light on T2wm, dark on DW
Calcium	Dark on all images
Fibrocellular with lipid	Dark on T2wm, light on T2wp
Gruel (necrotic core)	Dark on T2wp T2wm, dark on diffusion
Thrombus	Light on T2wp, light on diffusion
Fibrous cap	Fibrocellular or calcium over necrotic core

DW = Diffusion weighted; T2wm = maximally T2 weighted (TE 50ms); T2wp = partially T2 weighted (TE 30ms).

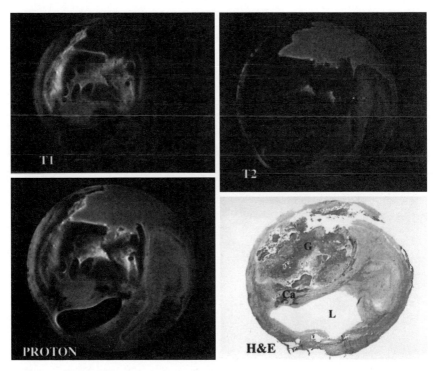

Figure 1. Proton density, T1 weighted, and T2 weighted images of a carotid artery plaque obtained at endarterectomy, together with the corresponding histopathologic section. The calcium (Ca), gruel (G), and lumen are marked on the histopathology.

therefore have a much higher signal to noise and image resolution. Recently, diffusion-weighted MRI has been shown to characterize thrombi.[13,14] Table 1 lists the plaque components together with their characteristic magnetic resonance (MR) appearance. Figures 1 and 2 show MR images of a carotid artery, together with the corresponding histopathology.

We recently tested the diagnostic accuracy of ex vivo carotid MRI in identifying plaque components. This work is summarized in Table 2.

There are several methodological issues involved in extending this work to in vivo. The signal to noise in a clinical magnet is less than it is in a high-resolution magnet. There are artifacts secondary to motion

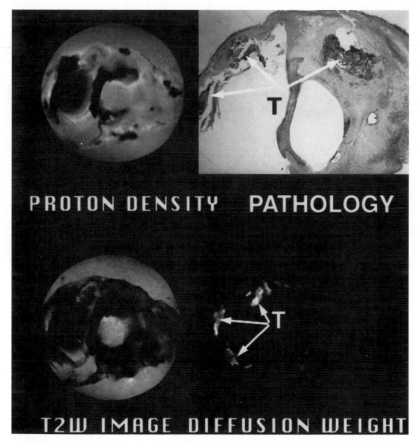

Figure 2. Proton density, T2-weighted, and diffusion-weighted image of a carotid artery plaque obtained at endarterectomy, together with the corresponding histopathology. Locations of thrombus (T) are identified on the histopathology and the diffusion-weighted image.

Table 2

Accuracy of Ex Vivo Carotid Magnetic Resonance Imaging in Identification of Plaque Components

	True positive	Sensitivity	True negative	Specificity
Calcium	66/66	100	0/0	
Fibrocellular	66/66	100	0/0	
Fibrocellular + lipid	47/47	100	18/19	95%
Gruel	61/61	100	5/5	100
Fibrous cap	61/61	100	5/5	100
Thrombus	43/51	84	15/15	100

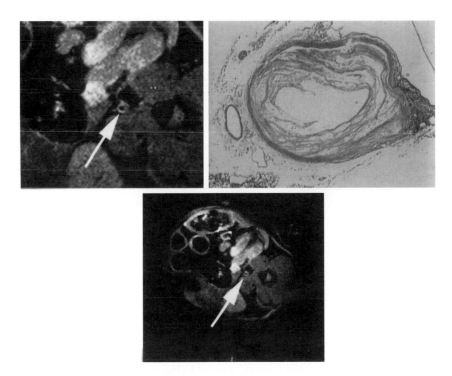

Figure 3. In vivo image of an apo E-deficient mouse, showing the site and size of an atherosclerotic plaque in the abdominal aorta. The histopathology is shown for comparison.

and flow. Therefore, close attention to detail, including optimizing the radiofrequency (RF) coil and pulse sequence, is necessary.[15] Recent data suggest, however, that such extension is feasible.[7,8]

Animal Models

MRI is useful for studying the development of atherosclerotic lesions in animal models. We recently extended our ability to image plaque to imaging transgenic mice (Fig. 3).[16] It is now possible to study the development and progression of atherosclerosis in different transgenic models of atherosclerosis.

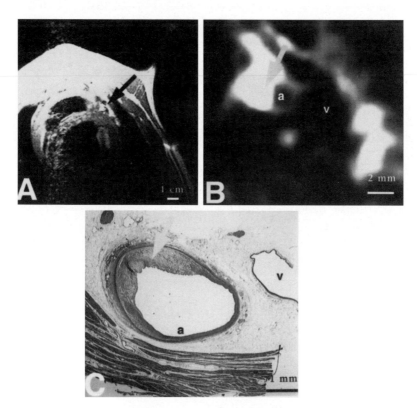

Figure 4. Panels **A** through **C** show a left anterior descending (LAD) lesion 3 months post percutaneous transluminal coronary angioplasty. **A.** A T1-weighted spin echo MR image (FOV 16 cm × 16 cm, 256 by 224, TE 16 ms, TR = 1 RR interval ~650 ms, 1.5 NEX, pixel size 625 by 714 microns) obtained transverse to the LAD. The black arrow points to the location of the LAD. **B.** An enlargement of the original MRI showing the LAD (a) and the surronding tissues including the anterior vein (v). **C.** A histopathological section corresponding to the MR image. The black arrows in **B** and **C** point to the postangioplasty fibrocellular lesion in the LAD wall.

Coronaries

The coronaries pose a unique problem. Cardiac motion complicates most standard techniques. As the vessel is only several millimeters in size, respiratory motion becomes a significant problem. We recently showed that if we suppress respiratory motion and gate to the cardiac cycle, we can image lesions in the wall of coronary vessels (Figs. 4 and 5).[17] Our model was a postpercutaneous transluminal coronary angioplasty injury model in the pig, rather than atherosclerosis. However, the ability to image the vessel wall suggests that atherosclerosis

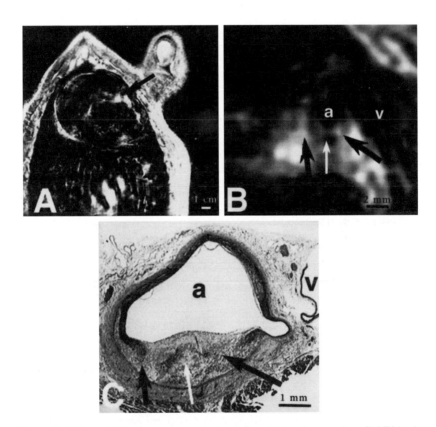

Figure 5. This set of images represents a left anterior descending (LAD) lesion just 2 weeks postpercutaneous transluminal coronary angioplasty. **A.** The MR image (FOV 20 cm × 20 cm, 256 by 192, TE 18 ms, TR = 1 RR interval ~ 700 ms, 1.0 NEX, pixel size 782 by 1140 microns) showing the location of the LAD (black arrrow). In **B** and **C**, the artery and vein are marked by an a and v, respectively. The black arrows in **B** and **C** denote the limits of the fibrocellular lesion in the LAD wall. The defect in the center of this LAD lesion (white arrow) corresponds to an organizing area of thrombus in the histopathology section.

can also be imaged. We are working on modifying the technique so that it can be applied to humans.

In summary, MRI has the unique ability to image and characterize plaque and its different components noninvasively in many different model systems.

References

1. Ambrose J, Tannenbaum M, Alexopoulos D, et al. Angiographic progression of coronary artery disease and the development of myocardial infarction. *J Am Coll Cardiol* 1988;12:56–62.
2. Falk E, Shah PK, Fuster V. Coronary plaque disruption. *Circulation* 1995; 92:657–671.
3. Topol EJ, Nissen SE. Our preoccupation with coronary luminology. *Circulation* 1995;92:2333–2342.
4. Toussaint JF, Southern JF, Fuster V, Kantor HL. T2-weighted contrast for NMR characterization of human atherosclerosis. *Arterioscl Thromb Vasc Biol* 1995;15(10):1533–1542.
5. Martin AJ, Gotlieb AI, Henkelman RM. High-resolution MR imaging of human arteries. *J Magn Reson Imaging* 1995;5:93–100.
6. Skinner MP, Yuan C, Mitsumori L, et al. Serial magnetic resonance imaging of experimental atherosclerosis detects lesion fine structure, progression and complications in vivo. *Nature Med* 1995;1:69–73.
7. Toussaint JF, LaMuraglia GR, Southern JF, et al. Magnetic resonance images lipid, fibrous, calcified, hemorrhagic, and thrombotic components of human atherosclerosis in vivo. *Circulation* 1996;94:932–938.
8. Wildy KS, Yuan C, Tsuruda JS, et al. Atherosclerosis of the carotid artery: Evaluation by magnetic resonance angiography. *J Magn Reson Imaging* 1996; 6(5):726–732.
9. Maynor CH, Charles HC, Herfkens RJ, et al. Chemical shift imaging of atherosclerosis at 7.0 Tesla. *Invest Radiol* 1988;24:52–60.
10. Pearlman JD, Zajicek J, Merickel MB, et al. High-resolution 1H NMR spectral signature from human atheroma. *Magn Reson Med* 1988;7:262–279.
11. Mohiaddin RH, Firmin DN, Underwood SR, et al. Chemical shift magnetic resonance imaging of human atheroma. *Br Heart J* 1989;62(2):81–89.
12. Vinitski S, Consigny PM, Shapiro MJ, et al. Magnetic resonance chemical shift imaging and spectroscopy of atherosclerotic plaque. *Invest Radiol* 1991; 26(8):703–714.
13. Shinnar M, Fallon J, Wehrli S, et al. Diffusion weighted imaging better characterizes atherosclerotic plaque and thrombus. *Circulation* 1996;94: I–345.
14. Toussaint JF, Southern JF, Fuster V, Kantor HL. Diffusion properties of human atherosclerosis and thrombosis measured by pulse field gradient NMR. *Arterioscler Thromb Vasc Biol* 1997;17:542–546.
15. Hayes CE, Mathis CM, Yuan C. Surface coil phased arrays for high-resolution imaging of the carotid arteries. *J Magn Reson Imaging* 1996;6(1):109–112.
16. Shinnar M, Dansky HM, Fayad ZA, et al. MRI characterization of vascular lesions in APO E deficient mice. *Circulation* 1997;96:I–110.
17. Shinnar M, Gallo R, Fayad ZA, et al. In vivo magnetic resonance imaging of post angioplasty coronary vessel wall lesions in pigs. *J Am Coll Cardiol* 1998;31:339A.

Chapter 9

Tissue Characterization of Human Atherosclerosis and Plaque Vulnerability by Nuclear Magnetic Resonance

Jean-François Toussaint, MD, PhD and Valentin Fuster, MD, PhD

Clinical assessment of human atherosclerosis progression depends predominantly on stenosis evaluation by conventional angiography or surface B-mode ultrasound. Angiographic studies, however, have demonstrated that luminal morphometry cannot predict the evolution of a plaque.[1] Intravascular ultrasound and angioscopy recently improved the observation of arterial walls, but these techniques are invasive and are limited in their ability to determine chemical composition.

Nuclear magnetic resonance (NMR), as a noninvasive biochemical imaging tool, can discriminate plaque components on the basis of chemical composition, molecular motion, diffusion, physical state, or water content. These differences may be especially important in determining the factors that contribute events related to plaque rupture; they depend strongly on two of the biochemical constituents: collagenous fibers and lipids.[2]

We developed several means of assessing plaque composition with NMR using ^{13}C-NMR spectroscopy,[3] T2 contrast,[4] or water diffusion imaging,[5] and applied these methods[6] to discriminate in vivo wall components in normal and atheromatous arteries. Identified regions in-

This work has been supported in part by the Harold M. English Fund from the Harvard Medical School, la Bourse Accelli de la Société Française de Cardiologie, l'Institut Electricité Santé, and le Fonds d'Etudes et de Recherche du Corps Médical des Hôpitaux de Paris.

clude: media, adventitia, perivascular fat, lipid-rich core, collagenous cap, and calcifications. Finally, we tested plaque resistance with in vitro models of angioplasty and atherectomy.[7]

Atheromatous Lipid Composition by Carbon-13 NMR Spectroscopy

Natural abundance ^{13}C-NMR spectroscopy allows the nondestructive characterization of lipid chemical composition. Because of its broad chemical shift band width, ^{13}C-NMR provides more information regarding chemical constituents than ^{1}H-NMR, and has been used for structural and dynamic studies of cholesteryl esters (CEs), triglycerides (TGs) and phospholipids (PLs). Hamilton et al[8] examined plasma lipoproteins and intact atherosclerotic plaques in humans, demonstrating that atheroma has spectral characteristics very similar to thermally denatured low-density lipoproteins (LDL), which suggests a comparable chemical composition. They emphasized the importance of CE phase transitions in determining the lipid state (liquid, smectic, or solid) and their spectral characteristics, and indicated that most of the atheromatous CE was derived from nonmetabolized lipoproteins.

With this technique, we demonstrated that the mean MUFA/PUFA ratio (monounsaturated versus polyunsaturated fatty acids) of lesions composed of uncomplicated, nonulcerated fibrous plaques was 1.15, while complex and more stenotic lesions had a 42% increased ratio. A decrease of the carbon 19 and 21 CE resonance could also be shown, with no significant variation of visible TG or PL as compared to the fatty acid pool. The ^{13}C peaks were predominantly derived from the mobile atheromatous lipids, which generate relatively narrow resonances.

These results suggest that the relation between MUFA/PUFA, C^{19}, C^{21}, and obstruction ratio did not apply to the total lipid content (including solid-state lipids such as free cholesterol crystals), but only to the mobile component. The importance of characterizing this component (the "soft" lipids) is explained by its probable contribution to plaque vulnerability and its role in the processes leading to plaque rupture through abnormal repartition of circumferential stress.

Alterations in fatty acid saturation and CEs in atheroma have been described and attributed to lipid and lipoprotein oxidation. This process has been previously studied with ^{1}H and ^{13}C-NMR by use of a model of LDL peroxidation.[9] These studies showed an increase in the MUFA/PUFA ratio as a result of oxidation, similar to our findings in lesions of increasing severity, resulting from a PUFA decrease without changes in MUFA.

Further support for the reduction in fatty acid saturation resulting from lipoprotein oxidation comes from other studies which describe the effects of oxidation on fatty acyl chain double bonds, demonstrating a 55% loss of polyunsaturated fatty acid chains,[10] with the production of reactive aldehydes and an increase in the content of thiobarbituric acids. The loss of PUFA has been ascribed to their low resistance to oxidation, and may have clinical implications with respect to atherosclerosis prevention. Their low content also influences the cytotoxic effects of oxidized LDL and alters the lipid phase transition and fluidity.

Our investigation also demonstrates a decrease in the resonance of the carbons 19 and 21 of the CEs. C19 and C21 are located on the edge of the cholesterol ring, and therefore have less restricted motion than inner-ring carbons, making them well suited for NMR analysis. This decrease of the C19, C21 peak of CE is consistent with previous studies[10] showing that the oxidation of the cholesterol moiety of lipoproteins caused a 55% decrease of cholesteryl esters. Another factor that explains the decrease of resonances from CEs in the most stenotic lesions could be the inhibition of the reesterification cycle by the cytotoxic effect of oxidized lipoproteins as described by Brown and Goldstein.[11] This inhibition leads to the accumulation of free cholesterol, which precipitates as monohydrate crystals, the hallmark of advanced lesions; these crystals have very short T2 relaxation times resulting from the solid phase, making them NMR-invisible.

These results demonstrate that the resonances from polyunsaturated fatty acyl chains and cholesteryl esters decreased as vessel obstruction increased, and suggest a loss of double bonds and a decrease of CEs in the mobile lipid pool when plaque progresses.

Plaque Structure by Proton MR Imaging

Through spectroscopy or imaging, NMR, as a noninvasive biochemical investigative tool, is capable of discriminating plaque components on the basis of chemical composition. This may be important for determining the factors that contribute to events related to plaque rupture, such as the distribution of circumferential stress,[12] plaque vulnerability,[2] or thrombogenicity,[13] which depend strongly on two of the biochemical constituents: collagenous fibers and lipids.

Previously, the characterization of atheroma by ^{1}H-NMR imaging had predominantly focused on the acquisition of the lipid signal, acquired with a T1w (T1-weighted) sequence by use of either a nonselective, a lipid-selective, a modified Dixon pulse, or a pattern recognition technique using multiple sequences.[14–18] These studies were conceived to image plaque lipids with long T2 and short T1 relaxation times, similar to adipocyte triglycerides. However, cholesterol and CEs are the predominant lipids in atherosclerotic plaques with NMR relaxation constants different than triglycerides, making standard lipid imaging techniques more problematic.

In our investigation we discriminated atherosclerotic plaque components in vitro using high- field, high-resolution ^{1}H-NMR imaging without frequency-selective sequences. Our spectral measurements showed a lipid/water peak ratio of 0.1 inside the atheromatous core. It is therefore important to consider that any chemical shift technique based on lipid frequency selection and aimed at imaging the lipid core of atherosclerotic plaque will face the inherent problem of a one-tenth lower signal to noise ratio than techniques based on water proton imaging. We also demonstrated that the atheromatous core, mostly composed of cholesterol and CEs in solid (crystal) or smectic (liquid-crystalline) state, was associated with a shortened water T2 when compared to collagenous cap and normal media; consequently in arterial walls, bright areas on T2w (T2-weighted) images from non–frequency-selective sequences do not correspond to lipid- rich regions, but to regions predominantly composed of fibers (collagen, elastin, and proteoglycan) either in media or in collagenous caps.

We confirmed previous results obtained at 7 Tesla by Maynor and colleagues,[19] who showed a lipid/water ratio of 1:9 in fibrous plaques with a water T2 of 23.6 ms and a lipid T2 of 17.3 ms. These investigators focused on the lipid regions as the regions of greatest histopathological interest. In our study,[4] we showed that lipid localization was possible through changes in water T2, and we identified collagen-rich layers in the same sequence. The importance of identifying these two components rests on their role in the process leading to plaque rupture through cap thinning and abnormal repartition of circumferential stress[12] which results in acute ischemic syndromes: myocardial infarction or strokes. It is therefore important to discriminate plaque with thin or incomplete caps, which may be more prone to rupture.

Short T2 Species

Several investigators have examined the lipid component using methods that suppress water, incorporate water and lipid in a multiparameter data set, or use chemical shift imaging (CSI) with long T2 suppression.[20,21] Pearlman et al[20] presented [1]H-spectra of atherosclerotic plaques at high field (6.3, 8.5, and 11.7 Tesla), though they did not evaluate water T2. We also showed that the T2 of atheromatous core lipids is shorter than the T2 of periadventitial lipids, which are mostly composed of adipocyte triglycerides in a liquid state. In this study, a short T2 component (T2 = 1.78 ms) corresponded to 14% of the NMR-visible lipid signal and represented a more ordered state, which was likely to be the crystalline and liquid-crystalline phase. A larger part of the visible lipids (86%) had a T2 of 22.4 ms, which corresponds to a less ordered state such as the liquid state. The ordered component likely resulted from core lipids with a low content of triglycerides and a high concentration of CEs and free cholesterol (the latter being either in a monohydrate crystal form or complexed with phospholipids).[4]

Two groups have recently addressed the issue of short T2 lipids and developed methods to improve in vitro imaging of the lipid component in atheromatous plaque. Altbach et al[22] examined an aortic plaque by use of a stimulated echo diffusion-weighted sequence and was able to improve water suppression and lipid visualization. More recent data from the same group illustrate the interest of diffusion weighting in lipid imaging.[23] This technique, however, also poses the problem of low signal-to-noise ratio and long acquisition times, which was not a limiting factor in the water imaging sequence used in our study.

Gold et al[21] implemented a back-projection technique with long T2 lipid suppression to image the short T2 lipid component. Although those investigators did not specifically calculate T2 for the different components, their sequence could detect species with a T2 between 150 ms and 9 ms. The development of this technique for in vivo studies will, however, be limited by low signal-to-noise ratio and a great increase in acquisition time necessitated by echocardiogram gating. These limitations do not apply for water imaging. We showed at 1.5 T that a contrast-to- noise ratio (CNR) of 40.5 could be produced for atheromatous core versus normal media for a total acquisition time of less than 5 minutes.[4]

Chemical Shift Imaging

Another approach to the direct imaging of plaque lipids was presented by Mohiaddin and colleagues,[16] who published the first application of a Dixon chemical shift selective sequence for the imaging of atherosclerotic lipids. They showed that histologic grade of lipid content correlates with the plaque signal intensity. This methodology demonstrated encouraging results for atherosclerosis imaging by magnetic resonance imaging.

Several factors may contribute to the shortening of water T2 in the atheromatous core. These include: (1) the susceptibility differences from the micellar structure of parietal lipoproteins; (2) the more numerous or more exposed hydrophilic sites resulting from lipoprotein oxidation[24]; (3) a longer contact time of the hydrophilic sites of CEs and the water molecules—either from $-C{=}0$ on the fatty acid chain (which may also explain the contrast between adventitia and media) or from $-OH$ of C10 and C18 on the cholesterol ring, with a further interchange between bound water layers and free water.

T1w images identify calcifications; these regions appear as low-intensity zones in all NMR sequences due to low water content.[14] CNR for calcified regions versus other components was higher in T1w images than in T2w images. Calcifications play an important role in plaque aging and arterial dysfunction, and their identification may add to our understanding of hemodynamics, regulation of stress distribution, and plaque aging associated with low vasoreactivity. Water T2 is shorter in the lipid-rich core of atherosclerotic plaques than in collagenous caps or normal media. This difference enables the generation of high contrast in T2w images and provides a unique method of discriminating collagenous from lipid-rich plaque regions.

Plaque Resistance and Vulnerability

Using T2 contrast, which combines morphometry and tissue characterization, we imaged in vitro the effects of cardiac interventional techniques. We tested the fibrous cap resistance to radial compression, investigated the consequences of balloon inflation on calcified and noncalcified plaques, and compared the effects of in vitro angioplasty and atherectomy on the fibrous components.[7]

Plaques were obtained at autopsy from human aortas, iliac, and femoral arteries. Calcified and noncalcified plaques underwent restrained angioplasty by radial compression. Group A consisted of plaques with a complete collagenous cap (corresponding to type Va lesions according to the new classification of the American Heart Association Vascular Committee[25]); group B plaques had no cap (corresponding to type IV lesions); group C consisted of calcified plaques; Group D plaques were fibrous and noncalcified lesions—they underwent directed atherectomy only. We also performed restrained angioplasty followed by directed atherectomy on half of the plaques of group A. All experiments were performed within 24 hours after autopsy.

Methods to Study Radial Compression

We performed in vitro angioplasty by radial compression on unfixed samples in a saline bath at 37°C.[7] One-centimeter long arterial segments were mounted in plastic tubes; this size was chosen to match the external vessel diameter in order to specifically study the compressive effect of angioplasty on the plaque components and to prevent dissection. A single balloon inflation at 6 atm was performed for the noncalcified plaques. For the calcified plaques two inflations were successively realized at 6 atm and 10 atm. We studied the effects of atherectomy using a 6-French Simpson digital vascular imaging (DVI) system.

Images were acquired at 9.4 T before and after the procedures, by use of conventional spin echo sequences: T1w: TR = 600 ms, TE = 3 ms; T2w: TR = 2 s, TE = 50 ms; field of view = 2 cm, resolution: $156 \times 156 \times 600$ μm. Using a computerized planimetry program, we measured the luminal area, the plaque area, the areas of collagenous cap and lipid core, the area surrounded by the external elastic lamina (EEL area), and the maximal cap thickness. We defined the obstruction ratio, which corresponds to the plaque burden in intravascular ultrasound studies as the ratio of the plaque area divided by the EEL area.[7]

Results of Balloon Compression and Atherectomy

For group A, no significant reduction was found after radial compression in plaque, cap, or lipid core. A slight increase in EEL area and luminal area was observed with a significant reduction of the obstruction ratio. The result of in vitro balloon compression on a type Va plaque from group A is shown in Figure 1. Radial compression did not alter plaque or cap in this eccentric lesion, but slightly enlarged luminal and EEL areas. This plaque with a complete collagenous cap was not modified, but the disease-free segment was stretched. The Sudan black staining performed after the procedure (Fig. 1, panel B) showed a thick undisturbed collagenous cap completely covering the deeper lipid core.

A significant plaque reduction was observed in group B plaques. This was mainly due to the reduction in lipid core, which was partly extruded into the lumen and partly redistributed into the wall. This reduction in plaque volume resulted in a significant increase in luminal area and reduction in obstruction ratio. EEL area did not change following compression. The result of compression on a fatty lesion is shown in Figure 2. The procedure resulted in a large reduction of plaque lipids, which were partially extruded on both sides of the balloon and partially redistributed inside the wall. The T2w images show a 30% reduction of plaque volume with no change of the EEL, resulting in a 60% luminal gain.

Figure 3 shows the result of compression on a calcified lesion from group C, with a large dissection at the shoulder of the plaque where a maximal stiffness gradient is usually found.

Atherectomy performed on group D lesions reduced collagenous

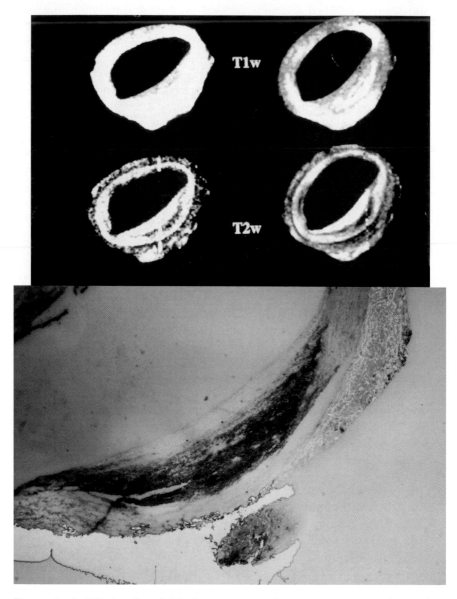

Figure 1. **A.** Effects of radial balloon compression on an eccentric femoral Va plaque. The left images are taken before the procedure, the right images afterward. The different layers are clearly differentiated by T2 contrast: collagenous cap and media in white, lipid core as a black layer under the cap, and adventitia in black surrounding the white media. The procedure does not alter plaque or cap, but enlarges the luminal area by 10%. **B.** Sudan Black staining showing the lipid infiltration in black under a complete thick collagenous cap.

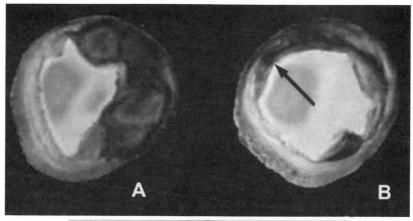

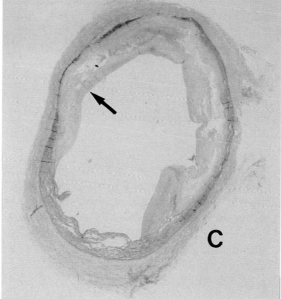

Figure 2. Results of in vitro angioplasty on a noncalcified fatty plaque without cap. **A.** T2w image taken before the procedure. Plaque volume in is 40 mm^3, lumen area is 36 mm^2 . **B.** T2w image taken after angioplasty. Black lipid-rich regions represent 87% of the plaque, and plaque volume is 28 mm^3, resulting from lipid extrusion and redistribution inside the wall as shown in the upper left segment (arrow). Lumen area is 56 mm^2. **C.** After angioplasty, the residual plaque is clearly seen on histology, with a large missing central portion and a semicircumferential lipid infiltration. The upper region of redistribution is shown by the arrow.

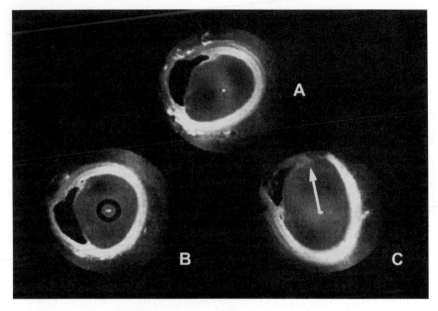

Figure 3. Radial compression of a calcified lesion. The angioplasty balloon is first inflated at 6 atmospheres during 5 min (**B**), then increased to 10 atm. At this point a large dissection appears at the shoulder of the plaque (arrow). The catheter appears as a central black circle in **B**. No change occurs after the first compression.

cap volume by 54% and plaque by 35%, resulting in a 20% luminal gain and a reduction of the obstruction ratio by 35%. The following are results of the successive procedures on fibrous plaques: collagenous cap and plaque volumes were unchanged by angioplasty, but were significantly reduced by 34% and 22%, respectively, during atherectomy; lumen and obstruction ratio were not affected by angioplasty but were significantly enlarged by atherectomy (7% and 24%, respectively), without change of the EEL area.

The effects of angioplasty followed by atherectomy on a fibrous lesion from group A are shown in Figure 4. Angioplasty did not affect the large collagenous cap and it did not change the lesion size. Instead, atherectomy produced lacerations and flaps on the luminal side of the cap.

MRI can image the effects of interventional procedures in atherosclerotic lesions. Radial compression on lesions with a complete cap does not alter plaque, whereas the luminal increase in vessels containing fatty plaques without cap results from plaque reduction through both redistribution into the wall and reduction of the lipid component. Although radial compression reduces stenosis in both groups, the con-

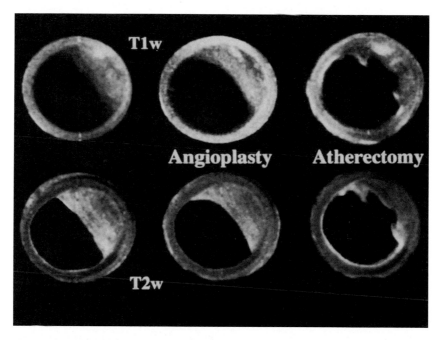

Figure 4. Effects of angioplasty followed by atherectomy on a fibrous lesion. Lipid core is minimal in this almost exclusively fibrous lesion. Angioplasty does not affect the collagenous cap. Atherectomy produces deep lacerations into the cap, reducing its volume by 27%.

sequences on the arterial wall in situ are quite different. This suggests differential effects of these procedures in vivo, depending on the type of plaque, which may be important to recognize and anticipate.

In fibrous plaques, directional atherectomy essentially removes collagenous layers with no specific effect of balloon compression on the collagenous components. After increasing pressure, calcified plaques rupture at the junction between calcification and the disease-free wall, where the gradient of circumferential stress should be maximal.

Fibrous Cap Resistance to Compression

The high resistance of the collagenous cap suggested that stenosis reduction during radial compression of fibrous plaques most likely results from stretching of the opposite disease-free side of the vessel wall, and not from a change in plaque structure, which was also shown in vitro by histologic examination,[26] and in vivo by coronary ultrasound.[27] In this latter study, this mechanism was responsible for almost 80% of the luminal gain.

Most of the plaque fractures during balloon angioplasty occur in the region of highest circumferential stress, usually at the shoulder of the plaque.[28] The shoulder is a junction site where the collagenous cap, which can be as much as five times stiffer than normal intima, produces a large stiffness gradient with the lipid core and thereby plays an important role in plaque susceptibility to rupture.[29] The resistance of a plaque to radial compression depends on the distribution of stress over the different plaque components. Lee et al[30] studied the stress-strain relation in dissected fibrous caps under uniaxial compression. They showed that plaques do not rupture under uniform compression if a cap occupies 50% of the lesion volume. Using a finite element analysis, they also demonstrated that variation of collagenous cap and lipid core thicknesses alter the distribution of circumferential stress, which determines plaque stability, in the vessel wall.[12]

In our investigation, we demonstrated that a thick complete collagenous cap was not altered in situ under a 6 atmosphere radial compression. This cap prevented any alteration of the underlying atheroma, and redistributed stress over the disease-free segments. In a clinical situation, one would expect that the effect of balloon inflation on such vessels would create a dissection of the intima-media that may be considered a mechanism of successful dilation.[31] Stretching of the disease-free segments rather than stretching of the plaque may be one mechanism of balloon angioplasty in lesions with a complete collagenous cap.[32]

Fatty Plaque and Lipid Redistribution

In our model,[7] compression reduced the volume of fatty plaques without complete caps by extruding the lipid core from the region of highest pressure into the lumen or into the shoulders of the plaque (Fig. 2). The most probable reason for this behavior is that lipids are less stiff than fibrous components,[33] and transmit stress and compression via redistribution.[29]

Our conclusions were not directly applicable to in vivo studies on plaques, but these results gave broad support to the contention that an intact collagenous cap largely reduces atheroma compressibility. This study, emphasizing the critical role of the collagenous cap, suggested that it may be important to characterize in vivo the chemical composition of atherosclerotic lesions before proceeding with an intravascular intervention. In order to predict plaque rupture for a particular patient, we must develop a biochemical imaging technique that is sensitive to the heterogeneous chemistry of a plaque and, particularly, capable of discriminating in vivo fibrous cap from lipid core. Recent technological developments in MRI may help to distinguish these components with high resolution in vivo and, therefore, improve our ability to select the most appropriate interventional method. Improving our comprehension of the three-dimensional response of atherosclerotic plaques to these procedures should limit the adverse effects of these plaques on the disease-free wall segments, and may also help to understand the relationship to restenosis.

Diffusion in Plaque Components

Diffusion of a fluid results from random translational motions. Measurement of displacements of water molecules by calculation of the apparent diffusion coefficient D can probe the microstructure of the environment in which these displacements take place. With a pulsed field gradient (PFG) sequence, NMR can measure water diffusion in atherosclerotic components and diffusion isotropy in the lipid core at the plaque shoulder (where destruction of the fibrous components could be larger under the action of macrophages metalloproteinases).[36] In the PFG experiment, water molecules are labeled by the Larmor precession frequencies of the proton spins at the hydrogen sites. These frequencies are made spatially dependent by the application of a magnetic field that varies with position. A series of six spin echo images was created at 9.4 T, with two diffusion gradients applied 1 ms apart from the nonselective refocusing pulse. Diffusion maps were produced for each sample and dimension using the equation:

$$\log(M/Mo) = - \ \gamma^2 \cdot G^2 \cdot \delta^2 \cdot (\Delta - \delta/3) \cdot D \tag{1}$$

where Mo = initial magnetization; γ = gyromagnetic ratio; G = diffusion gradient amplitude; δ = diffusion gradient duration; $(\Delta = t + \delta)$ = interval between the two diffusion gradients or diffusion time; and D = apparent diffusion coefficient. Using this method, we demonstrated that water diffusion is limited and that it behaves isotropically in the lipid core of atheromatous plaques[5]; D values were much lower in that region than in any of the other components of normal or diseased arterial walls. The mechanisms for altered diffusion in such atheromatous structures are not known, but they may result from the presence of oxidized lipoproteins, which restrict diffusion by allowing water penetration into their micellar structure, or from the presence of lipids in the smectic phase that may structure water to a higher degree than matrix proteoglycans or proteins do. The alteration of water diffusion in lipid cores may help to further discriminate this major component of susceptible plaques by NMR.

D was similar in collagenous cap and media. This result, along with their similar T2s,[4] provided another argument for biophysical similarity in tissue structure between these two arterial components. The entangled network of protein matrix produced by smooth muscle cells may explain this similarity.

Magnetic Resonance Imaging and High-Frequency Ultrasound Characterize Plaque Vulnerability

We also compared parametric images of atheromatous lesions with MRI T2 maps at 3 Tesla and ultrasound attenuation maps at 50 MHz.[34,35] This study revealed a significant difference between media and collagen T2 and attenuation values, and between aortic and iliac media T2s, which we had not previously noticed at other field strengths; this suggested that 3T MRI may allow better discrimination between these components than lower field images. These results also indicated that both techniques could be used to separate lipid cores from collagenous cap and normal media in vitro, both having a strong potential for in vivo characterization of vulnerable plaques.

In Vivo MR Imaging of Carotid Atheroma

A recent study showed the usefulness of MRI in describing progression of experimental atherosclerosis, and its ability to image in vivo plaque components such as fibrous caps, necrotic cores, and intraplaque hemorrhage resulting from balloon injury to the abdominal aorta, in six cholesterol-fed rabbits.[37] In order to study human plaque structure in situ, we imaged advanced lesions in carotid arteries in patients referred for endarterectomy.[6] The relaxation constant T2 of various plaque components in vivo were calculated before operation and compared with these values obtained in vitro after surgery. MR images of the arterial wall characterizing atherosclerosis were obtained from T1w and T2w sequences and CSI with lipid suppression at 1.5 T. In this investigation atherosclerotic plaque components in vivo were discriminated by use of MRI in a clinical imager with routinely available pulse sequences. These data demonstrated that T2 contrast allows the fine description of normal and pathological walls (Fig. 5) and the quantification of the plaque size, which may both provide a better idea of the local stage of the disease by its parietal and luminal components and predict more closely the evolution of stenoses.[38]

The capability to discriminate atheromatous components allows for large-scale clinical studies of plaque progression, regression, and

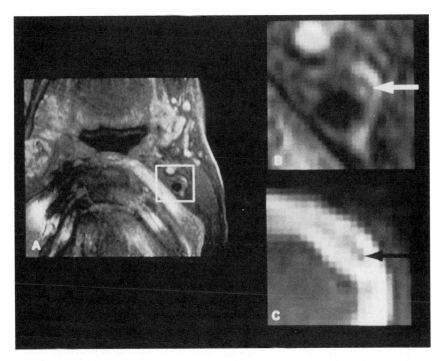

Figure 5. Left common carotid lesion: **A, B.** T2w transaxial in vivo images (with magnification in **B**). From lumen (in black) to adventitia, three successive layers are defined: two long T2 layers (56.4 ms, and 54.2 ms) with high signal intensity surround a short T2 region (32.1 ms, white arrow) with lower signal. **C.** In vitro T2w axial image with two high-intensity layers surrounding a low-intensity region. Histology confirmed the infiltration of extracellular lipids in the atheromatous core (central region, arrows) delimited by a fibrous cap and media.

stabilization, and their effects on clinical events. This may improve our understanding of the slow evolution of atherosclerosis in the early decades of life, and may provide a basis for screening young patients. Longitudinal studies of vascular interventional therapies may also benefit from these results.[7] The combination of MR angiography for luminal morphometry, three-dimensional velocity mapping for the analysis of peristenotic bloodflow stream lines, TOF echo-planar MRI for the determination of flow reserve in terminal arteries, perfusion measurement based on T1 changes and determination of circumferential stress,[39–43] and tissue characterization sequences may provide a complete description of the atherosclerotic process and its dynamic consequences. Finally, identification of intraplaque hemorrhage and acute thrombosis allows for the study of the cascade of events that lead from plaque rupture to arterial thrombosis, acute ischemia, and infarction[2]; this may provide newer methods for prediction and prevention of these life-threatening events.

This tool may also allow for the study of deep injury, plaque growth (edge versus shoulder), arterial remodeling and compensatory enlargement concepts, and all of the dynamic processes in animal models of rupture and thrombosis. With dietary or pharmacological studies, it may avoid unnecessary and costly histologic sampling, and may finally provide new grounds for intravascular imaging.

References

1. Little WC, Constantinescu M, Applegate RJ, et al. Can coronarography angiography predict the site of subsequent myocardial infarction in patients with mild-to-moderate coronary artery disease? *Circulation* 1988;78: 1157–1166.
2. Falk E. Why do plaques rupture? *Circulation* 1992;86:III30–III42.
3. Toussaint JF, Southern JF, Fuster V, Kantor HL. ^{13}C-NMR spectroscopy of human atherosclerotic lesions: Relation between fatty acid saturation, cholesteryl ester content, and luminal obstruction. *Arterioscler Thromb* 1994; 14:1951–1957.
4. Toussaint JF, Southern JF, Fuster V, Kantor HL. T2 Contrast for NMR characterization of human atherosclerosis. *Arterioscler Thromb Vasc Biol* 1995; 15:1533–1542.
5. Toussaint JF, Southern JF, Fuster V, Kantor HL. Diffusion properties of human atherosclerosis and thrombosis measured by pulse field gradient NMR. *Arterioscler Thromb Vasc Biol* 1997;17:542–546.
6. Toussaint JF, Southern JF, LaMuraglia GM, et al. Magnetic resonance images lipid, fibrous, calcified, hemorrhagic, and thrombotic components of human atherosclerosis in vivo. *Circulation* 1996;94:932–938.
7. Toussaint JF, Southern JF, Fuster V, Kantor HL. Comparative effects of angioplasty and atherectomy on human atherosclerotic plaques studied by high field NMR imaging. *J Am Coll Cardiol* 1994;23:387A.
8. Hamilton JA, Cordes EH. Lipid dynamics in human low density lipoproteins and human aortic tissue with fibrous plaques. A study by high field 13C-NMR spectroscopy. *J Biol Chem* 1979;254:5435–5441.
9. Bradamante S, Barenghi L, Guidici GA, Vergani C. Free radicals promote modifications in plasma high-density lipoprotein: Nuclear magnetic resonance analysis. *Free Radic Biol Med* 1992;12:193–203.
10. Jialal I, Chait A. Differences in the metabolism of oxidatively modified low density lipoprotein and acetylated low density lipoprotein by human endothelial cells. *J Lipid Res* 1989;30:1561–1568.
11. Brown MS, Goldstein JL. Lipoprotein metabolism in the macrophage: Implications for cholesterol deposition in atherosclerosis. *Annu Rev Biochem* 1983;52:223–261.
12. Cheng GC, Loree HM, Kamm RD, et al. Distribution of circumferential stress in ruptured and stable atherosclerotic lesions. *Circulation* 1993;87: 1179–1187.
13. Davies MJ, Richardson PD, Woolf N, et al. Risk of thrombosis in human

atherosclerotic plaque: Role of extracellular lipid, macrophage, and smooth muscle cell content. *Br Heart J* 1993;69:377–381.

14. Kaufman L, Crooks LE, Sheldon PE, et al. Evaluation of NMR imaging for detection and quantification of obstructions in vessels. *Invest Radiol* 1982; 17:554–560.

15. Herfkens RJ, Higgins CB, Hricak H, et al. Nuclear magnetic resonance imaging of atherosclerotic disease. *Radiology* 1983;148:161–166.

16. Mohiaddin RH, Firmin DN, Underwood SR, et al. Chemical shift magnetic resonance imaging of human atheroma. *Br Heart J* 1989;62:81–89.

17. Vinitski S, Consigny PM, Shapiro MJ, et al. Magnetic resonance chemical shift imaging and spectroscopy of atherosclerotic plaque. *Invest Radiol* 1991; 26:703–714.

18. Merickel MB, Carman CS, Brookeman JR, et al. Identification and 3-D quantification of atherosclerosis using magnetic resonance imaging. *Comput Biol Med* 1988;18:89–102.

19. Maynor CH, Charles HC, Herfkens RJ, et al. Chemical shift imaging of atherosclerosis at 7.0 Tesla. *Invest Radiol* 1988;24:52–60.

20. Pearlman JD, Zajicek J, Merickel MB, et al. High-resolution 1H-NMR spectral signature from human atheroma. *Magn Reson Med* 1988;7:262–279.

21. Gold GE, Pauly JM, Glover GH, et al. Characterization of atherosclerosis with a 1.5T imaging system. *J Magn Reson Imaging* 1993;3:399–407.

22. Altbach MI, Mattingly MA, Brown MF, Gmitro AF. Magnetic resonance imaging of lipid deposits in human atheroma via a stimulated-echo diffusion-weight technique. *Magn Reson Med* 1991;20:319–326.

23. Altbach MI, Trouard TP, Theilmann RJ, et al. A diffusion-weighted projection reconstruction method for detecting atherosclerotic lipids at 1.5 Tesla. *Proc Int Soc Magn Reson Med* 1997;2:794.

24. Witztum JL, Steinberg D. Role of oxidized low density lipoprotein in atherogenesis. *J Clin Invest* 1991;88:1785–1792.

25. Fuster V. Lewis A Conner Memorial Lecture. Mechanisms leading to myocardial infarction: Insigths from studies of vascular biology. *Circulation* 1994;90:2126–2146.

26. Virmani R, Farb A, Burke AP. Coronary angioplasty from the perspective of atherosclerotic plaque: Morphologic predictors of immediate success and restenosis. *Am Heart J* 1994;127:163–179.

27. Braden GA, Herrington DM, Downes TR, et al. Qualitative and quantitative contrasts in the mechanisms of lumen enlargement by coronary balloon angioplasty and directional coronary atherectomy. *J Am Coll Cardiol* 1994; 23:40–48.

28. Lee RT, Loree HM, Cheng GC, et al. Computational structure analysis based on intravascular ultrasound imaging before in vitro angioplasty: Prediction of plaque fracture location. *J Am Coll Cardiol* 1993;21:777–782.

29. Richardson PD, Davies MJ, Born GVR. Influence of plaque configuration and stress distribution on fissuring of coronary atherosclerotic plaques. *Lancet* 1989;2:941–944.

30. Lee RT, Grodsinsky AJ, Frank EH, et al. Structure-dependent dynamic mechanical behavior of fibrous caps from human atherosclerosis plaques. *Circulation* 1991;83:1764–1770.

31. Waller BF, Orr CM, Pinkerton CA, et al. Coronary balloon angioplasty dissections: "The good, the bad, and the ugly." *J Am Coll Cardiol* 1992;20: 701–706.

32. Hjemdal-Monsen CE, Ambrose JA, Borrico S, et al. Angiographic patterns

of balloon inflation during percutaneous transluminal coronary angioplasty: Role of pressure-diameter curves in studying distensibility and elasticity of the stenotic lesion and the mechanism of dilation. *J Am Coll Cardiol* 1990;16:569–575.

33. Loree HM, Tobias BJ, Gibson LJ, et al. Mechanical properties of model atherosclerotic lesion lipid pools. *Arterioscler Thromb* 1994;14:230–234.

34. Raynaud JS, Bridal S, Toussaint JF, et al. Characterization of atherosclerotic plaque components by high-resolution quantitative MR and US imaging. *Magn Reson Imaging* 1998. In press.

35. Raynaud JS, Toussaint JF, Bridal SL, et al. MRI and US parametric images characterize atherosclerotic plaque vulnerability: Proc Int Soc Magn Reson Med. 5th meeting. April 1997.

36. Libby P. Molecular bases of the acute coronary syndromes. *Circulation* 1995; 91:2844–2850.

37. Skinner MP, Yuan C, Mitsumori L, et al. Serial MRI of experimental atherosclerosis detects lesion fine structure, progression, and complications in vivo. *Nat Med* 1995;1:69–73.

38. Topol EJ, Nissen SE. Our preoccupation with luminology: The dissociation between clinical and angiographic findings in ischemic heart disease. *Circulation* 1995;92:2333–2342.

39. Buonocore MH. Estimation of total coronary artery flow using measurements of flow in the ascending aorta. *Magn Reson Med* 1994;32:602–611.

40. Poncelet BP, Weisskoff RM, Wedeen VJ, et al. Time of flight quantification of coronary flow with echo-planar MRI. *Magn Reson Med* 1993;30:447–457.

41. Detre JA, Leigh JS, Williams DS, Koretsky AP. Perfusion imaging. *Magn Reson Med* 1992;23:37–45 .

42. Oyre S, Ringgaard S, Erlandsen M, et al. Automatic accurate in vivo determination of blood flow, wall shear stress, and subpixel vessel wall position in the common carotid artery throughout the entire heart cycle by MRI. *Circulation* 1997;96(8):I-50. Abstract.

43. Yuan C, Tsuruda JS, Beach KN, et al. Techniques for high-resolution MR imaging of atherosclerotic plaque. *J Magn Reson Imaging* 1994,4:43–49.

Chapter 10

Coronary and Carotid Magnetic Resonance Imaging

Robert R. Edelman, MD

In magnetic resonance (MR) images, flowing blood has an appearance that is distinct from that of stationary tissue. This property can be used to particular advantage for diagnosis of vascular disorders that affect the neurovascular system and coronary arteries. The gold standard for diagnosis of carotid and coronary artery disease is x-ray angiography, an invasive, costly, and potentially hazardous procedure. Magnetic resonance imaging (MRI) has already supplanted a substantial portion of the x-ray angiograms done for extracranial carotid artery disease, and progress is being made toward making coronary MRI a clinical reality. This chapter reviews the basic principles underlying the MRI appearance of flowing blood, the techniques used to image blood flow and render angiogram-like MR images, and the results from clinical studies to date.

Blood may appear bright or dark, depending on the imaging technique used. On spin-echo images, blood vessels usually appear dark. With spin-echo pulse sequences, a pair (90°, 180°) of section-selective radiofrequency (RF) pulses is used to produce an MR signal. If blood flows out of the plane of section in the time interval between successive RF pulses, the result is an absence of signal called a *flow void*.[1] The flow void can be emphasized by use of thin sections or long echo time. In a *fast spin-echo* sequence, a long train of echoes is acquired by using a series of 180° RF pulses; as a result, wash-out effects are even more substantial than with spin-echo techniques (Fig. 1). Other methods for creating a flow void include presaturation, which involves application of an additional RF pulse outside the plane of section in order to suppress the signal intensity of inflowing blood, dephasing gradients, and preinversion pulses to null the blood signal.

From: Fuster, V (ed). *The Vulnerable Atherosclerotic Plaque: Understanding, Identification, and Modification.* Armonk, NY: Futura Publishing Company, Inc.; © 1999.

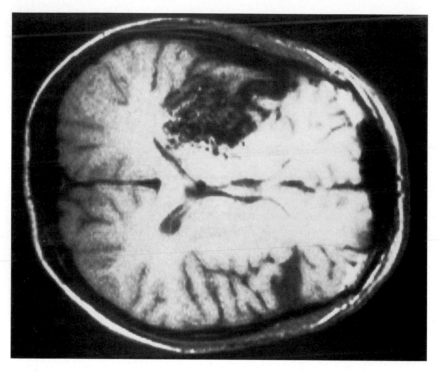

Figure 1. Axial spin-echo MRI of the brain shows a large arteriovenous malformation. Wash-out effects are largely responsible for the extensive signal voids within the vessels of the malformation.

In order to create bright blood images, *gradient-echo* pulse sequences are used. In a gradient-echo sequence, only a single RF pulse is applied during each sequence repetition, so no signal is lost due to wash-out effects, as occurs with spin-echo. Data for images on which blood is bright can be acquired as series of overlapping thin sections (sequential two-dimensional [2-D]) or as one or more thick volumes (three-dimensional [3-D]). Each sequence has advantages, as discussed later in this chapter. Bright-blood techniques can be subcategorized into time-of-flight[1] and phase contrast.[2] The basis of time-of-flight techniques is that positive flow contrast is generated by inflow effects, whereas the background is saturated by the rapid repeated application of RF pulses. The basis for phase contrast, another class of MR angiography techniques, is that the flow of blood along a magnetic field gradient causes a shift in the phase of the MR signal. With phase contrast, pairs of images are acquired that have different sensitivities to flow. These are then subtracted to cancel background signal, leaving only the signal from flowing blood. Phase contrast also permits flow quantification,[3] since the phase shift is proportional to the velocity.

The present method of choice for MR angiography involves the combination of breath-hold 3-D gradient-echo sequences with short time to repetition/time to echo (TR/TE) and administration of a gadolinium chelate, typically in a double dose.[4,5] The contrast agent shortens the T1 to a low value (eg, <50 ms), so that the blood appears bright irrespective of flow patterns or velocities. The 3-D acquisition is advantageous for displaying detailed vessel anatomy and reducing artifacts.

Maximum Intensity Projection

The heart of MR angiography is the ability to portray blood vessels in a projective format similar to that of x-ray angiography. Currently, projection images are created by postprocessing images acquired by a 2-D or 3-D gradient-echo sequence. Although image processing can be postponed until after the patient has left the MR suite, it is best done while the patient is still within the magnet so that additional scans can be obtained if needed. The images are most commonly processed by use of a maximum intensity projection algorithm (Fig. 2).[6,7] With this algorithm, the brightest pixels along a user-defined direction are extracted to create a projection image. Areas with poor flow contrast, including the edges of blood vessels and small vessels with slow flow, may be obscured by overlap with brighter stationary tissue.[8] By reducing the pixel size and suppressing stationary signal intensity, the quality of intracranial MR angiography can be improved substantially. The reduction in pixel size is accomplished with use of a large (eg, 256×512) acquisition matrix; background suppression is accomplished with use of magnetization transfer pulses.[9–11] These are off-resonance RF pulses that preferentially saturate tissues that contain large amounts of macromolecules, including brain and muscle. Blood, which contains a paucity of macromolecules, is affected less, so that flow contrast is improved.

Flow Artifacts

A variety of artifacts, caused by phase or magnitude variations in the MR signal, afflict MR angiography (Fig. 3). Within a voxel, blood protons flowing at different velocities accumulate a range or dispersion of phase shifts. Complex flow can produce signal loss due to intraview phase dispersion (ie, it occurs during each repetition of the pulse sequence), ghost artifacts from view-to-view signal variations (ie, occurring over multiple sequence repetitions), and flow displacement errors

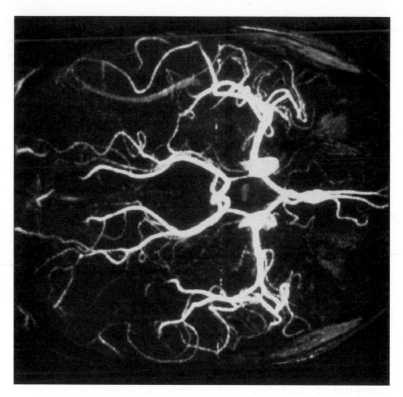

Figure 2. Maximum intensity projection image of the circle of Willis created from an axial 3-D MRA acquisition. Magnetization transfer pulses were used to suppress background signal intensity and better depict small branch vessels.

relating to the time delay between RF excitation and frequency-encoding or between phase- and frequency-encoding. These effects tend to falsely exaggerate the severity of a stenosis, and are worst with 2-D MR angiography. A short TE minimizes flow displacement and phase dispersion artifacts; phase dispersion is further decreased by minimizing the voxel size (eg, by using thin sections). Small voxels and short TE are most easily obtained with 3-D time-of-flight methods. The biggest drawback of the thick volumes used with 3-D is that slow or recirculating flow can become saturated. The advantages of both 2-D and 3-D techniques are gained with a series of thin-slab 3-D acquisitions. The sequential 3-D (or multiple overlapping thin-slab acquisition [MOTSA]) technique gives better flow enhancement than single-slab 3-D techniques and less dephasing than 2-D techniques.[12] The method has some drawbacks as well. For instance, the nonrectangular profile of the 3-D slabs necessitates use of substantial overlap (up to 50%) of

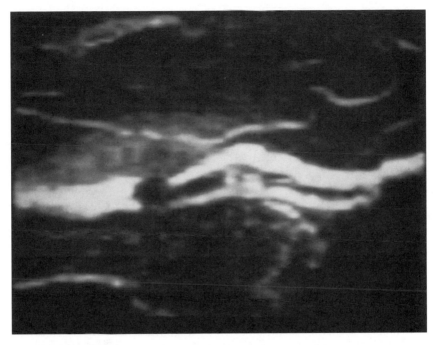

Figure 3. MIP from 2-D time-of-flight acquisition in a patient with severe stenoses of the internal and external carotid arteries. The signal voids are artifactual
due to dephasing effects with rapid, pulsatile blood flow.

adjacent slabs, so that total scan time is increased compared with single-
slab 3-D. Moreover, signal intensity variations within the individual
slabs, due to saturation effects, cause an annoying "venetian blind"
artifact. With sequential 2-D or 3-D acquisitions, slight patient motion
can generate discontinuities in the vessel contour that can be mistaken
for stenosis or fibromuscular dysplasia.

Neurovascular Applications

MR angiography is best established for the diagnosis of extracranial carotid bifurcation disease. A major incentive for the development
of a noninvasive means for evaluating the carotid bifurcation came
from the North American Symptomatic Carotid Endarterectomy Trial,
which showed that carotid endarterectomy significantly reduces the
prevalence of stroke in symptomatic patients with stenosis in which
the diameter of the affected vessel is narrowed 70% or more.[13] The
prevalence of major morbidity associated with conventional angiogra-

phy is 0.5% to 3.0%. Duplex sonography is accurate but operator-dependent, and few surgeons are willing to operate solely on the basis of a sonographic study. Occlusions cannot always be differentiated from critical stenoses. Moreover, tandem intracranial stenoses, which may preclude endarterectomy, are not accessible without the additional use of transcranial Doppler sonography or other noninvasive tests.

From a technical standpoint, MR angiography of the carotid bifurcation is aided by the paucity of motion artifacts and the availability of surface coils for the neck. Dedicated head and neck MR angiography coils are becoming available that permit efficient imaging of the aortic arch through the circle of Willis, without the need for multiple coil placements. Most studies to date have shown excellent sensitivity but variable specificity for MR angiographic detection of disease of the carotid bifurcation, depending on the equipment and pulse sequence used. Recent studies, in which 3-D sequences with short echo times were used to evaluate extracranial carotid stenoses, found highly significant correlations (r values ranging >0.9) for diameters of stenoses measured by using MR angiography and x-ray angiography (Fig. 4).[14,15] Ultimately, 2-D and 3-D time-of-flight techniques are both necessary for optimal evaluation. Because 3-D techniques are less sensitive to turbulence than 2-D techniques are, the grading of carotid stenoses based on findings by 3-D time-of-flight sequences correlates better with x-ray angiography findings.

In order to differentiate a severe stenosis from an occlusion, one could use a 3-D phase-contrast MR angiogram made sensitive to low velocity flow by use of a small velocity-encoding sensitivity (VENC), but the acquisition is time consuming. As a result, 2-D time of flight is more commonly used to depict slow flow, particularly in the differentiation of an occlusion from a critical stenosis. Evidence is mounting that this differentiation can be reliably made by using MR angiography, although no large studies specifically addressing this problem have yet been published. In our experience, imaging of both the intra- and extracranial carotid circulations should be done to help solve this problem.

MRI is an accurate method for detection of carotid and vertebral dissections,[16] although in the vertebrobasilar system x-ray angiography sometimes is preferred because of its better spatial resolution and proven ability to show subtle lesions. Similar to x-ray angiography, in MR angiography the dissected vessel typically appears tapered; however, shine-through from paramagnetic methemoglobin can create an artifactual widening of the lumen in maximum intensity projection images. Since intramural blood appears bright in spin-echo images, and flow effects cause the intraluminal blood to appear dark, the addition of a spin-echo sequence resolves any confusion.

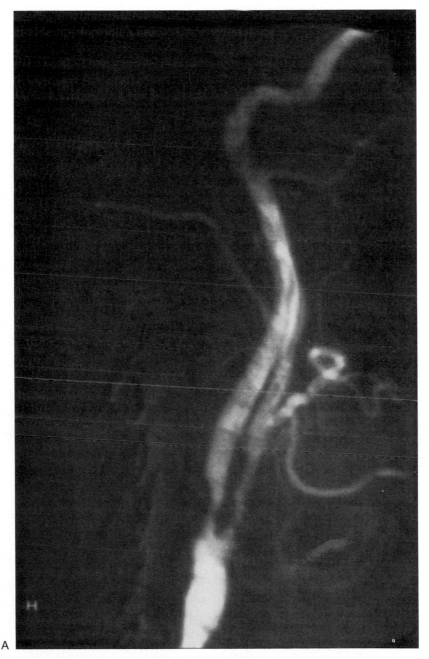

A

Figure 4. Same patient as Figure 3. **A.** Intra-arterial DSA study. **B.** MIP of 3-D MR angiogram. The stenoses are accurately depicted, in contrast with the 2-D MR angiogram method. *(continued)*

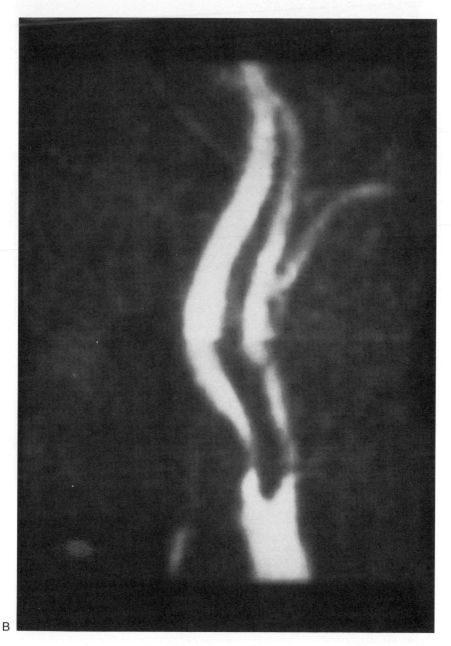

Figure 4. *(continued)*

The combination of duplex sonography and MR angiography, with x-ray angiography reserved for discordant cases, has been shown to be the most cost-effective approach for presurgical evaluation of extracranial carotid bifurcation disease.[17] It appears increasingly likely that the combination of noninvasive MR angiography and duplex sonography will eventually replace x-ray angiography in most patients with disease of the carotid bifurcation; however, this degree of accuracy assumes use of state-of-the-art equipment and of radiologists experienced in the interpretation of MR angiography. As yet, the accuracy of MR angiography in the evaluation of the carotid and vertebral origins off the aortic arch is not known.

Use of MR angiography in order to screen asymptomatic patients for intracranial aneurysms remains controversial. In one series, the accuracy of detection was 95%, but some small (≤ 5 mm) aneurysms were missed.[17a] The complication rate from such small aneurysms is low. Whether this sensitivity is acceptable will depend on the institution-dependent biases of the referring clinicians, and must be balanced against the potential morbidity associated with x-ray angiography. High-resolution imaging with targeted maximum intensity projections of critical regions such as the middle cerebral bifurcations, basilar tip, and carotid siphons is essential to maintain accuracy. MR angiography is not an acceptable substitute for x-ray angiography in patients with subarachnoid hemorrhage, although it may be a helpful adjunct to define the bleeding site. MR angiography is sensitive to intracranial vascular malformations and can be used to determine the volume of persistent nidus after radiosurgery, but it cannot substitute for x-ray angiography in defining feeder vessels and shunting. Administration of a paramagnetic contrast agent is sometimes useful for giving better definition of the nidus.

Coronary Artery Magnetic Resonace Imaging

Cardiovascular disease remains the leading cause of death in the United States, with an estimated 1.2 million myocardial infarctions and 600,000 deaths per year attributed to coronary artery disease.[18] Minimally invasive tests for myocardial ischemia include single photon emission tomography (SPECT)[19,20] and positron emission tomography (PET).[21,22] These tests reveal perfusion abnormalities, but do not depict the coronary artery stenoses that cause them, nor do they provide direct measurements of coronary artery blood flow. The gold standard for evaluation of the coronary arteries is contrast angiography, with over 500,000 diagnostic cardiac catheterizations performed annually in the United States. Despite the development of multiple noninvasive tests for the detection of myocardial ischemia, up to 20% of these coronary angiograms reveal insignificant coronary artery disease.[23] Information derived from such angiograms, however, is the standard by which mechanical interventions and many medical therapies are planned. In addition, prognostic information is also gained from data regarding coronary artery patency.

Hospital charges alone for cardiac catheterizations have been estimated at over $1.8 billion, annually. In addition, coronary angiography carries with it a low, though finite, major complication rate—death (0.12% to 0.20%), cerebrovascular accident (0.03% to 0.20%), myocardial infarction (0.0% to 0.25%); and minor complication rate—vascular complication, local infection (0.57% to 1.6%), or arrhythmias (0.30% to 0.63%).[24–26] The high cost and associated risk make routine coronary angiography inappropriate for use as a screening test. Furthermore, while semiquantitative techniques exist for estimating the flow restriction caused by a coronary artery stenosis based on the conventional angiogram,[27] they do not provide a quantitative measure of coronary artery blood flow.

The ability to perform noninvasive coronary angiography would represent a major improvement in patient care. Information regarding coronary anatomy could then be acquired with minimal risk, as well as in those patients in whom coronary angiography is relatively contraindicated[28] due to severe allergic history to radiographic contrast agents, fever with documented infection, bleeding diatheses, or recent gastrointestinal bleeding or cerebrovascular accident. Follow-up angiographic information in patients undergoing revascularization procedures could also be more readily obtained.

MRI is well suited for evaluating the heart, with excellent soft-tissue contrast and the ability to image the heart in double-oblique tomographic sections. Complex cardiac anatomy[29] and systolic function[30] have already been elucidated with use of MRI techniques. MR angiography is currently being used in several clinical applications, including screening for intracranial aneurysms[31] and detection of stenoses of the extracranial carotid arteries,[32] vertebro-basilar system, and renal arteries.[33] Furthermore, MR techniques that are sensitive to blood flow are capable of assessing the velocity of blood within a small lumen.[34] In order to apply MR angiographic techniques to the coronary arteries, substantial technical obstacles must be overcome. These challenges include minimizing the effects of respiratory and cardiac motion that preclude reliable visualization of the coronary arteries, and the development of sequences that allow for both high spatial resolution and high signal-to-noise, given the small size of the coronary vessels.

Human coronary arteries are small in caliber. The left main coronary artery is typically 4 to 6 mm in diameter,[35] while the left anterior descending and left circumflex coronary arteries are generally 3 to 4 mm at their origins and taper distally. The right coronary artery, supplying less myocardium, is smaller than the left main, and is typically 3 to 4 mm proximally. High-resolution MR angiography of arteries of similar caliber (renal artery, brain) to epicardial coronary vessels has been successful, but reproducible coronary angiography has remained elusive due to the effects of significant cardiac and respiratory motion. Standard electrocardiogram-gated, spin-echo, and gradient-echo cine images only occasionally show portions of the coronary arteries, and these images are not adequate for detailed evaluation.[36]

Given these anatomic and physiological constraints, there are several obvious challenges for in vivo coronary artery imaging. Combined respiratory and cardiac gating using spin-echo techniques is possible, but this would markedly prolong scan duration and be impractical to implement on a clinical basis. Blurring from respiratory motion can be eliminated by using breath-hold techniques, but simultaneous cardiac gating is also necessary. Furthermore, data must be acquired during a very small portion of the cardiac cycle to minimize blurring due to the rotational and translational motion of the heart, a situation which precludes image acquisition with use of standard techniques.

Ultrafast imaging techniques are essential to the future of cardiac and pulmonary MRI, and are useful in a variety of other clinical applications. The speed with which an MR image can be acquired is increasing as the technology improves. The scan time for a spin-echo image is typically on the order of 5 to 15 minutes. During this time, the data may be degraded by cardiac or respiratory motion, or by gross patient movement. Recently, so-called "turbo" spin-echo or "fast" spin-echo pulse sequences have been implemented. Scan times (as little as 1.5 minutes for a T2-weighted screening study of the brain) and signal-to-noise are improved, and 512^2 spatial resolution can be obtained in reasonable scan times. Nonetheless, scan times are still long compared with the time allowable for a breath-hold, so that images are still sensitive to respiratory and cardiac motion. Gradient-echo pulse sequences reduce scan times further, to as little as 3 to 20 seconds, thereby permitting acquisition of an entire image in a single breath-hold. Gradient-echo techniques have proved valuable for T1-weighted imaging of the abdomen. Finally, turboFLASH sequences are a speeded-up version of gradient-echo sequences. An image may be obtained in less than 1 second. TurboFLASH images are insensitive to respiratory motion, and are recommended for patients who cannot cooperate for breath-holding. In addition, various prepulses can be applied to alter tissue contrast.

There are several fast imaging methods that have been used for coronary artery imaging. Three-dimensional gradient-echo methods[37] permit thin sections and short TE, thereby minimizing partial volume averaging and flow-related dephasing. With 3-D approaches, however, saturation effects are more severe than with 2-D approaches, resulting in suboptimal flow contrast, particularly in the setting of low flow velocities. Unfortunately, long scan time for 3-D acquisitions (at least several minutes for ECG-gated studies) precludes breath-holding, so that significant blurring from respiratory motion will occur.

Subtraction methods also have potential value for coronary artery imaging. One approach involves the interleaved acquisition of a pair of projection (thick section) images, of which one has a spatially localized inversion pulse applied to the aortic root to tag the coronary inflow.[38] Since only the signal intensity of the coronary arteries is altered by the inversion pulse, background and cardiac chamber signals are eliminated by image subtraction. Potential drawbacks of this method are the need for prolonged breath-holding periods (eg, 24 seconds or longer), inadvertent saturation of other structures such as blood within the left atrium, dependence of flow contrast on the RR interval, and potential misregistration resulting in imperfect subtraction. The method also assumes that blood within the major epicardial coronary arteries is completely displaced within one RR interval by blood from the aortic root. The use of a thick section also has the drawback of increased intravoxel dephasing compared with the use of thin sections. Nonetheless, encouraging preliminary results have been demonstrated in healthy volunteers.

With use of a conventional whole-body MR imaging system, a standard gradient-echo sequence, and a high-resolution (eg, 256×128) acquisition matrix, an image cannot be obtained in less than a few hundred milliseconds. This is obviously too long to freeze cardiac motion and avoid motion artifacts. Instead, the acquisition can be "segmented" into blocks of phase-encoding steps that are then interleaved to create an image. Segmentation within a single breath-hold of 12 to 15 seconds can reduce the time for data acquisition within each cardiac cycle to 100 ms or less, which is adequate to minimize cardiac motion artifacts.

We optimized segmented gradient-echo sequences to permit acquisition of high-resolution, ECG-gated cine images within a single end-expiratory breath-hold.[40] Eight phase-encoding steps were acquired in rapid sequence, constituting one segment. One segment was acquired during each heart beat by use of prospective ECG triggering and delay in sequence initiation so as to acquire the data in mid-diastole. Sixteen segments were interleaved so as to complete a 128×256 matrix, requiring 16 heart beats. Scan time was typically 12 to 16 seconds, permitting imaging within a single breath-hold. Cine imaging

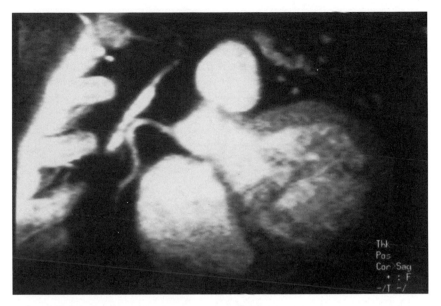

Figure 5. Breath-hold oblique, fat-suppressed, ECG-triggered, segmented tur-boFLASH image of the proximal right coronary artery.

was also feasible by acquisition of multiple segments within each breath-hold.

Despite their small caliber, images of the proximal coronary arteries were consistently obtained (Fig. 5). Since the proximal coronary arteries are embedded in epicardial fat, we applied chemical shift-selective (CHESS) fat saturation pulses prior to each segment. We obtained a large improvement in flow contrast/noise for the coronary arteries, due to the reduction in fat signal intensity. With this technique, the proximal portions of the left main, left anterior descending, and right coronary arteries were routinely seen. Nowadays, a four-element body phased array coil is used; this provides a major improvement in image quality for the heart compared with prior studies using the body coil or surface coils.

We have begun clinical studies of MR coronary angiography (Fig. 6).[41] Sensitivity and specificity for coronary artery disease are in the 80% to 90% range, which is comparable to thallium scintigraphy. One problem has been poor flow contrast resulting from slow flow distal to a severe stenosis, making it difficult to distinguish from an occlusion. This problem might be ameliorated by the use of contrast agents. Blood pool contrast agents that could greatly improve the quality of coronary artery images are currently under development. Flow velocity mea-

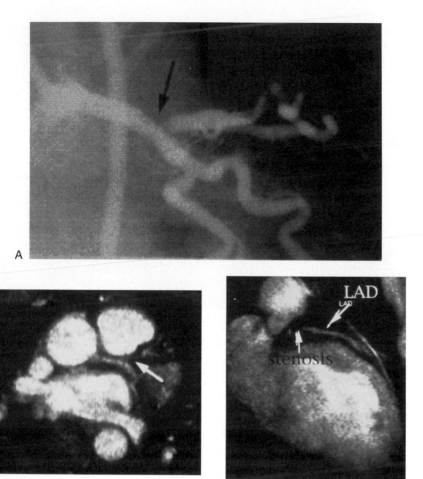

Figure 6. MR angiogram in a patient with proximal left anterior descending (LAD) stenosis. **A.** X-ray cineangiogram. **B.** Breath-hold axial (left) and oblique (right) coronal fat-suppressed segmented turboFLASH images show similar findings.

surements can be done pre- and post-administration of a vasodilator, such as adenosine, to obtain a measure of flow reserve and to help determine the physiological significance of a coronary stenosis.[42]

The biggest recent development was the introduction of navigator gating and correction to eliminate the need for breath-holding. For navigator gating, MR data are only accumulated for image reconstruction when the navigator echo indicates that the interface of interest is within a certain operator-defined range. In this respect, navigator echoes perform a similar function to the bellows used for respiratory gating, but in our experience, provide more consistent results. Because much data are rejected, acquisition times are typically increased by a factor of four or more, depending on breathing patterns. However, if a fast imaging sequence such as segmented gradient-recalled echo (GRE) is used, scan times are still reasonable, on the order of a few minutes at most. Image sharpness is as good as with breath-holding. Since navigator echoes permit signal averaging, signal-to-noise is increased and higher in-plane spatial resolution can be obtained (eg, 0.5 mm). Moreover, navigator echoes ensure a consistent cardiac position from image to image, thereby minimizing misregistration artifact if one wishes to process a projection image.

The navigator gating technique discards data that are acquired when the diaphragm is incorrectly positioned and, thus, increases scan time. Adaptive correction of image location using real-time navigator measurement of diaphragm position is a potential method for reducing slice registration errors.[43] This method dynamically repositions the slice so as to follow the movement of the diaphragm and thus have the slice in a constant relation to the tissue of interest, despite its motion. This technique, called *navigator correction*, can be combined with navigator gating to improve the efficiency of data acquisition.

Although our work to date has focused on 2-D acquisitions, 3-D acquisitions may offer certain advantages. The slices (or partitions) are truly contiguous, residual motion artifacts tend to be averaged with the acquisition of multiple acquisitions, as they would using multiple signal averages, and very thin sections (eg, 1 to 2 mm) are readily obtained. On the other hand, breath-holding is not feasible unless ultrafast imaging techniques such as echo-planar are used. However, breath-hold segmented 3-D echo-planar suffers from limited signal-to-noise. The best approach is to use a combination of navigator gating and correction with 3-D segmented GRE. This permits the acquisition of artifact-free 3-D volumes within a reasonable acquisition period (eg, a 16-partition volume can be acquired in approximately 4 to 5 minutes, depending on breathing patterns).

References

1. Edelman RR, Mattle HP, Wallner B, et al. Extracranial carotid arteries: Evaluation with black blood MR angiography. *Radiology* 1990;177:45–50.
1. Keller P. Time-of-flight magnetic resonance angiography. *Neuroimaging Clin N Am* 1992;4:639–656.
2. Dumoulin CL. Phase contrast MR angiography techniques. *Magn Reson Imaging Clin N Am* 1995;3:399–411.
3. Walker MF, Souza SP, Dumoulin CL. Quantitative flow measurement in phase contrast MR angiography. *J Comput Assist Tomogr* 1988;12:304–313.

4. Prince MR. Gadolinium-enhanced MR aortography. *Radiology* 1994;191: 155–164.
5. Prince MR. Body MR angiography with gadolinium contrast agents. *Magn Reson Imaging Clin Am* 1996;4(1):11–24.
6. Saloner D. MRA: Principles and display. In Higgins CB, Hricak H, Helms CA eds: *Magnetic Resonance Imaging of the Body*. Philadelphia: Lippincott-Raven Publishers; 1997:1345–1368.
7. Laub G. Displays for MR angiography. *Magn Reson Med* 1990;14:222–229.
8. Anderson C, Saloner D, Tsuruda J, et al. Artifacts in maximum intensity projection display of MR angiograms. *AJR Am J Roentgenol* 1990;154: 623–629.
9. Edelman RR, Ahn SS, Chien D, et al. Improved time-of-flight MR angiography of the brain with magnetization transfer contrast. *Radiology* 1992;184: 395–399.
10. Atkinson D, Brant-Zawadzki M, Purdy D, et al. Improved MR angiography: Magnetization transfer suppression with variable flip angle excitation and increased resolution. *Radiology* 1994;190:890–894.
11. Furst G, Hofer M, Steinmetz H, et al. Intracranial stenoocclusive disease: MR angiography with magnetization transfer and variable flip angle. *AJNR Am J Neuroradiol* 1996;17:1749–1757.
12. Blatter DD, Parker DL, Robison RO. Cerebral MR angiography with multiple overlapping thin slab acquisition. *Radiology* 1991;179:805–811.
13. Collaborators NASCET. Beneficial effect of carotid endarterectomy in symptomatic patients with high-grade carotid stenosis. *N Engl J Med* 1991; 325:445–453.
14. Anderson CM, Saloner D, Lee RE, et al. Assessment of carotid artery stenosis by MR angiography: Comparison with X-ray angiography and color-coded Doppler ultrasound. *AJNR Am J Neuroradiol* 1992;13:989–1003.
15. Patel MR, Kuntz KM, Klufas RA, et al. Preoperative assessment of the carotid bifurcation: Can magnetic resonance angiography and duplex ultrasonography replace contrast arteriography? *Stroke* 1995;26:1753–1758.
16. Klufas RA, Hsu L, Barnes PD, et al. Dissection of the carotid and vertebral arteries: Imaging with MR angiography. *AJR Am J Roentgenol* 1995;164: 673–677.
17. Kent C, Kuntz KM, Patel MR, et al. Perioperative imaging strategies for carotid endarterectomy: An analysis of morbidity and cost-effectiveness in symptomatic patients. *JAMA* 1995;274:888–893.
17a. Huston J III, Nichols DA, Luetmer PH, et al. Blinded prospective evaluation of sensitivity of MR angiography to known intracranial aneurysms: Importance of aneurysm size. *AJNR* 1994;15:1607–1614.
18. Assessment of coronary artery disease. In Yang SS, Bentivoglio LG, Maranhao V, Goldberg H eds: *Cardiac Catheterization Data to Hemodynamic Parameters, 3rd Ed*. Philadelphia: F.A. Davis; 1988:256.
19. Holman BL, Moore SC, Shulkin PM, et al. Quantitation of perfused myocardial mass using Tl-201 and emission computed tomography. *Invest Radiol* 1983;18:322.
20. Cladwell JH, Williams DL, Harp GD, et al. Quantitation of size of relative myocardial perfusion defect by single-photon emission computed tomography. *Circulation* 1984;70:1048–1056.
21. Marshall RC, Tillisch JH, Phelps ME, et al. Identifcation and differentiation of resting myocardial ischemia and infarction in man with positron computed tomography, F-18 labeled fluorodeoxyglucose and N-13 ammonia. *Circulation* 1983;67:766–778.

22. Brunken R, Tillisch JH, Scwaiger M, et al. Regional perfusion, glucose metabolism and wall motion in patients with chronic electrocardiographic Q-wave infarctions: Evidence of persistence of viable tissue in some infarct regions by positron emission tomography. *Circulation* 1986;73:951–962.
23. Johnson LW, Lozner EC, Johnson D, et al. Coronary arteriography 1984–1987: A report of the registry of the Society for Cardiac Angiography and Interventions. I. Results and complications. *Cathet Cardiovasc Design* 1989;17:5–10.
24. Davis K, Kennedy JW, Kemp HG, et al. Complications of coronary arteriography from the collaborative study of Coronary Artery Surgery (CASS). *Circulation* 1979;59:1105.
25. Kennedy JW, and the Registry Committee of the Society for Cardiac Angiography. Complications associated with cardiac catheterization and angiography. *Cathet Cardiovasc Diagn* 1982;8:5.
26. Wyman RM, Safian RD, Portway V, et al. Current complications of diagnostic and therapeutic cardiac catheterization. *J Am Coll Cardiol* 1988;12:1400.
27. Gould KL. Detecting and assessing severity of coronary artery disease in humans. *Cardiovasc Intervent Radiol* 1990;13:5–13.
28. Guidelines for coronary angiography. A report of the American College of Cardiology/American Heart Association Task Force on Assessment of Diagnostic and Therapeutic Cardiovascular Procedures (Subcommittee on Coronary Angiography). *Circulation* 1987;76:963A.
29. Didier D, Higgins CB, Fisher MR, et al. Congenital heart disease: Gated MR imaging in 72 patients. *Radiology* 1986;158:227–235.
30. Higgins CB, Holt W, Pflugfelder P, Sechtem U. Functional evaluation of the heart with magnetic resonance imaging. *Magn Reson Med* 1988;6:121–139.
31. Ruggieri PM, Laub GA, Masaryk TJ, Modic MT. Intracranial circulation: Pulse-sequence considerations in three-dimensional (volume) MR angiography. *Radiology* 1989;171:785–791.
32. Masaryk TJ, Modic MT, Ruggieri PM, et al. Three-dimensional (volume) gradient-echo imaging of the carotid bifurcation: Preliminary clinical experience. *Radiology* 1989;171:801–806.
33. Kent KC, Edelman RR, Kim D, et al. Magnetic resonance imaging: A reliable test for the evaluation of proximal atherosclerotic renal arterial stenosis. *J Vasc Surg* 1991;13:311–318.
34. Mattle H, Edelman RR, Reis MA, et al. Middle cerebral artery: Determination of flow velocities with MR angiography. *Radiology* 1991;181:527–530.
35. Paulin S. Coronary angiography. A technical, anatomic and clinical study. *Acta Radiologica* 1964;(suppl):125–137.
36. Paulin S, von Schulthess GK, Fossel E, Krayenbuehl HP. MR imaging of the aortic root and proximal coronary arteries. *Am J Radiol* 1987;148:665–670.
37. Paschal CB, Haacke EM, Adler LP, et al. *Proceedings of the 9th Annual Meeting of the Society of Magnetic Resonance in Medicine.* August 18–24, 1990; New York; 278.
38. Wang SJ, Hu BS, Macovski A, Nishimura DG. Coronary angiography using fast selective inversion recovery. *Magn Reson Med* 1991;18:417–423.
39. Chien D, Anderson CM, Lee RE. MR angiography: Basic principles. In: Edelman RR, Hesselink JR Zlatkin ME eds: *Clinical Magnetic Resonance Imaging, 2nd Edition.* Philadelphia: W.B. Saunders Co.; 1996:271–301.
40. Edelman RR, Manning WJ, Burstein D, Paulin S. Coronary arteries: Breath-hold MR angiography. *Radiology* 1991;181:641–643.
41. Manning WJ, Li W, Edelman RR. A preliminary report comparing magnetic

resonance coronary angiography with conventional angiography. *N Engl J Med* 1993;328:828–832.

42. Edelman RR, Manning WJ, Gervino E, Li W. Flow velocity quantifcation in human coronary arteries with fast, breath-hold MR angiography. *J Magn Reson Imaging* 1993;3:699–703.

43. Grimm RC, Rossman PJ, Reiderer SJ, Ehman RL, Real-time adaptive motion correction using navigator echoes. *In Proc SMR, 3rd Annual Meeting, Nice, 1995.* 741.

Chapter 11

Aortic Arch Vulnerable Plaques

Pierre Amarenco, MD and Ariel Cohen, MD

Anatomically, the arch of the aorta is a precerebral artery. There-fore, complicated atherosclerotic plaques of this artery located proximal to the ostium of the left subclavian artery may constitute a threat for the brain. In up to 40% of cases, either the cause of brain infarction is unknown or the findings moderate internal carotid artery occlusion (ICAO) stenosis (<70%) or minor cardiac abnormalities, such as patent foramen ovale, which cannot be accepted as the definite cause.[1] Simi-larly, it has been shown that patients with retinal cholesterol emboli do not have more frequent ipsilateral carotid stenosis than controls,[2,3] and hence the source of retinal embolism should be located further down in the arterial tree. Until now, complicated atherosclerotic disease of the aortic arch had not been routinely considered as possibly causal in patients with brain infarction of unknown cause or with retinal cho-lesterol emboli.

With the advent of transesophageal echocardiography, clinicians can now detect plaques in the aortic arch.[4,5] If one accepts that a causal link between brain infarcts and complicated plaques with highly mobile thrombi in the lumen of the aortic arch,[4] particularly in patients with otherwise unexplained stroke or stroke following aortography[6] or aor-tic cannulation for cardiopulmonary bypass,[7-10] it is likely, then by contrast, other plaques without mobile components might merely be markers for diffuse atherosclerosis and, hence, for the true cause of ischemic stroke. Alternatively, they may well be a cause, and we are therefore justified to question the potential clinical importance of such lesions and the best way to identify vulnerable plaques. Several recent works have established a statistical link between the presence of athero-sclerotic disease in the aortic arch and ischemic stroke.[11-20]

From: Fuster, V (ed). *The Vulnerable Atherosclerotic Plaque: Understanding, Identification, and Modification.* Armonk, NY: Futura Publishing Company, Inc.; © 1999.

Case Control Studies

Atherosclerosis in the aortic arch is obviously a marker of generalized atherosclerosis. Several recent studies reinforce the notion that plaques in the aortic arch are independent risk factors for brain ischemia (Table 1). The main morphological parameters that were studied to identify vulnerable plaques were ulcerations at autopsy and plaque thickness at trasesophageal echocardiography (TEE), followed by other morphological parameters such as surface irregularities, calcifications, hypoechoic plaques (suggestive of thrombus), and mobile thrombus floating in the lumen of the aortic arch.

Ulcerated Plaques at Autopsy

In our autopsy study, performed in the laboratory of Neuropathology at La Salpêtrière hospital in 500 consecutive patients, we and others

Table 1

Prevalence and Risk of Ischemic Stroke in the Presence of Large Protruding Plaques in the Aortic Arch in Case-Control Studies

Case-control studies		N =	Patients	Controls	Adjusted odds ratio
Autopsy		239	28%	5%	4.0 [95% CI, 2.1–7.8]
Amarenco et al[3] ulcerated plaques (UP)		40	68%	34%	5.8 [95% CI, 1.1–31.7]
Khathibzadeh et al[50] UP, thrombi, debris					
Transesophageal echocardiography		122	27%	9%	3.2 [95% CI, 1.6–6.5]
Tunick et al[92]	PI ≥5 mm	250	14.4%	2.0%	9.1 [95% CI, 3.3–25.2]
Amarenco et al[2]	PI ≥4 mm	215	21.4%	3.5%	8.2 [95% CI, 3.0–22.4]
Jones et al[45]	PI ≥5 mm	42	48%	22%	not done
Nihoyannopoulos et al[65]	PI not measure	49	32.7%	7%	not done
Stone et al[82]	PI ≥5 mm	106	26%	13%	2.6 [95% CI, 1.1–5.9]
Di Tullio et al[31]	PI ≥5 mm				
Intraoperative epiaortic echo Dávilla-Román et al[27]	PI ≥3 mm	158	26.6%	18.1%*	1.65 [95% CI, 1.1–2.4]

* 88.3% of patients in this study underwent coronary artery bypass grafting, explaining this high rate of aortic plaques in the control group.

found ulcerated plaques in the aortic arch in 28% of patients with cerebrovascular disease and in only 5% of patients with other neurological disease.[12] This difference was very significant and after adjustment for age, sex, and hypertension, we found an odds ratio of 4.0 (95% CI, 2.1 to 7.8). When we compared the frequency of ulcerated plaques in the aortic arch in patients with brain infarct of unknown cause with those suffering infarcts of known etiology, we also found a very significant difference (61% versus 28%, adjusted odds ratio 5.7; 95% CI, 2.4 to 13.6). The presence of ulcerated plaques in the aortic arch was not correlated to the presence of internal carotid artery stenosis or atrial fibrillation.[12] These two last points suggest that ulcerated plaques in this autopsy series may have been causally related to brain infarction of unknown etiology. One other very important points of this study was the observation that among the 75 patients who had ulcerated plaques in the aortic arch, only 2 were less than 60 years of age and 73 (97%) were 60 years old or older.[12]

Recently Khathibzadeh et al[23] studied 120 consecutive autopsies, 40 of which had cerebral, visceral, or lower-limb embolisms at pathological examination. They were able to confirm an association between ulcerated plaques, mural thrombi, or both in the aortic arch and arterial embolism. Ulcerated plaques, mural thrombi, or both in the aortic arch or in the descending aorta were found in 25 patients (69%) with cerebral infarction. Interestingly, 9 patients among the 12 with cerebral infarction that had not been diagnosed clinically had ulcerated plaques in the aortic arch, and 28 patients with cerebral infarction had silent visceral embolisms at pathological examination.

Plaque Thickness

In 1991, Tunick and colleagues[11] reported a retrospective study, based on the recruitment of their echocardiography laboratory, comparing the frequency of plaques 5 mm or greater in thickness in the thoracic aorta in 12 patients referred because of emboli and in 12 patients referred for other cardiological reasons. They found such large plaques in 27% of the patients who had an embolic event and in 9% of those who had no emboli. After adjustment for principal risk factors, the odds ratio was 3.2 (95% CI 1.6 to 6.5). The results of this study were not adjusted for the presence of other potential causes of brain infarct or peripheral emboli.

In a prospective case-control study[13] in which we used transesophageal echocardiography in 250 consecutively admitted patients, aged over 60 years, with brain infarcts, we found a frequency of plaques in the aortic arch that was significantly different from that in controls. In

Table 2

Risk of Cerebral Infarct as a Function of Thickness of Atherosclerotic Plaques in the Ascending Aorta and Proximal Arch

Wall thickness	Patients % (n°)	Controls % (n°)	Crude OR [95% CI]	Adjusted OR† [95% CI]	P Value
<1 mm††	39.6 (99)	75.6 (189)	1	1	-
1 to 1.9 mm*	11.2 (28)	6.4 (16)	3.3 [1.7 ; 6.5]	4.4 [2.1–8.9]	<0.001
2 to 2.9 mm*	22.4 (56)	10.4 (26)	4.1 [2.4 ; 7.0]	5.0 [2.7–9.0]	<0.001
3 to 3.9 mm*	12.4 (31)	5.6 (14)	4.2 [2.2 ; 8.3]	3.4 [1.5–7.4]	<0.001
≥4 mm	14.4 (36)	2.0 (5)	13.8 [5.2 ; 36.1]	9.1 [3.3–25.2]	<0.001

† After controlling for age, sex, hypertension, cigarette smoking, high serum cholesterol, diabetes, past myocardial infarction, and atrial fibrillation; †† reference category; * the adjusted risk of plaques 1–3.9 mm is 4.4 (95 percent confidence interval, 2.8 to 6.8); CI = confidence interval; OR = odds ratio. From Reference 13.

this study we looked at the risk according to the plaque thickness. We found that the risk of brain infarct attached to aortic arch plaques located proximal to the left subclavian artery ostium increased with the thickness of plaques (Table 2).

This large increase was observed only in lesions of 4 mm or greater that were located proximal to the left subclavian artery ostium in the ascending aorta or proximal arch; it was not seen in those distal to the left subclavian artery ostium in the distal arch or descending aorta. The increase in the risk of ischemic stroke associated with plaques of 4 mm or greater in the proximal arch was independent of the presence of the two major risk factors for stroke in the elderly, ie, carotid stenosis and atrial fibrillation. The frequency of plaques of 4 mm or greater in the proximal arch did not differ according to the degree of carotid stenosis, and the frequency of such plaques was lower in patients with atrial fibrillation than in those without atrial fibrillation. Plaques of 4 mm or greater in thickness located proximal to the left subclavian artery ostium were also associated with an abrupt increase in the risk of stroke among patients who had ischemic strokes with no apparent cause. Furthermore, the presence of a mobile component of the plaque was associated with an odds ratio of 14 among patients with ischemic stroke of unknown cause.

These results were strengthened by another case-control study performed the same year in Australia by Jones and colleagues,[14] who found a 7.1-fold increase in the risk of ischemic stroke in the presence of "complex atheroma" in the aortic arch. The singularity of this study was that the authors compared patients with brain infarcts or transient ischemic attacks with a population-based control group that included only healthy volunteers. Of 304 consecutive patients with a first-ever ischemic stroke, the investigators included 215 (of whom 20 had only transient ischemic attacks), and 202 healthy volunteers for TEE examination; 94% of patients with ischemic stroke and 78% of control subjects also had carotid imaging. They found "simple" plaques less than 5 mm thick and smooth in the ascending aorta and aortic arch in 33% of patients and 22% of controls, and "complex" plaques greater than 5 mm thick or any plaques with irregular surface or with mobile components in 22% of patients and 4% of controls. In a further analysis, using a more objective measure of atheroma severity and comparing patients and controls with plaques 5 mm thick or greater or plaques less than 5 mm thick, rather than "simple" and "complex" plaques, they found an adjusted odds ratio of 8.2 (95% CI, 3.0 to 22.4) for plaques 5 mm thick or greater and 2.2 (95% CI, 1.2 to 4.1) for plaques less than 5 mm. They also found mobile protruding atheroma in the aortic arch in 11 patients and in only 1 control subject (crude OR, 10.8; 95% CI, 1.4 to 84.7). However, they did not confirm a significant association between complex aortic arch plaques and ischemic stroke of unknown origin (20% in patients with stroke of unknown origin and 23% in patients with ischemic stroke with a known cause).[14]

Dávila-Román and colleagues[10] studied a consecutive series of 1334 cardiac patients 50 years old or older who were undergoing open heart surgery.[10] This study was very important because they used an intraoperative epiaortic ultrasonography device (not transesophageal echocardiography) that allows assessment of the entire length of the ascending aorta from the root of the aorta to the level of the proximal arch, a region which is difficult to image with TEE (which shows mainly the aortic arch). The ascending aorta is also more likely to be a donor site for brain embolism than more distal regions of the aorta. Among 1200 patients who underwent epiaortic ultrasonography, 158 had a previous embolic event and 1042 were free of embolic event. They found plaques greater than or equal to 3 mm in the ascending aorta in 26.6% of patients who had a previous neurological event and in 18.1% in the "control" subjects who were free of neurological events. Most of these patients (88.3%) were undergoing coronary artery bypass grafting, which easily explains the high rate of protruding plaques in the control group. Multivariate analysis showed that significant predictors of previous neurological ischemic events were hypertension (OR = 1.81), ascending aorta atherosclerosis (OR = 1.65), atrial fibrillation (OR = 1.54), and, in the subset of 789 patients who were evaluated for carotid artery disease with ultrasound, severe carotid stenosis (OR = 2.7).

Nihoyannopoulos et al[15] prospectively studied the aortas of 152 consecutive patients older than 40 years who were referred to be examined for atherosclerosis of the thoracic aorta. Lesions in the aorta were classified into fixed atherosclerotic lesions and mobile lesions. In addition, duplex ultrasound of carotid arteries was performed in all patients with distinction between obstructive lesion (stenosis >50%) and nonobstructive lesion (stenosis <50%). Among the whole group of 152 patients, 44 (29%) had at least one major atheromatous lesion in the thoracic aorta. Atherosclerotic plaques were located in the horizontal portion of the aortic arch in 20 of these 44 patients (45%), in the ascending aorta in 7 patients (16%), and in the descending aorta in 17 patients (39%). All but two patients with major atherosclerotic lesions in the descending aorta also had other smaller lesions at the horizontal portion. Only 3 of the 44 (8%) patients had mobile lesions. Atherosclerotic plaques in the thoracic aorta were present in 20 of 42 (48%) patients with embolic event, and in 24 of 110 (22%) patients without embolic events ($P<0.001$). Among the 152 patients, 26 had atherosclerotic lesions in the carotid arteries, including 7 with >50% stenosis, all associated with extensive atherosclerotic disease in the thoracic aorta, 19 with <50% stenosis, 16 with plaques in the aorta, and 3 without plaque.

Stone et al[16] studied with TEE 49 consecutive patients aged 40 years or older with ischemic stroke and 57 age-matched control subjects without stroke. They found protruding plaque greater than or equal to 5 mm in 16 (32.7%) patients and in 4 (7%) control subjects.

More recently Di Tullio and colleagues[17] studied 106 patients and 114 stroke-free control subjects and found large ($\geq$0.5cm) protruding atheroma in the proximal aortic arch in the stroke patients more frequently than in the controls (26% versus 13%), particularly in patients 60 years or older with unexplained stroke (22% versus 8% in controls). After multivariate analysis, proximal aortic atheroma was found to be independently associated with stroke (adjusted odds ratio 2.6, 95% CI, 1.1 to 5.9).

Thus clearly, the thickness of plaques in the aortic arch identifies vulnerable plaques.

Other Morphological Parameters: Calcification, Plaque Surface Irregularities, Hypoechoic Plaque, and Mobile Thrombi

Interestingly, in their study, Stone et al[16] used video calipers to try to distinguish ulceration within plaques and adherent mobile debris. Ulcers were defined, with use of a multiplane transducer, as craters greater than or equal to 2 mm in depth and width. The 49 patients were divided into 23 with unexplained ischemic stroke and 26 with ischemic stroke with a known cause. Ulcerated plaques were significantly more frequent in patients with unexplained ischemic stroke (39%) than in patients with a known cause (8%) and in control subjects (7%) ($P<0.001$).[16] This was an important study because it was the first attempt to find out the clinical importance of what can be interpreted as ulceration at TEE examination. Although numbers were small, the authors believed that these results concurred with what has been found at autopsy with ulcerated plaques in the same groups of patients with brain infarcts of unknown cause.[12]

As Stone et al[16] found, Di Tullio et al[17] noted that ulcerated (using the same definition for ulceration) and mobile atherosclerotic lesions were also more frequent in patients than in controls (12% versus 5%; $P<0.06$). They also found that differences were entirely attributable to patients 60 years or older, and concluded that the absence of carotid stenosis does not exclude aortic atheromas as a potential cause for ischemic stroke.[17]

In our French Study of Aortic Plaques in Stroke (FAPS),[20] the case-

Table 3

Risk of Brain Infarction as a Function of Morphological Characteristics of Atherosclerotic Plaques in the Ascending Aorta and Proximal Arch in 338 Patients as Compared with 357 Controls

Wall thickness	Crude OR [95% CI]	P Value	Adjusted OR† [95% CI]	P Value
Calcifications	**2.9** [2.1 ; 4.2]	<0.001	**2.3** [1.6 ; 3.3]	<0.001
Irregular surface	**4.3** [2.5 ; 7.1]	<0.001	**3.4** [2.0 ; 5.7]	<0.001
Thickness ≥4 mm	**7.6** [3.4 ; 17.2]	<0.001	**5.4** [2.3 ; 12.4]	<0.001
Thickness ≥4 mm with calcifications	**6.9** [3.0 ; 15.9]	<0.001	**2.2** [0.8 ; 5.9]	=0.095
Thickness ≥4 mm with irregular surface	**11.3** [4.0 ; 32.2]	<0.001	**7.4** [2.6 ; 21.8]	<0.001
Thickness ≥4 mm without calcifications	∞ [7.0 ; ∞]	<0.001		

† Adjusted for age, sex, peripheral vascular diseases, tabacco consumption, and hypertension; CI = confidence interval; OR = odds ratio. Data from the FAPS study.[20]

control analysis showed that calcifications and surface irregularities suggestive of ulcerations were independently associated with brain infarction, but plaque thickness still had the strongest association (Table 3). When we combined plaque thickness and calcification, plaque thickness and surface irregularities, then plaque thickness and no calcification, the strongest association was found in patients with plaques greater than 4 mm and no calcification.

Prospective Studies

Plaque Thickness

Plaque thickness was also the most well-studied morphological parameter, prospectively (Table 4).

Tunick et al[18] found an annual event rate of 33% in patients who had protruding plaques greater than or equal to 5 mm in the thoracic aorta as compared with 7% in matched controls. This study focused not on plaques that were located in the aortic arch, but those in the entire thoracic aorta. The difference between the two groups was not significant concerning brain and retinal emboli only (7 versus 3 events in patients and controls, respectively). In a study of 33 patients at 1 year, Montgomery et al[19] found that 24% had died, and at follow-up TEE examination they found that severe lesions were dynamic, with formation of new mobile components in 61% of cases, while there was resolution of specific previously documented mobile lesions in up to 70% of cases.

The FAPS study followed 331 consecutive patients admitted to the hospital for brain infarct for 2 to 4 years.[20] All patients had transesophageal echocardiography at presentation. The annual incidence of recurrent brain infarcts was 11.9 per 100 patient-years of follow-up in patients with aortic arch plaques greater than or equal to 4 mm, as compared with 3.5 in patients with plaques from 1 mm to 3.9 mm, and with 2.8 in patients with no plaque. The incidence of all vascular events (combining stroke, myocardial infarction, peripheral emboli, and vascular death) was, respectively, 26 as compared with 9.1 and 5.9 per 100 patient-years of follow-up (Fig. 1). In patients with cryptogenic brain infarcts at entry and with plaques greater than or equal to 4 mm in thickness, the event rates per 100 patient-years of follow-up were 16 for recurrent brain infarct and 26 for all vascular events.

Multivariate analysis showed that aortic arch plaques 4 mm or greater in thickness were significant predictors of new brain infarcts, independent from the presence of carotid stenosis, atrial fibrillation,

Table 4

Risk of New Vascular Events in Patients with Large Protruding Plaques as Compared with Control Subjects

Follow-up studies	Patients	Controls	Relative risk
Tunick et al[18] 42 pts	PI ≥5 mm	No atheroma	
Mean follow-up 14 months			
Stroke + MI + peripheral emboli	33% at 2 yrs	7% at 2 yrs	4.3 [95% CI, 1.2–15.0]
Stroke + retina	16% at 2 yrs	7% at 2 yrs	
FAPS study[20*] 331 pts	PI≥4 mm	No atheroma	
788 person-years of follow-up			
Stroke + MI + peripheral emboli	26 p.100 p-y	5.9 p.100 p-y	3.5 [95% CI, 2.1–5.9]
Stroke	11.9 p.100 p-y	2.8 p.100 p-y	3.8 [95% CI, 1.8–7.8]
Mtusch et al[24] 183 pts			
241 person-years of follow-up	PI ≥5 mm or Mobile	PI <5 mm	
Stroke + peripheral emboli	Thrombi	4.1 p.100 p-y	4.3 [95% CI, 1.5–12.0]
Previously symptomatic patients:	13.8 p.100 p-y		
Stroke + peripheral emboli	15.9 p. 100 p-y	7.1 p.100	
Dávila-Román et al[10]	PI ≥5 mm	No atheroma	
1800 pts	30% at 1 yr	9% at 1 yr	1.7 [95% CI, 1.4–2.0]
All events	11% at 1 yr	3% at 1 yr	1.6 [95% CI, 1.2–3.2]
Neurological events			

*For the estimated risk at 1, 2, 3, and 4 years, see the Kaplan-Meier curve and make projections on axis (Figs. 1 and 2). MI = myocardial infarction.

and peripheral artery disease, with a relative risk of 3.8 (95% confidence interval, 1.8 to 7.8; $P<0.002$). The significant difference observed between the three Kaplan-Meier curves (Figs. 1 and 2), according to the aortic plaque thickness, is a further strong argument for a causality link between plaques greater than or equal to 4 mm in thickness and brain infarcts in some of these patients. However, this study also showed that the presence of plaques greater than or equal to 4 mm in thickness in the aortic arch is a strong and independent predictor of all vascular events with a relative risk of 3.5 (95% confidence interval, 2.1 to 5.9; $P<0.001$).[20] These observations led to the conclusion that

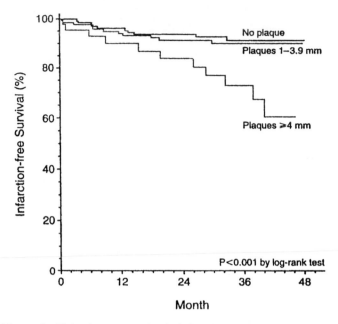

Figure 1. Risk of recurrent brain infarction. From Reference 20.

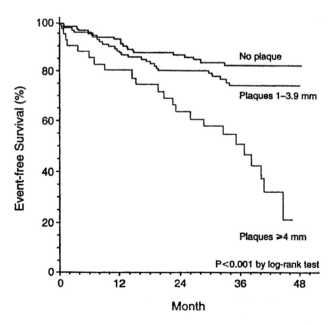

Figure 2. Risk of new vascular events (combining brain infarcts, myocardial infarctions, peripheral events, and vascular deaths). From Reference 20.

Table 5

Risk of New Vascular Events* in Patients with Plaques ≥4 Mm in the Aortic Arch Proximal to the Take-off of the Left Subclavian Artery**

Plaques ≥4 mm	Relative risk	P value
New vascular events		
Calcifications	4.1 [2.0–8.5]	<0.001
No calcifications	9.6 [3.9–24.0]	<0.001

*Brain infarction, myocardial infarction, peripheral emboli, or vascular death; **according to the presence or the lack of calcification of plaques. From Reference 25.

plaques greater than or equal to 4 mm in the aortic arch are, above all, good markers for generalized atherosclerosis that could be used to select patients at high vascular risk in therapeutic trial.

Other Morphological Parameters

In the FAPS study[20] we found that among morphological parameters such as plaque thickness, surface irregularities, calcifications, and hypoechoic plaques suggestive of thrombus, plaque thickness greater than 4 mm still had the highest event rate. When we combined plaque thickness and hypoechoic plaques or surface irregularities, we found no additive prognostic value compared with only the thickness of plaques greater than 4. However, we found a very significant prognostic additive value when we compared plaques greater than 4 mm with no calcification to plaques greater than 4 mm (Table 5).[25]

Thus, plaques greater than or equal to 4 mm in the aortic arch, as detected with TEE, are markers for a high risk of recurrent brain infarcts and mainly for other vascular events. Surface irregularities, hypoechoic appearance of plaques, and the presence of calcification have little or no additive prognostic value, but plaques 4 mm or greater with no calcifications are much more predictive of new vascular events than are plaques 4 mm or greater with calcification. The relative benefits and risks of therapeutic interventions should now be evaluated in patients with such plaques.

The Etiologic Burden of Aortic Arch Plaques 4 mm Thick or Greater in Ischemic Stroke

Thus, aortic arch plaques greater or equal to 4 mm are new strong, independent risk factors for brain infarcts, with a possible causal link.

Table 6

Prevalence of Mobile Thrombi in the Lumen of the Aortic Arch in Consecutive Series

Origin of series	Sample size	Mobile thrombi	Percentage of mobile thrombi
Consecutive ischemic stroke pts			
Toyoda et al 1992 (embolic stroke)	62	3	4.8%
Nihoyannopoulos et al 1993[15]	152	3	2%
Jones et al 1994[14] (unselected pts)	202	11	5.4%
Amarenco et al 1994[13] (unselected pts)	250	7	2.8%
Stone et al 1995[16] (unselected pts)	49	2	4.1%
Consecutive TEE performed in an echolab	122	11	9.0%
Tunick et al 1991[11]	556	11	2.0%
Karalis et al 1991[5]	600	5	0.8%
Mitchell et al 1992[21]	335	8	2.4%
Mitusch et al 1995[22]			
Embolic events or unexplained brain infarction	122	11	9.0%
Tunick et al 1991[11] (embolic events)	44	11	25.0%
Karalis et al 1991[5] (embolic events)	183	7	4%
Horowitz et al 1992 (embolic stroke)	42	3	7.1%
Nihoyannopoulos et al 1993[15] (embolic events)	78	6	7.7%
Amarenco et al 1994[13] (unexplained brain infarct)	23	2	8.7%
Stone et al 1995[16] (unexplained brain infarct)	80	5	6.3%
Mitusch et al 1995[22] (embolic events)			

Plaques greater than or equal to 4 mm are present in one third of patients with cryptogenic stroke, who account themselves for one third of the total ischemic stroke population aged 60 years or older.[13] Some of these patients have complicated plaques with pedunculated and mobile thrombotic components, which constitute a permanent threat for brain emboli. This can be expected in 1 of 10 patients with cryptogenic stroke (Table 6).[13] The attributable risk of plaques 4 mm or greater is 12.6% with a confidence interval of 7.6 to 17.6%. This means that the etiologic part of plaques 4 mm or greater could be as high as in nonvalvular atrial fibrillation or severe stenosis of internal carotid artery origin.

The Missing Link

Aortic arch atherosclerotic disease is probably an underestimated source of emboli. It could account for a greater or lesser part of these brain infarcts of unknown cause, with no carotid or cardiac source of emboli (Table 6). Clinicians should be aware that this location of atherosclerotic disease is rare in people under 60 years of age. It mainly involves patients older than 60 years of age and is actually frequent in people in their eighties. Transesophageal echocardiography is accurate, safe, and well tolerated for the examination of the aortic arch, even in very old patients over 85 years of age. Future clinical trials and practical implications for patients should be important considerations.

References

1. Sacco RL, Ellenberg JH, Mohr JP, et al. Infarcts of undetermined cause: The NINCDS stroke data bank. *Ann Neurol* 1989;25:382–390.
2. Bruno A, Russell PW, Jones WL, et al. Concomitants of asymptomatic retinal cholesterol emboli. *Stroke* 1992;23:900–902.
3. Bruno A, Jones WL, Austin JK, et al. Vascular outcome in men with asymptomatic retinal cholesterol emboli. A cohort study. *Ann Intern Med* 1995; 122:249–253.
4. Tunick PA, Kronzon I. Protruding atherosclerotic plaque in the aortic arch of patients with systemic embolization: A new finding seen by transesophageal echocardiography. *Am Heart J* 1990;120:658–660.
5. Karalis DG, Chandrasekaran K, Victor MF, et al. Recognition and embolic potential of intraaortic atherosclerotic debris. *J Am Coll Cardiol* 1991;17: 73–78.
6. Ramirez G, O'Neill WM, Lambert R, Bloomer A. Cholesterol embolization, a complication of angiography. *Arch Intern Med* 1978;138:1430–1432.
7. Gardner TJ, Horneffer PJ, Manolio TA, et al. Stroke following coronary artery bypass grafting: A ten-year study. *Ann Thorac Surg* 1985;40:574–580.
8. McKibbin DW, Bukley BH, Green WR, et al. Fatal cerebral atheromatous embolization after cardiopulmonary bypass. *J Thorac Cardiovasc Surg* 1976; 71:741–745.
9. Katz ES, Tunick PA, Rusinek H, et al. Protruding aortic atheromas predict stroke in elderly patients undergoing cardiopulmonary bypass: Experience with intraoperative transesophageal echocardiography. *J Am Coll Cardiol* 1992;20:70–77.
10. Dávila-Román VG, Barzilai B, Wareing TH, et al. Atherosclerosis of the ascending aorta. Prevalence and role as independant predictor of cerebrovascular events in cardiac patients. *Stroke* 1994;25:2010–2016.
11. Tunick PA, Perez JL, Kronzon I. Protruding atheromas in the thoracic aorta and systemic embolization. *Ann Intern Med* 1991;115:423–427.
12. Amarenco P, Duyckaerts C, Tzourio C, et al. The prevalence of ulcerated plaques in the aortic arch in patients with stroke. *N Engl J Med* 1992;326: 221–225.
13. Amarenco P, Cohen A, Tzourio C, et al. Atherosclerotic disease of the aortic arch and the risk of ischemic stroke. *N Engl J Med* 1994;331:1474–1479.
14. Jones EF, Kalman JM, Calafiore P, et al. Proximal aortic atheroma. An independent risk factor for cerebral ischemia. *Stroke* 1995;26:218–224.
15. Nihoyannopoulos P, Joshi J, Athanasopoulos G, Oakley CM. Detection of atherosclerotic lesions in the aorta by transesophageal echography. *Am J Cardiol* 1993;71:1208–1212.
16. Stone DA, Hawke MW, LaMonte M, et al. Ulcerated atherosclerotic plaques

in the thoracic aorta are associated with cryptogenic stroke: A multiplane trasesophageal echocardiographic study. *Am Heart J* 1995;130:105–108.

17. Di Tullio MR, Sacco RL, Gersony D, et al. Aortic atheromas and acute ischemic stroke: A transesophageal echocardiographic study in an ethnically mixed population. *Neurology* 1996;46:1560–1566.

18. Tunick PA, Rosenzweig BP, Katz ES, et al. High risk for vascular events in patients with protruding aortic atheromas: A prospective study. *J Am Coll Cardiol* 1994;23:1085–1090.

19. Montgomery DH, Ververis JJ, McGorisk G, et al. Natural history of severe atheromatous disease of the thoracic aorta: A transesophageal echocardiographic study. *J Am Coll Cardiol* 1996;27:95–101.

20. The French Study of Aortic Plaques in Stroke Group. Atherosclerotic disease of the aortic arch as a risk factor for reccurrent ischemic stroke. *N Engl J Med* 1996;334:1216–1221.

21. Mitchell MM, Frankville DD, Weinger MB, Dittrich HC. Detection of thoracic atheroma with transesophageal echocardiography in patients without symptoms of embolism. *Am Heart J* 1991;122:1768–1771.

22. Mitusch R, Stierle U, Kummer-Kloess D, et al. Systemic embolism in aortic arch atheromatosis. *Eur Heart J* 1994;15:1373–1380.

23. Khathibzadeh M, Mitusch R, Stierle U, et al. Aortic atherosclerotic plaques as a source of systemic embolism. *J Am Coll Cardiol* 1996;27:664–669.

24. Mitusch R, Doherty C, Wucherpfennig H, et al. Vascular events during follow-up in patients with aortic arch atherosclerosis. *Stroke* 1997;28:36–39.

25. Cohen A, Tzourio C, Bertrand B, et al, on behalf of the FAPS investigators. Aortic plaque morphology and vascular events. A follow-up study in patients with ischemic stroke. *Circulation* 1997;96:3838–3841.

Chapter 12

Radioisotopic Imaging of Atheroma

Shankar Vallabhajosula, PhD

Introduction

Quantitative assessment of atherosclerotic or atherothrombotic disease during its natural history and following therapeutic interventions is important in order to understand the progression and stabilization of the disease and to select appropriate medical or surgical interventions. A number of invasive and noninvasive imaging techniques, such as angiography, intravascular ultrasound, and magnetic resonance, are now available to detect and display different characteristics of vascular lesions of clinical and/or research interest.[1] The choice and appropriateness of each imaging technique, however, depends on its diagnostic efficacy and, most importantly, on the type of questions asked.[1] Most of the standard techniques identify some of the morphological parameters of the atherosclerosis and provide qualitative or semiquantitative assessment of the relative risk associated with the disease. These standard techniques, however, do not characterize plaque composition or correlate the image parameters with histopathological lesion types, which more accurately reflect clinical relevance.

In the last 20 years, many radiotracers have been developed based on a number of molecules and cells involved in atherogenesis. Many investigators have studied the potential diagnostic utility of these radiotracers to image atherosclerotic lesions in animal models.[2-5] These radiotracers were primarily designed to image atherosclerotic lesions (Table 1) and provide plaque composition, or to detect the intra-arterial thrombus associated with these lesions (Table 2). The characteristics and requirements of an ideal radiotracer to image atherosclerosis and

From: Fuster, V (ed). *The Vulnerable Atherosclerotic Plaque: Understanding, Identification, and Modification.* Armonk, NY: Futura Publishing Company, Inc.; © 1999.

Table 1

Radiotracers for Imaging Atherosclerosis

Low-density lipoprotein (LDL):	^{123}I-LDL, ^{111}In-DTPA-LDL, ^{99m}Tc-LDL, ^{99m}Tc-oxidized-LDL
Immunoglobulins: Nonspecific	^{111}In-DTPA-IgG (bind to FC receptors on macrophages)
Specific	^{111}In-Z2D3 F(ab')2, IgM (monoclonal) (against smooth muscle cells)
	^{131}I-anti-ICAM-1, IgG (monoclonal) (against endothelial adhesion molecule)
Peptides:	^{123}I-SP-4, ^{99m}Tc-P199 and ^{99m}Tc-P215 (peptides based on apo-B)
Monocytes:	^{111}In-Monocytes
Metabolic tracer:	^{18}F-Fluorodeoxyglucose (FDG) (may reflect macrophage density)

atherothrombosis are described in Table 3. Based on these criteria, a single radiotracer is not ideally suited for imaging atherosclerosis or providing the prognostic and clinical indicators necessary for medical and surgical interventions. Preliminary clinical evaluations of some of these tracers were performed in patients with carotid atherosclerotic disease. Very few clinical studies, however, have been performed to correlate in vivo imaging data with histopathology of plaques. The

Table 2

Radiotracers for Imaging Intra-Arterial Thrombosis

Platelets:	^{111}In-platelets, ^{99m}Tc-HMPAO-platelets
Fibrinogen:	^{123}I-Fibrinogen
Plasminogen activator:	^{131}I or ^{123}I-[DLT-PPACK]-t-PA
Specific monoclonal IgG:	^{99m}Tc-S-12-IgG Fab' (against GP GMP-140 on activated platelets)
	^{99m}Tc-T2G1, IgG Fab' (against fibrin only)
Peptides:	^{99m}Tc-P280, ^{99m}Tc-P748, ^{99m}Tc-RP-431 (against GP IIb/IIIa receptor on activated platelets)
	^{123}I-Disintegrins (against GP IIb/IIIa receptor on act. platelets)

Table 3

Characteristics of an Ideal Radiotracer to Image Atherosclerosis

1. Detect the presence of disease, and the radiotracers must be specific for lipid core, macrophage density, or thrombus.
2. Detect lesions in coronary, carotid, and ileo-femoral arteries.
3. Assess progression-regression of atherosclerosis.
4. Predict clinically significant events.
5. Provide prognostic indicators in "population studies."
6. Tracer must have high specificity and sensitivity.
7. Tracer must have faster blood clearance and high target/background (T/B) ratios.
8. Tracer must have a kit formulation to prepare instantly.

advantages and disadvantages of some of these radiotracers are discussed below:

Radiotracers for Imaging Atherosclerosis

Low-Density Lipoproteins

Atherogenic molecules such as plasma low-density lipoproteins (LDLs) accumulate in the arterial lesions. In a balloon-catheter de-endothelialized aorta of a rabbit, focal LDL accumulation is predominantly seen in the edges of regenerating endothelial islands.[6] Based on this observation, Lees and coworkers[7] first developed radioiodinated LDL and demonstrated the potential diagnostic utility for imaging carotid atherosclerotic lesions in patients. Subsequently, several investigators labeled LDL with a number of radionuclides with different physical half- lives, such as Iodine 123, Technetium 99m, and Indium 111, and demonstrated the uptake in atherosclerotic lesions in a variety of hypercholesterolemic rabbit models[2,8,9] and in patients.[10–14] In patients with carotid atherosclerosis, the uptake of [99mTc] LDL was seen in soft lesions rich in macrophages, while the mature fibro-calcific plaques did not accumulate radiolabeled LDL.[10,11] In two clinical studies, the tendon xanthomas in hypercholesterolemic patients and the expanded bone marrow in myeloproliferative patients also showed intense uptake of [99mTc] LDL that correlated with increased macrophage content in these tissues.[12,13] Even though the potential for diagnostic imaging of radioiodinated LDL and [99mTc] LDL was demonstrated in patients with carotid and femoral atherosclerosis, clinical utility of this technique remains elusive. In coronary arteries, ^{99m}Tc LDL imaging does not detect lesions for two reasons: the absolute and specific uptake of radiotracer in the lesion is very low (<0.1% of the injected dose), and the blood pool activity is very high due to slow plasma clearance of the radiotracer.

Monocyte-derived macrophages in atheroma appear to sequester oxidized LDL more efficiently than native LDL. Therefore, oxidized LDL labeled with ^{99m}Tc would be expected to be more selective than radiolabeled native LDL for imaging atherosclerotic lesions in vivo. This hypothesis was recently tested in a clinical study with patients who were candidates for carotid endarterectomy.[15] Both planar and single photon emission computed tomography (SPECT) imaging studies were performed in the same subject, with both tracers. Technetium 99m uptake in carotid lesions was slightly greater with oxidized LDL (ox-LDL) than with native LDL. There were no significant differences, however, between the two tracers regarding lesion delectability, even though the blood clearance of LDL was enhanced due to oxidation.[15] Similar results were also reported in animal studies, where the aortic focal uptake of modified LDL was similar to that of native LDL, suggesting that the focal uptake of LDL in arterial lesions is mediated by specific oxidation-independent patterns of charge and polarity.[16]

Peptides

Lipoproteins are large molecules and, consequently, clear from circulation very slowly. By contrast, peptides are very small molecules (normally 10 to 20 amino acids), which clear from the circulation very rapidly and therefore provide high target/background ratios within minutes postinjection. Two different classes of peptide molecules have been evaluated as potential atherosclerosis-imaging agents: peptides based on the apo-B portion of LDL, and endothelin analogues. Specific cellular uptake of LDL by fibroblasts and hepatocytes involves the classic LDL receptor, which recognizes a particular portion of apo-B. This LDL receptor-binding domain, however, is not involved in focal accumulation of LDL by monocyte macrophages in atheroma, since homozygous familial hypercholesterolemic (FH) patients with absent LDL receptors also develop atherosclerotic lesions. Therefore, a synthetic peptide (SP-4) was developed,[17] and radioiodinated SP-4 showed significant accumulation in experimental atherosclerotic lesions.[18] Since then, other synthetic peptides were developed (P-199 and P-215) which can be radiolabeled with [99m]Tc.[19] The principle advantage of ^{99m}Tc-labeled peptides compared to ^{99m}Tc LDL is that with ^{99m}Tc-labeled peptides, imaging can be performed within 1 hour postinjection, as the peptides clear much faster than LDL from the circulation. In pilot studies involving patients with carotid atherosclerotic lesions documented by ultrasound, ^{99m}Tc-P215 SPECT images showed some uptake in the atherosclerotic lesions immediately postinjection.[20] The diagnostic value of this tracer, however, is not yet evaluated in well-controlled clinical trials.

In conditions associated with endothelial cell injury, the peptide endothelin has been shown to be present in vascular smooth muscle cells and endothelial cells of human atherosclerotic lesions. Radioiodinated endothelin has been shown to accumulate in experimentally induced arterial wall injuries in rabbits.[21] A number of endothelin derivatives were recently labeled with ^{99m}Tc and have been shown to accumulate in significant amounts in experimental atherosclerotic lesions in rabbits.[22] The diagnostic significance and clinical utility of these peptides, however, has not been well established.

Immunoglobulins

Macrophage-derived foam cells are present in abundant quantity in the fatty streaks and vulnerable plaques. These cells specifically express cell surface Fc receptors. It has been hypothesized that radiolabeled immunoglobulin G (IgG), which contains an Fc subunit, would be an appropriate radiotracer to image macrophage density in the atherosclerotic lesions.[23] The potential diagnostic value of ^{111}In-labeled polyclonal human IgG was evaluated in patients with carotid atherosclerosis. Indium 111-IgG identified 86% of the lesions shown by ultrasonography. However, it did not correlate with plaque morphology and clinical stage of the disease as shown by ultrasound.[24] Indium 111-IgG imaging studies in Watanabe Heritable Hyperlipidemic Rabbits (WHHR) also failed to detect the early lesions in the aorta. In addition, treatment of the rabbits with antioxidants and a hypolipidemic drug did not reduce the lesion uptake of the radiotracer.[25] The images obtained even after 4 to 5 days postinjection would not provide adequate target/blood ratios to visualize coronary artery lesions, since the plasma clearance of the tracer is very slow. The clinical and animal data clearly suggest that the accumulation of the tracer in the lesion may be nonspecific, and radiolabeled IgG may not be an appropriate radiotracer to image and identify vulnerable atherosclerotic lesions.

In order to circumvent the problem of nonspecific localization of IgG, monoclonal antibodies were developed against different cells and antigens present in the atherosclerotic lesions. Smooth muscle cell proliferation is one of the major consequences of atherosclerotic disease. The targeting of these cells with a specific radiolabeled antibody is expected to image metabolically active atherosclerotic lesions. A mouse/human chimeric monoclonal antibody fragment, Z2D3 F (ab')$_2$ IgM, was developed with specificity for an antigen associated with smooth muscle cells.[26] Indium-111-(DTPA-PL)-Z2D3 F (ab')$_2$ IgM negative charge-modified antibody fragments were shown to localize in experimental atherosclerotic lesions.[27]

Amino malonic acid (AMA) has been isolated from human atherosclerotic plaques. This molecule has possible calcium binding properties and is crucial in progressive stages of the atherosclerotic process for inclusion of monocyte intimal recruitment and foam cell production. Radioiodinated monoclonal antibody against AMA (^{131}I-AMA) has been shown to localize in experimental atherosclerotic lesions.[28]

Radiotracers to Image Intra-Arterial Thrombus

In coronary, cerebral, and peripheral vascular beds, atherothrombotic events underlie acute clinical vascular syndromes. Identification of the ruptured plaque or of the clinically so-called "culprit lesion" is crucial for clinical management and therapeutic intervention. Loscalzo and Rocco[29] have clearly pointed out that the lack of a simple, relatively noninvasive method for identifying an acute atherothrombotic process is a notable deficiency in current cardiovascular practice. The search for thrombus-specific agents began almost two decades ago, and three principle elements of thrombus have been selected as targets for developing radiotracers. These include fibrin, platelets, and fibrinolytic molecules (Table 2). Radiotracers that would localize in forming thrombi will be ideal for imaging fresh propagating thrombi. The relative advantages and clinical utility of these tracers is discussed below.

Platelets

Platelets have been implicated in the pathogenesis of atherosclerosis. They play an important role in the initial steps of lesion development by adhering to subendothelial connective tissue. Platelet mural thrombi have been associated with lesion formation during all phases of the disease; massive thrombi, in particular, are seen in advanced lesions. Autologous platelets can be labeled efficiently with ^{111}In or ^{99m}Tc lipophilic complexes.[30,31] Platelets labeled with ^{111}In have been evaluated as radiotracers for the detection of complicated unstable plaques because radiolabeled platelets were presumed to accumulate only in an active thrombus that is being formed. A number of clinical studies have shown ^{111}In-platelet uptake in atherosclerotic lesions of carotid and femoral arteries and in the abdominal aorta.[3,32] Several groups of investigators recently reevaluated the potential diagnostic and clinical utility of ^{111}In-platelet imaging technique in patients with carotid atherosclerosis.[33,34] The ^{111}In-platelet uptake in the carotid arteries did not correlate with clinical symptomatology, angiographic or ultrasound results, or pharmacological intervention. In a recent review, however, it was pointed out that platelet scintigraphy has a sensitivity of 43% to 73% and a specificity of 87% to 100% compared with angiographic abnormalities.[32] In a recent clinical study consisting of 60 patients with carotid atherosclerosis who were not receiving antithrombotic medication, ^{111}In-platelet uptake was shown to be significantly greater in ulcerated plaques characterized by B-mode ultrasonography.[34] In spite of this optimistic clinical finding, ^{111}In-platelet imaging has significant limitations. Due to slow clearance of platelets from circulation, imaging has to be performed at least 48 hours after reinjection of platelets. The count density in the image is very poor due to the limitations on the amount of radioactivity that can be injected. Finally, like radiolabeled LDL, ^{111}In platelets are also not useful for detection of vulnerable plaques in the coronary arteries due to very high blood pool activity.

Proteins

Radioiodinated fibrinogen was the first scintigraphic agent used successfully to detect thrombus.[2] The tracer localizes only in actively growing thrombus but requires delayed imaging (several days) for optimal diagnostic accuracy because the plasma clearance of the tracer is very slow. In addition, the thrombus/blood ratios are suboptimal for the detection of intra-arterial lesions because arterial thrombi are not rich in fibrin. Fibronectin is a relatively large glycoprotein (440 kDa), known to interact with fibrin, collagen, and proteoglycans. It is present in atherosclerotic lesions of the intima, especially in developing fibrous plaques. Iodine 131-labeled fibronectin is taken up by the de-endothelialized lesions in rabbit aortas.[36] There are no reported clinical studies with this tracer. Since blood clearance of the tracer is very slow, optimal imaging time might be 2 to 3 days postinjection and the diagnostic potential of this tracer might be low and similar to ^{111}In-labeled polyclonal IgG.

Within hours after acute thrombus formation, a number of fibrin degradation products are formed. Fibrin fragment E_1 is a 60-kDa fragment of human fibrin that binds specifically to fibrin polymers but not to fibrin monomer or fibrinogen.[37] Both ^{123}I and ^{99m}Tc-labeled fibrin fragment E_1 have shown excellent thrombus uptake in vivo in a canine deep-vein thrombosis (DVT) model. Images can be obtained within 1 hour postinjection; thrombus/blood ratios are higher than fibrinogen and platelets, since the blood pool activity is minimal.[37] The tracer has not yet been tested in an intra-arterial thrombus animal model or in patients.

Annexin V is a human protein (36 kDa) of 319 amino acids that binds with very high affinity to phosphatidylserine moiety that is exposed on activated platelets.[38] Since there is no circulating pool of annexin V, and platelets in circulation are quiescent, the plasma clearance of this protein is very rapid compared to fibrinogen, fibronectin, and immunoglobulins. Technetium 99m-labeled annexin V has shown intense localization in an acute porcine left atrial thrombus within 2 hours postinjection. The thrombus/blood ratios of 14 to 22 suggest that this tracer has a great potential for intra-arterial thrombus detection.[39]

Immunoglobulins

In the last two decades, a number of radiolabeled antibodies against platelets and fibrin have been evaluated, in animal models and in patients, as potential thrombus imaging agents.[2,37,40] To date, however, no radiolabeled antibody has been approved by the Food and Drug Administration specifically for thrombus detection. Recent animal and clinical studies have indicated the potential utility of certain new radiolabeled immunoglobulins. Monoclonal antibodies have been developed against two sites which become exposed on activated platelets: glycoprotein IIb/IIIa, (fibrinogen receptor), and glycoprotein GMP-140 (the α-granule membrane glycoprotein). The antibody, S-12, is specific for GMP-140 and is expressed on activated platelets only.[40] Technetium 99m-labeled S-12 Fab' fragment has shown significant localization in an acute animal model with intra-arterial thrombi rich in platelets.[40] Secretion of platelet α-granule contents such as platelet-derived growth factor (PDGF) and platelet factor-4 occurs at lower thrombin concentrations, while high thrombin concentrations secrete serotonin from the dense granules. Therefore, it is hypothesized that Tc 99m-S-12 Fab' antibody uptake in an arterial lesion would be a marker for PDGF release and thus would reflect postangioplasty hyperproliferative response.[40]

Antifibrin antibodies (T2G1s) bind specifically to fibrin but not to circulating fibrinogen or fibrin degradation products. Animal and human studies have demonstrated the uptake of radiolabeled T2G1 antibody in both venous and intra-arterial thrombi where there is an active fibrin deposition.[41] Technetium 99m-labeled T2G1 antifibrin antibody Fab' fragments in patients were recently evaluated in order to detect arterial thrombosis, and the results were compared to ^{111}In-platelet thrombus uptake in the same patients.[42] The study demonstrated that T2G1 antibody scintigraphy was less likely to detect chronic thrombi than ^{111}In-platelets.

Peptides

In the last 2 to 3 years, radiolabeled thrombus-binding peptides have shown excellent potential for detection of active thrombi in animal models. A number of synthetic peptides have been prepared, and the targeting sequence of the peptides was derived from the primary binding region of the fibrinogen molecule, which binds to the glycoprotein IIb/IIIa (fibrinogen receptor) on activated platelets. The advantage of peptides is that they have rapid blood clearance and are less immunogenic than immunoglobulins. In a canine model of DVT, ^{123}I-bitistatin,[43] ^{99m}Tc-P280,[44] ^{99m}Tc-P748,[45] and ^{99m}Tc-RP431[46] demonstrated significant thrombus uptake within 1 to 2 hours postinjection. In a canine model of intra-arterial thrombus, ^{99m}Tc-P748 localized in thrombus within minutes following injection and showed excellent thrombus/blood ratios, similar to those of ^{111}In-platelets.[47]

[99m]Tc-P280: Clinical Studies

Atherosclerotic disease at the carotid artery bifurcation has been established as a source of cerebral ischemic stroke and transient cerebral ischemic attack.[48] Clinical and ultrasound evidence suggests that carotid plaque activity (CPA) is an important factor in thromboembolic cerebral ischemia, in addition to the degree of stenosis.[49,50] Since ^{99m}Tc-labeled peptides have demonstrated localization in arterial thrombus of animal models, we examined the potential diagnostic utility of ^{99m}Tc-P280 peptide to image thrombus activity associated with atherosclerotic plaque in patients with carotid artery atherosclerosis.[51]

Nine patients were injected with 20 mCi of Tc-P280, and SPECT imaging of the neck was performed at 15 and 90 minutes. The peptide imaging studies showed asymmetric localization of ^{99m}Tc activity in all patients (Figure 1). The intensity of ^{99m}Tc uptake was compared to the contralateral side and was qualitatively graded as diffuse, mild, or moderate. Ultrasound studies were performed to assess the degree of the complexity of CPA. Based on duplex studies, thrombus involvement was suggested in 9 of 18 carotid arteries. Tc-P280 imaging showed moderate uptake in 6 of 9 (67%) of these carotid arteries. In addition, five more carotid arteries showed moderate peptide uptake, while duplex studies indicated no thrombus involvement. The peptide localiza-

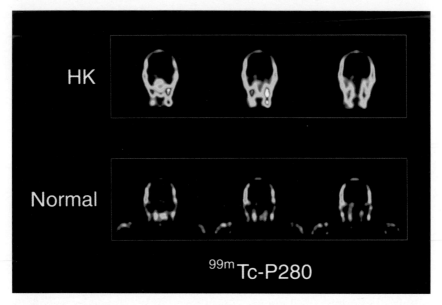

Figure 1. Single photon emission computed tomography (SPECT) images of ^{99m}Tc-P280 peptide in a patient (HK) with carotid atherosclerosis and a normal subject. The images of the neck were obtained 90 minutes postinjection of the radiotracer. In the normal subject there is minimal uptake of radiotracer activity in the area of carotid arteries. In the patient, greater uptake of activity is seen in the area of left carotid artery bifurcation compared to contralateral side. Duplex studies of the patient demonstrate bilateral carotid artery stenosis with a heterogenous proliferative mural ulcerative plaque at the left carotid bifurcation.

tion in the carotid lesions, however, was independent of percent stenosis. These preliminary results (unpublished data) suggest that ^{99m}Tc-P280 imaging appears to identify intra-arterial thrombi associated with atherosclerosis and may potentially be useful for detecting the majority of propagating CPA, which may or may not be indicated by ultrasound studies.[51] Correlation of imaging results with lesion histopathology is necessary in order to determine the clinical significance of these studies and the potential diagnostic value of ^{99m}Tc-P280 studies for intra-arterial thrombus detection.

Positron Emission Tomography

The conventional nuclear medicine gamma cameras have a resolution of 1.0 to 1.5 cm for planar and SPECT imaging techniques. In contrast, the state-of-the-art positron emission tomography (PET) cameras provide 4- to 5-mm resolution. In addition, a number of biochemicals and metabolic substrates can be labeled with positron-emitting radionuclides such as carbon 11 and fluorine 18, which might provide better radiotracers to image functional status of atherosclerotic lesions.

Fluorine 18-labeled fluorodeoxyglucose (FDG), an analogue of glucose, has been used extensively as a radiotracer to estimate glucose metabolic rates of brain, heart, and tumor.[52,53] This analogue competes with glucose for transport into the cell and, subsequently, for phosphorylation within the cell. Unlike glucose-6-phosphate, FDG-6-phosphate is not metabolized further and is trapped within the cell. While investigating the mechanisms of FDG accumulation in tumor tissue, Kubota and colleagues[54] recently reported that within the tumor, the uptake of deoxyglucose by macrophages was higher than by tumor cells, and the uptake of FDG by macrophages is believed to be caused by an enhanced rate of glucose use. Since atherosclerotic lesions are rich in macrophages, we hypothesized that FDG-PET imaging of atherosclerosis may provide a noninvasive test to image and quantitate the extent of macrophage content in an atherosclerotic lesion.

To test the validity of this hypothesis, we performed PET imaging studies in a rabbit model of atherosclerosis.[55] Rabbits fed a high-cholesterol diet (1%) for 1 to 2 months become hypercholesterolemic (HC) and develop "fatty streaks" in the ascending aorta, especially in the aortic arch. HC rabbits and normal rabbits were injected with 0.8 to 1.0 mCi of [18F]FDG, intravenously. Thirty minutes postinjection, FDG-PET images of rabbit chests were obtained for 10 minutes with use of a GE 4000 brain PET camera. These preliminary studies (unpublished results) demonstrated intense uptake of FDG by the fatty streaks in HC rabbits compared to normal rabbit aortas (Figure 2, panel A). The animals were sacrificed immediately and the aortas were carefully isolated from the rabbits. Ex-vivo FDG-PET images of the HC and normal rabbit aortas (Figure 2, panel B) also showed significant accumulation of FDG in the aortic arch of HC rabbits only.

We previously showed[8,56] that [99mTc]-labeled native and oxidized-LDL preparations localize in fatty streaks of HC rabbits. The major disadvantage of these tracers is that the blood clearance is very slow; as a result, aorta/blood ratios are suboptimal and not ideal for imaging studies. In contrast, the absolute aortic uptake (percent injected dose/gram of tissue) of FDG in HC rabbits was slightly more than radiolabeled LDL preparations (Figure 3, panel A). In addition, FDG clears from circulation very rapidly and minimal activity is present in blood at 30 minutes postinjection. As a result, aorta/blood ratios are six to 10 times higher than [99mTc]-labeled LDL preparations (Figure 3, panel B).

These results clearly suggest that FDG accumulates in atherosclerotic lesions and shows significant potential as a noninvasive marker for the macrophage density in the vulnerable atherosclerotic lesion.

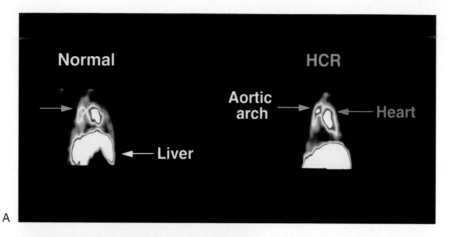

A

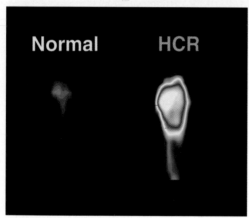

B

Figure 2. A. Positron emission tomographic (PET) images of normal and hypercholesterolemic rabbit (HCR). The images were obtained 30 minutes postinjection of ^{18}F-fluorodeoxyglucose (FDG). The uptake of FDG in the aortic arch of the HCR was significantly higher compared to that in the normal rabbit. **B.** PET images of normal and HCR aortas. The images of the isolated aortas was obtained ex-vivo. The uptake of FDG in the aortic arch of the HCR was significantly higher compared to that in the normal rabbit.

Since FDG clears from circulation rapidly, FDG-PET scans may provide excellent image quality with very high target/background ratios within 1 hour postinjection.

Conclusions

In the last 20 years, many radiotracers were developed for noninvasive nuclear scintigraphic technique to detect and display different characteristics of vascular lesions of clinical and/or research interest. Many of the tracers were developed based on a number of molecules and cells involved in atherogenesis and thrombosis. Proteins labeled with radioiodine, ^{99m}Tc, or ^{111}In were evaluated to image atheroscle-

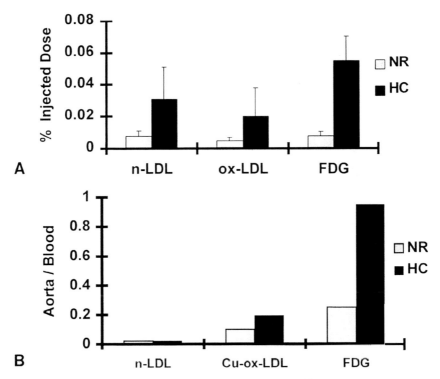

Figure 3. **A.** The uptake (percent injected dose) of ^{18}F-fluorodeoxyglucose (FDG) in normal (NL) and hypercholesterolemic (HC) rabbit aortas: Comparison with ^{99m}Tc-native-LDL and ^{99m}Tc-oxidized-LDL. **B.** Aorta/blood ratios of FDG, ^{99m}Tc-native-LDL, and ^{99m}Tc-oxidized-LDL in normal NL and HC rabbit aortas.

rotic lesions. These include lipoproteins (native LDL and oxidized LDL) and specific and nonspecific immunoglobulins against macrophages, smooth muscle cells, or endothelial adhesion molecules. These tracers showed significant uptake in experimental atherosclerotic lesions. The limited clinical trials, however, could not demonstrate clinical utility, due to slower clearance of radiotracers from circulation and poor target/background ratios. Radiolabeled peptides and metabolic tracers such as FDG, which show faster clearance from circulation and appear to provide higher contrast than radiolabeled proteins, were recently introduced. Similarly, for detecting intra-arterial thrombus, radiolabeled antifibrin antibody fragments and peptides (which bind to glycoprotein IIb/IIIa receptors on activated platelets) clear faster from circulation compared to radiolabeled platelets, and offer significant clinical potential for imaging atherothrombosis. At this time, however, no single radiotracer is ideally suited to image atherosclerosis and provide the prognostic and clinical indicators necessary for medical and surgical interventions. Radiolabeled peptides, antibody fragments, and metabolic tracers like FDG appear to offer new opportunities for noninvasive imaging of atherosclerosis and atherothrombosis. Recent advances in molecular biology have shown the potential significance of many molecules such as PDGF, transforming growth factor- B, interleukin 1 (IL-1), IL-4, and tumor necrosis factor in the pathogenesis of atherosclerosis and response to the injury of arterial wall. Radiolabeled antibody molecules against these biochemicals may also provide an excellent opportunity for noninvasive imaging of atherosclerosis. Therefore, a clear understanding of the cellular and biochemical composition of the vulnerable plaques (and the mechanisms involved in plaque rupture) are crucial for the development of nuclear scintigraphic techniques needed to (1) identify clinically relevant "unstable vulnerable plaques"; (2) quantitate the natural progression of atherosclerotic disease; and finally (3) assess the therapeutic effectiveness of various drugs on the stabilization and regression of plaques.

References

1. Vallabhajosula S, Fuster V. Atherosclerosis: Imaging techniques and the evolving role of nuclear medicine. *J Nucl Med* 1997;38:1788–1796.
2. Sinzinger H, Virgolini I. Nuclear medicine and atherosclerosis. *Eur J Nucl Med* 1990;17:160–178.
3. Kritz H, Underwood SR, Sinzinger H. Imaging of atherosclerosis (Part II). *Wien Klin Wochenschr* 1996;108:87–97.
4. Borer JS. Atherosclerosis imaging: Pathophysiological assessment for a new era. *J Nucl Med* 1993;34:1321–1324.
5. Strauss WH. Imaging atherosclerosis—A worthy challenge. *J Nucl Cardiol* 1996;3:278–280.
6. Chang MY, Lees AM, Lees RS, et al. Time course of ^{125}I-labeled LDL accumulation in the healing, balloon-de-endothelialized rabbit aorta. *Arterioscler Thromb* 1992;12:1088–1098.
7. Lees RS, Lees AM, Strauss HW. External imaging of human atherosclerosis. *J Nucl Med* 1983;24:154–156.
8. Vallabhajosula S, Paidi M, Badimon JJ, et al. Radiotracers for low density lipoprotein biodistribution studies in vivo: Technetium-99m low density lipoprotein versus radioiodinated low density lipoprotein preparations. *J Nucl Med* 1988;29:1237–1245.
9. Rosen JM, Butler SP, Meinken GE, et al. Indium-111 labeled LDL: A potential agent for imaging atherosclerotic disease and lipoprotein distribution. *J Nucl Med* 1990;31:343–350.
10. Lees AM, Lees RS, Schoen FJ, et al. Imaging human atherosclerosis with ^{99m}Tc-labeled low density lipoproteins. *Atherosclerosis* 1988;8:461–468.
11. Virgolini I, Rauscha F, Lupattelli G, et al. Autologous low-density lipoprotein labeling allows characterization of human atherosclerotic lesions in

vivo as to presence of foam cells and endothelial coverage. *Eur J Nucl Med* 1991;18:948–951.

12. Vallabhajosula S, Goldsmith SJ. ^{99m}Tc-low density lipoprotein: Intracellularly trapped radiotracer for non-invasive imaging of LDL metabolism in vivo. *Semin Nucl Med* 1990;20:68–79.

13. Ginsberg HN, Goldsmith SJ, Vallabhajosula S. Non-invasive imaging of [99m]Technetium-labeled low density lipoptoein uptake by tendon xanthomas in hypercholesterolemic subjects. *Arteriosclerosis* 1990;10:256–262.

14. Pirich C, Sinzinger H. Evidence for lipid regression in humans in vivo performed by ^{123}I-low-density lipoprotein scintiscanning. *Ann N Y Acad Sci* 1995, 748: 613–621.

15. Luliano L, Signore A, Vallabhajosula S, et al. Preparation and biodistribution of [99m]Technetium labeled oxidized LDL in man. *Atherosclerosis* 1996; 126:131–141.

16. Chang MY, Lees AM, Lees RS. Low density lipoprotein modification and arterial wall accumulation in a rabbit model of atherosclerosis. *Biochemistry* 1993;32:8518–8524.

17. Shih I-L, Lees RS, Chang MY, Lees AM. Focal accumulation of an apolipoprotein B-based synthetic oligopeptide in the healing rabbit arterial wall. *Proc Natl Acad Sci U S A* 1990;87:1436–1440.

18. Hardoff R, Braegelmann F, Zanzanico P, et al. External imaging of atherosclerosis in rabbits using an ^{123}I-labeled synthetic peptide fragment. *J Clin Pharmacol* 1993;33:1039–1047.

19. Vallabhajosula S, Ali KSM, Goldsmith SJ, et al. Evaluation of Tc-99m labeled peptides for imaging atherosclerotic lesions in vivo. *J Nucl Med* 1993;34: 66P.

20. Lees RS, Lees AM. Radiopharmaceutical imaging of atherosclerosis. In Fuster V ed: *Syndromes of Atherosclerosis: Correlations of Clinical Imaging and Pathology.* Armonk, NY. Futura Publishing Company, Inc; 1996: 369–385–401.

21. Prat L, Torres G, Carrio I, et al. Polyclonal ^{111}In-IgG, ^{125}I-LDL and ^{125}I-endothelin-1 accumulation in experimental arterial wall injury. *Eur J Nucl Med* 1993;20:1141–1145.

22. Dinkelborg LM, Hilger CS, Semmier W. Endothelin derivatives for imaging of atherosclerosis. *J Nucl Med* 1995;36:102P.

23. Fischman AJ, Rubin RH, Khaw BA, et al. Radionuclide imaging of experimental atherosclerosis with nonspecific polyclonal immunoglobulin G. *J Nucl Med* 1989;30:1095–1100.

24. Sinzinger H, Rodrigues M, Kritz H. Radioisotopic imaging of atheroma. In: Fuster V ed: *Syndromes of Atherosclerosis: Correlations of Clinical Imaging and Pathology.* Armonk, NY: Futura Publishing Company, Inc.; 1996: 369–383.

25. Demacker PNM, Dormans TPJ, Koenders EB, Corstens FHM. Evaluation of indium-111- polyclonal immunoglobulin G to quantitate atherosclerosis in Watanabe Heritable Hyperlipidemic rabbits with scintigraphy: Effect of age and treatment with antioxidants or ethinylestradiol. *J Nucl Med* 1993; 34:1316–1321.

26. Narula J, Petrov A, Bianchi C, et al. Noninvasive localization of experimental atherosclerotic lesions with mouse/human chimeric Z2D3 F(ab')2 specific for the proliferating smooth muscle cells of human atheroma. Imaging with conventional and negative charge-modified antibody fragments. *Circulation* 1995;92:474–484.

27. Carrio I, Pieri P, Prat L, et al. In-111 Chimeric negative-charged Z2D3 PL-F(ab')$_2$ in the detection of atherosclerotic plaques. *J Nucl Med* 1995;36:133P. Abstract.

28. Chakrabarti M, Cheng K, Spicer KM, et al. Biodistribution and radiopharmacokinetics of ^{131}I-Ama monoclonal antibody in atherosclerotic rabbits. *Nucl Med Biol* 1995;22:693–697.

29. Loscalzo J, Rocco TP. Imaging arterial thrombi. An elusive goal. *Circulation* 1992;85:382–385.

30. Vallabhajosula S, Machac J, Goldsmith SJ, et al. Indium-111 platelet kinetics in normal human subjects: Tropolone versus oxine. *J Nucl Med* 1986;27: 1669–1674.

31. Becker W, Borst U, Krahe T, Borner W. Tc-99m-HMPAO labeled human platelets: In vitro and in vivo results. *Eur J Nucl Med* 1989;15:296–301.

32. Smyth JV, Dodd PDF, Walker MG. Indium-111 platelet scintigraphy in vascular disease. *Br J Surg* 1995;82;588–595.

33. Minar E, Ehringer H, Dudczak R, et al. Indium-111-labeled platelet scintigraphy in carotid atherosclerosis. *Stroke* 1989;20:27–33.

34. Moriwaki H, Matsumoto M, Handa N, et al. Functional and anatomic evaluation of carotid atherosclerosis. A combined study of In-111 platelet scintigraphy and B-mode ultrasonography. *Arterioscler Thromb Vasc Biol* 1995;15: 2234–2240.

35. Mettinger KL, Larsson S, Ericson K, Casseborn S. Detection of atherosclerotic plaques in carotid arteries by the use of ^{123}I-fibrinogen. *Lancet* 1978; 1(8058):242–244.

36. Uehara A, Isaka Y, Hashikawa K, et al. Iodine-131-labeled fibronectin: Potential agent for imaging atherosclerotic lesion and thrombus. *J Nucl Med* 1988;29:1264–1267.

37. Knight LC. Scintigraphic methods for detecting vascular thrombus. *J Nucl Med* 1993;34:554–561.

38. Thiagarajan P, Tait JF. Binding of annexin V, placental anicoagulant protein I to platelets. Evidence for phosphatidylserine exposure in the procoagulant response of activated platelets. *J Biol Chem* 1990;265:17420–17423.

39. Stratton JR, Dewhurst TA, Kasina S, et al. Selective uptake of radiolabeled annexin V on acute porcine left atrial thrombi. *Circulation* 1995;92: 3113–3121.

40. Miller DD. Radionuclide labeled monoclonal antibody imaging of atherosclerosis and vascular injury. In: Fuster V ed: *Syndromes of Atherosclerosis: Correlations of Clinical Imaging and Pathology.* Armonk, NY: Futura Publishing Company, Inc.; 1996:403–416.

41. Seabold JE, Rosebrough SF. Will a radiolabeled antibody replace In-111-platelets to detect active thrombus? [Editorial] *J Nucl Med* 1994;35: 1738–1740.

42. Stratton JR, Cerqueira MD, Dewhurst TA, Kohler TR. Imaging arterial thrombosis in humans: Comparison of technetium-99m-labeled monoclonal antifibrin antibodies and indium-111-labeled- platelets. *J Nucl Med* 1994;35:1731–1737.

43. Knight LC, Maurer AH, Romano JE, et al. Comparison of iodine-123-disintegrins for imaging thrombi and emboli in a canine model. *J Nucl Med* 1996; 37:476–482.

44. Lister-James J, Lister-James J, Knight LC, et al. Thrombus imaging with a technetium-99m- labeled activated platelet receptor-binding peptide. *J Nucl Med* 1996;37:775–781.

45. Lister-James J, Vallabhajosula S, Moyer BR, et al. Thrombus imaging using Technetioum-99m- labeled, activated platelet receptor-binding peptides: Pre-clinical evaluation of ^{99m}Tc-P748. *J Nucl Med* 1997;38:105–111.

46. Barrett JA, Bresnick M, Crocker A, et al. RP431, a potential thrombus imaging agent. *J Nucl Med* 1995;36:16P.

47. Vallabhajosula S, Lister-James J, Dean RT, et al. Technetium-99m-P748, platelet specific techtide[tm] for imaging arterial thrombus: Preclinical studies in a canine model of intra-arterial thrombus. *J Nucl Med* 1996;37:152p.

48. Kohler TR. Imaging of carotid artery lesions: A surgeon's view. In Fuster V ed: *Syndromes of Atherosclerosis: Correlations of Clinical Imaging and Pathology.* Armonk, NY: Futura Publishing Company, Inc.; 1996:205–223.

49. Weinberger J, Ramos L, Ambrose JA, Fuster V. Morphologic and dynamic changes of atherosclerotic plaque at the carotid artery bifuration: Sequential imaging by real-time B-mode ultrasonography. *J Am Coll Cardiol* 1988;12: 1515–1521.

50. Patel MR, Kuntz KM, Klufas RA, et al. Preoperative assessment of the carotid bifurcation. Can magnetic resonance angiography and duplex ultrasonography replace contrast arteriography? *Stroke* 1995;26:1753–1758.

51. Vallabhajosula S, Weinberger J, Machac J, et al. Technetium-99m P280, activated platelet specific techtide[tm]: Phase II clinical studies in patients with carotid atherosclerosis. *J Nucl Med* 1996;37:272p.

52. Phelps ME, Hoffman EJ, Selin C, et al. Investigation of 18F-2-deoxyglucose for the measurement of myocardial glucose metabolism. *J Nucl Med* 1978; 19:1311–1319.

53. Strauss LG, Conti PS. The applications of PET in clinical oncology. *J Nucl Med* 1991;32:623–648.

54. Kubota R, Kubota K, Yamada S, et al. Microautoradiographic study for the differentiation of intratumoral macrophages, granulation tissues and cancer cells by the dynamics of fluorine-18- fluorodeoxyglucose uptake. *J Nucl Med* 1994;35:104–112.

55. Vallabhajosula J, Machac K, Knesaurek J, et al. Imaging atherosclerotic macrophage density by positron emission tomography using F-18-fluorodeoxyglucose (FDG). *J Nucl Med* 1996;37:38p.

56. Ali KSM, Vallabhajosula S, Censi C, et al. Biodistribution and imaging of Tc-99m-native-LDL and oxidized-LDL. *J Nucl Med* 1993;34:67P.

Chapter 13

Thermography

Ward Casscells, MD, Mark David, MD,
Greg Bearman, PhD, Fred Clubb, Jr., PhD, DVM,
and James T. Willerson, MD

A frustrating problem in modern cardiology is that people who feel well and have no known cardiovascular disease continue to die suddenly of a first myocardial infarction or cardiac arrest. Usually, these patients have not been seen by a cardiologist. Therefore many cardiologists do not recognize the magnitude of the problem. Ten years ago, Ambrose and colleagues[1] and, separately, Little and colleagues[2] pointed out that angiograms of patients who experience myocardial infarction frequently show an occlusive thrombus in an area that is not "significantly" stenosed from a hemodynamic standpoint. Most of the plaques confer a 50% to 70% stenosis angiographically, which may be an overestimate, since thrombolysis is often incomplete; and in those patients who had angiograms in the 6 months prior to their infarction, the stenosis at the site that subsequently occluded was typically 50% or less.[3–6]

Pathological studies have described thrombosis on more substantial plaques, reflecting the fact that angiography underestimates the amount of intramural plaque.[3,4,6] Autopsy studies have also demonstrated that the plaques that rupture are typically inflamed with a thin fibrous cap.[7] The thinness of the cap has been attributed to a paucity of smooth muscle cells—which produce the collagen—perhaps due to apoptosis.[8] Active digestion of the plaque by enzymes released from macrophages, and perhaps from smooth muscle cells, has also been demonstrated in experimental models and in human atherosclerotic

Supported in part by NHLBI grant No. 1RO1 HL50179-01, NHLBI Grant No. 1RO1 HL54839-01A1, Training Grant T32HL07591, State of Texas House Bill #1, Article III, Education, 75th Legislative Session, and U. S. Army Grant No. DAMD17-98-1-8002.

From: Fuster, V (ed). *The Vulnerable Atherosclerotic Plaque: Understanding, Identification, and Modification.* Armonk, NY: Futura Publishing Company, Inc.; © 1999.

specimens.[6] The two explanations for plaque thinning are not mutually exclusive. Plaques with this morphology represent a minority of plaques.

Given the rapid improvement in prognosis in patients with coronary atherosclerosis in the past two decades—to the point where annual mortality is down to 1% to 3% in many series—the important public health problem now is in identifying patients who are sick but don't know it. This might be achieved by noninvasive and inexpensive techniques to identify plaque vulnerability, perhaps in conjunction with techniques to identify systemic inflammatory and hemostatic conditions.[9]

Invasive techniques to identify vulnerable plaques would also enable us to test the increasingly popular hypothesis that prognosis is, to a large extent, plaque-specific.[10] Numerous studies indicate that strong prognostic variables, such as a depressed left ventricular ejection fraction, apply to only a minority of patients. This leaves the majority of patients without an adverse prognostic variable, yet these patients account, in the aggregate, for the majority of deaths. Hence, our ability to give a prognosis to a particular patient is limited.

Longitudinal studies of individual lesions in the same patient have demonstrated that several can progress while others regress, and others remain unchanged over time. The influence of laminar flow and shear can perhaps explain some of this lesion-specific variability in outcome, but techniques that might identify plaque vulnerability on the basis of cap thinness, such as intravascular ultrasound, have not yet proven practical,[5] perhaps because the cap thickness at the time of rupture is estimated to be 50 μm on average.[3,4,6]

We recently proposed that inflamed plaques might give off more heat than noninflamed plaques.[11] Inflammation has long been known to be characterized by heat (*calor, tumor, rubor* and *dolor* being the classic features of inflammation), though it is not known whether the heat is produced by inflammatory cells or by the parenchymal cells in inflamed organs.

We further reasoned that heat detection would permit the localization not only of the superficial inflammation, which characterizes the denuded and eroded plaques (which account for approximately 40% of myocardial infarctions and sudden deaths), but also plaques thought to be vulnerable due to inflammation beneath a thin fibrous cap. We reasoned that the temperature of the cap would be proportional to the density and metabolic activity of the inflammatory cells and to their proximity to the surface.

Methods

We studied 26 atherosclerotic plaques removed from 26 patients at the time of carotid endarterectomy performed for symptoms or for severe angiographic stenosis. With the approval of the Institutional Review Board of the St. Luke's Episcopal Hospital and the Texas Heart Institute, specimens were collected in the operating room and immediately inspected by the pathologist (FC) prior to examination with a 24-gauge needle thermistor (Cole-Parmer Model No. 8402-20, resolution 0.1°C.; time constant 0.15 sec) in a 37° chamber. The specimens were examined at approximately 2-mm intervals, yielding approximately 30 measurements per plaque. This enabled a background temperature to be established with, in general, 10 zones per plaque, showing variations of more than 0.2°C. For each plaque, the background temperature in two other zones (most of which were warmer than background) were marked with colorfast dye of different colors for subsequent localization on tissue sections. The tissues were then fixed in 10% formalin, cut and embedded to reveal the intima and media, and processed for routine histology followed by staining with haematoxylon and eosin or Masson's trichrome or immunostaining for macrophages with the HAM-56 and KP1 (CD68) antibodies from Dako.

Under a Nikon microscope (SMZ-U Nikon Optiphot-2) the cell density was measured in a 300×400-μm region beneath the marked regions, using the program NIH Image, Version 1.43.

In another series of experiments, with the permission of the University of Texas Animal Care and Use Committee, 1-year-old Watanabe hypercholesterolemic rabbits were anesthetized and the aortas were removed. They were quickly rinsed, studied by use of the thermistor technique described above, and subjected to routine photography and infrared photography with a Mark 5 Flexi-Therm IR camera (Westbury, NY).

Results

As shown in Figure 1, the temperature of the lumen surface in living human carotid endarterectomy specimens varied within the same specimen by as much as 4°C. The thermistor's characteristics and the reproducibility of the temperatures at these locations were excellent (always 0.2°C or less), and all of the specimens demonstrated differences of 0.3°C or more between their warmest and coolest measured locations.

Not shown is the fact that the cells closest to the surface, presumably contributing the bulk of the heat, were mostly macrophages, as determined by immunohistology with several antibodies to human macrophages, including HAM-56 and KP-1, and electron microscopy.

The deeper the clusters of cells with respect to the surface, the lower the temperature at the surface. The analysis arbitrarily included both acellular and hypocellular caps, since so few caps are completely

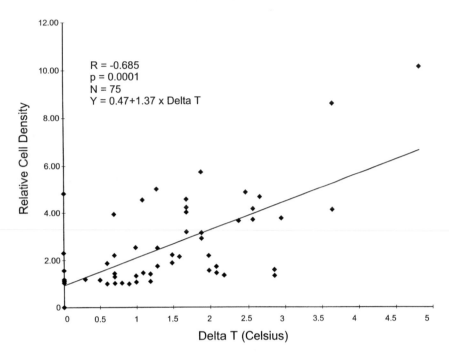

Figure 1. Temperature differences correlate with the underlying cell density in living human carotid atherectomy specimens. Specimens from 26 patients were measured with a needle thermistor at approximately 30 locations on the luminal surface of each plaque, and grouped into approximately 10 isothermal zones. The coolest zone was designated the background temperature. That and the zone of median temperature and zone of hottest temperature are plotted (ie, 78 points for 26 patients). Twenty-four points are at the intercept of the vertical axis.

acellular, and no distinction was made between endothelialized and nonendothelialized caps, nor was a distinction made between regions with just a cluster of cells that might act as a point source of heat versus regions with a layer of diffuse cellularity beneath the surface. Finally, no distinction was made between inflammatory and smooth muscle cells. Nevertheless, there was a statistically significant inverse relationship between cell depth (essentially, cap thickness) and surface temperature (Fig. 2). Figure 3 illustrates some of the marked variability in histology that limits a more exact analysis.

Similar relationships of heat to cell density and cell depth were found in Watanabe-heritable hypercholesterolemic rabbits, as shown in Figures 4 and 5.

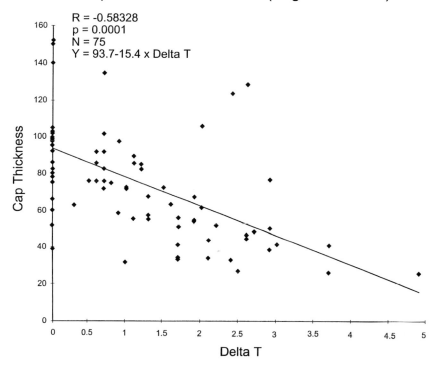

Figure 2. The temperature at the surface of living human carotid endarterectomy specimens is inversely proportional to the depth of the underlying cells. The specimens were obtained and measured as described in Figure 1. The thickness of the cap (defined as an acellular or hypocellular fibrous region at the lumen, with or without overlying endothelium) was measured from vertical sections through the plaque and analyzed using the NIH Image Program.

An infrared camera which correlated with mercury-bulb thermometry (Fig. 6) showed living atherosclerotic rabbit aortic tissue with remarkable thermal heterogeneity (Fig. 7). In another explanted aortic segment, similar heterogeneity was documented with use of the needle thermistor (Fig. 8).

Discussion

The present results demonstrate that living human and rabbit atherosclerotic plaques exhibit thermal heterogeneity on their luminal surface, and this relates well to the depth of underlying cells, most of

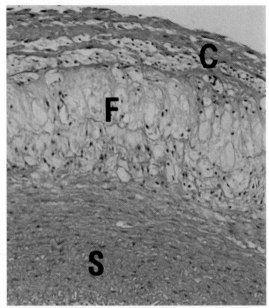

A

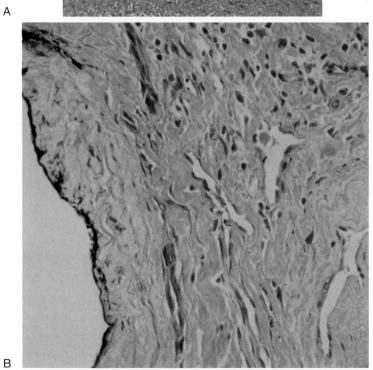

B

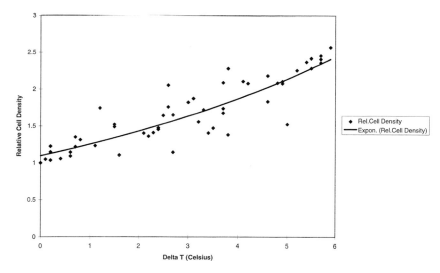

Figure 4. Relation of temperature to the density of underlying cells in living Watanabe rabbit aorta tissue examined ex vivo, using the methods of Figure 1. R = 0.88025; *P*<0.0001; y = 1.03 + 0.22 (Delta T).

which are macrophages. It is likely that lesions with inflammatory cells on the surface are dangerous because of the thrombotic tendency of these cells and the lack of antithrombotic and vasorelaxing endothelium. It is also likely that thin caps with inflammatory cells in or beneath the caps are at risk of rupture. However, we cannot yet conclude that a hot plaque indeed goes on to rupture. This will require prospective studies, and these will be challenging because of the lack of a universally accepted animal model of plaque rupture. Nevertheless, there

◄───

Figure 3. A. Photomicrograph of a warm specimen with a denuded and partially infiltrated cap of approximately 50 μm in thickness (C) overlying a region of foam cells (F), which in turn overlies a zone of smooth muscle cells. This particular plaque is relatively devoid of vasa vasorum and has little in the way of a necrotic core (pultaceous debris). No thrombus is evident at the surface, despite the lack of endothelium (H&E stain). **B.** Higher-power view of a Masson trichrome-stained specimen of the same temperature and cap thickness as in **A**, but this specimen is characterized by angiogenesis and non–foam-cell macrophages beneath the cap, and the endothelium (obscured by the application of colorfast dye) was intact. As in **A**, there is little in the way of a necrotic core, except for an amorphous region at the lower left corner. Which of the two plaques is more dangerous, and what impact the differences in angiogenesis and foam-cell content have, are questions for future research.

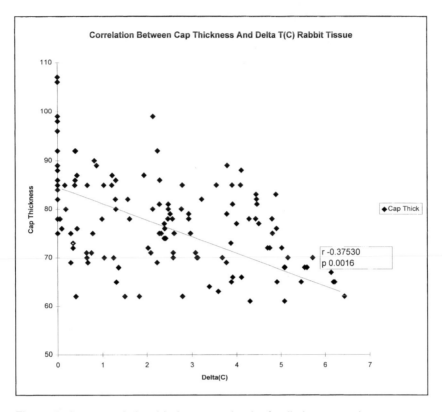

Figure 5. Inverse relationship between depth of cell clusters and temperature at the luminal surface of living Watanabe rabbit aorta, by use of a needle thermistor, as described in Figure 2.

may be utility in a technique that could address the risk of plaque rupture—the cause of approximately 60% of myocardial infarctions and an unknown number of strokes[3]—and also help predict the risk of thrombosis due to endothelial denudation and superficial inflammation and erosion (the underlying substrate in 30% to 40% of fatal myocardial infarctions).[3] Thermal techniques could conceivably be combined with ultrasound catheters, or newer techniques, such as optical coherence tomography,[12] to provide both functional and anatomic information. Noninvasive studies, such as positron tomography and magnetic resonance imaging, could also conceivably be adapted to provide similar information, since inflammatory cells avidly consume glucose, and it should be possible to image them using 18- fluorodeoxyglucose. Thermal magnetic resonance imaging has been used in some animal models to follow heat therapy for experimental tumors, but the

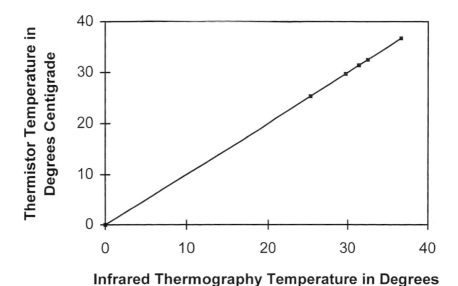

Figure 6. Graph showing the close correlation between infrared temperature measurements and mercury bulb thermometer measurements of beakers of water at various temperatures.

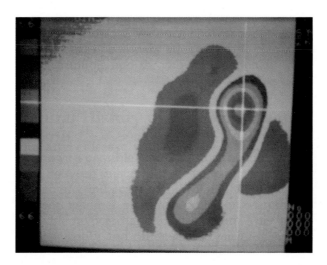

Figure 7. Infrared photomicrograph of living aortic tissue (luminal surface) of a Watanabe-heritable hypercholesterolemic rabbit.

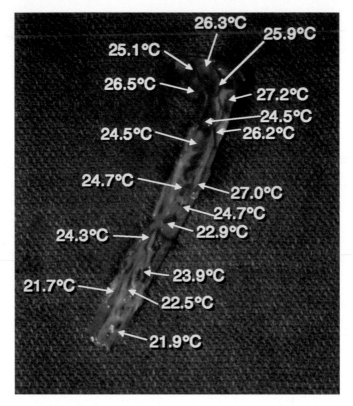

Figure 8. Temperature differences in living aorta (ex vivo) of a Watanabe-heritable hypercholesterolemic rabbit, as determined with use of a needle thermistor.

current thermal resolution is in the range of 1° to 3°C, which exceeds the thermal heterogeneity of many human carotid plaques.

Potential Therapeutic Implications

If it can be shown that hot plaques do indeed go on to develop superficial thrombosis and/or rupture, they conceivably could be treated with angioplasty on the grounds that rupture and/or thrombosis is better performed in a safe, controlled environment, such as the cardiac catheterization laboratory, where patients can be treated with heparin, ticlopidine, stenting, etc., rather than at a random time outside the hospital.

Therapies other than angioplasty and stenting also suggest themselves. These might include local treatment with anti-inflammatory drugs, antibiotics,[13] or cytokines, such as TGF β-1, which is anti-inflammatory while at the same time stimulates smooth muscle cell proliferation and matrix secretion. Yet another treatment might be gentle heating to invoke apoptosis of microphages. Treatments such as these may temporarily stabilize the patient until atherosclerotic regression in response to statins, aspirin, antioxidants, ACE inhibitors, and lifestyle changes can take hold.

It has not escaped our notice that macrophage density has been found by Moreno et al[14] to be the best cellular predictor of restenosis. Therefore, heat-localizing techniques might also be useful to predict lesions at risk of restenosis. Heat localization may also aid in predicting the rate of progression of inflammatory aneurysms.[15,16]

References

1. Ambrose JA, Tannenbaum MA, Alexopoulos D, et al. Angiographic progression of coronary artery disease in the development of myocardial infarction. *J Am Coll Cardiol* 1988;12:56–62.
2. Little WC, Constaninescu M, Applegate RJ, et al. Can coronary angiography predict the site of a subsequent myocardial infarction in patients with mild to moderate coronary artery disease? *Circulation* 1988;78:1157–1166.
3. Burke AP, Farb A, Malcom GT, et al. Coronary risk factors and plaque morphology in men with coronary disease who died suddenly. *N Engl J Med* 1997;336:1276–1281.
4. Mann JM, Davies MJ. Vulnerable plaque. *Circulation* 1996;94:928–931.
5. de Feyter PJ, Ozaki Y, Baptista J, et al. Ischemia-related lesion characteristics in patients with stable or unstable angina. *Circulation* 1995;93:1408–1413.
6. Falk E, Shah Pk, Fuster V. Coronary plaque disruption. *Circulation* 1995; 92:657–671.
7. Van der Wal AC, Becker AE, van der Loos CM, Das PK. Site of intimal rupture or erosion of thrombosed coronary atherosclerotic plaques is characterized by an inflammatory process irrespective of the dominant plaque morphology. *Circulation* 1994;89:36–44.
8. Libby P, Geng YJ, Aikawa M, et al. Macrophages and atherosclerotic plaque stability. *Curr Opin Lipidology* 1996;7:330–335.
9. Davies MJ. Detecting vulnerable coronary plaques. *Lancet* 1996;347:1422.
10. Lee RT, Libby P. The unstable atheroma. *Arterioscler Thromb Vasc Biol* 1997; 17:1859–1867.
11. Casscells W, Hathorn B, David M, et al. Thermal detection of cellular infiltrates in living atherosclerotic plaques: Possible implications for plaque rupture and thrombosis. *Lancet* 1996;347:1447–1449.
12. Brezinski ME, Tearney GJ, Bouma BE, et al. Optical coherence tomography for optical biopsy: Properties and demonstration of vascular pathology. *Circulation* 1996;93:1206–1213.
13. Gupta S, Leatham EW, Carrington D, et al. Elevated Chlamydia pneumoniae antibodies, cardiovascular events, and azithromycin in male survivors of myocardial infarction. *Circulation* 1997;96:404–407.
14. Moreno PR, Bernardi VH, Lopez-Cuellar J, et al. Macrophage infiltration

predicts restenosis after coronary intervention in patients with unstable angina. *Circulation* 1996;94:3089–3102.

15. Dobrin PB, Baumgartner N, Anidjar S, et al. Inflammatory aspects of experimental aneurysms: Effect of methylprednisolone and cyclosporine. *Ann N Y Acad Sci* 1996;800:74–88.

16. Freestone T, Turner RJ, Coady A, et al. Inflammation and matrix metalloproteinases in the enlarging abdominal aortic aneurysm. *Arterioscler Thromb Vasc Biol* 1995;15:1145.

Chapter 14

Cardiovascular Imaging with Optical Coherence Tomography

Mark E. Brezinski, MD, PhD, Guillermo J. Tearney, PhD, James F. Southern, MD, PhD, and James G. Fujimoto, PhD

Introduction

Several groups have now shown that most myocardial infarctions result from the rupture of mild to moderately sized cholesterol-laden plaques in the coronary arteries, followed by thrombosis and vessel occlusion.[1-4] In general, with currently available imaging technologies these lesions cannot be characterized prior to rupture.[4,5] A clinical need exists for an imaging technology that is capable of assessing tissue microstructure near the level of histopathology. Optical coherence tomography (OCT), a recently developed technology capable of micron scale imaging, appears promising for ultrahigh resolution, intravascular imaging, and the diagnosis of high-risk coronary lesions.[6,7]

OCT is analogous to ultrasound, measuring the intensity of backreflected infrared light rather than acoustic waves.[6] With OCT, low-coherence light, which can be viewed for illustrative purposes as analogous to a train of pulses, is directed at the sample (Fig. 1). The time for light to be reflected back from the sample, or ECHO delay time, is used to measure distances. However, due to the high speeds associated with the propagation of light, the ECHO delay time cannot be measured

Supported in part by grants to M.E.B. from the Whittaker Foundation and the National Institutes of Health and to J.G.F. from the National Institutes of Health, the Medical Free Electron Laser Program, Office of Naval Research, the Air Force Office of Scientific Research, the Joint Services Electronics Program.

From: Fuster, V (ed). *The Vulnerable Atherosclerotic Plaque: Understanding, Identification, and Modification.* Armonk, NY: Futura Publishing Company, Inc.; © 1999.

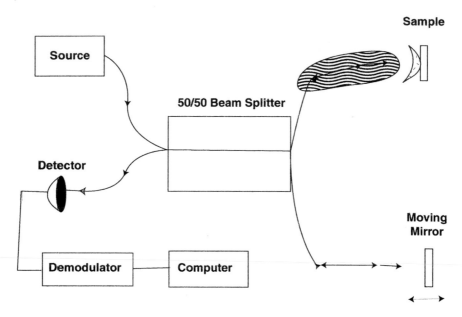

Figure 1. Schematic of the optical coherence tomography system. Shaded area is region within the catheter.

electronically. Therefore, a technique known as *low-coherence interferometry*, which requires a reference arm, must be used.

The principles behind low-coherence interferometry are illustrated in Figure 1. With interferometry, light emitted by the source is split evenly down two fibers, one directed at the sample and one toward a mirror. These are designated the sample arm and the reference arm, respectively. Light reflects off the mirror and from within the sample. Backreflected light in both arms is recombined in the beam splitter. If reflected light from each arm arrives at the beam splitter almost simultaneously (specifically, nearly matched in group delay), interference will occur. OCT measures the intensity of interference, which is used to represent backscattering or backreflecting intensity. To obtain interference data from different depths within the tissue, the path light travels (optical pathlength) in the reference arm must be varied. This is achieved in original OCT systems by translating the reference mirror. The result is a plot of backreflection intensity as a function of depth. Once data are obtained in a single axial plane, the beam is scanned across the sample to produce two- and three-dimensional data sets.

Although OCT was originally used to image the transparent tissue of the eye, recent advances have allowed imaging in nontransparent tissue (see below).[6-12] Several features of OCT suggest its potential for high-resolution intravascular imaging. First, although penetration is generally less than 3 mm, the use of light allows extremely high resolutions to be achieved. OCT images at the subcellular level (4 μm) have now been obtained.[13] Second, the fiber-based design allows relatively straightforward integration with catheters and endoscopes. A 2.9-French OCT imaging catheter has been developed which, unlike ultrasound, contains no transducer within the catheter body, making it relatively inexpensive.[14] Third, unlike ultrasound, OCT requires no transducing medium and can be performed through air or saline. Fourth, OCT is compact and portable, an important consideration within the tight confines of the catheterization laboratory. Finally, unlike magnetic resonance imaging (MRI) or computed tomography (CT), OCT can be performed at or near real time. Current systems exist at 4 to 8 frames per second, but video rates are likely attainable with future modifications.[15]

In this chapter the historical application of OCT to imaging in transparent tissue is briefly discussed. Then, the advances leading to imaging in nontransparent tissue, particularly the cardiovascular system, are described, followed by a short discussion on the potential limitations for in vivo cardiovascular imaging. The chapter concludes with an expanded technical discussion in the *Technical Appendix*.

Imaging in Transparent Tissue

The initial results on OCT, published in *Science* in 1991, demonstrated tomographic imaging of the human retina in vitro.[6] The work was performed as a collaborative effort between James Fujimoto, PhD, of the Department of Electrical Engineering at MIT, Eric Swanson from the Optical Communications Group at M.I.T. Lincoln Laboratory, and Carmen A. Puliafito, MD, of New England Eye Center. An OCT prototype system suitable for performing preliminary clinical studies was developed and, in 1993, obtained the first in vivo OCT images in transparent tissue of human subjects. Studies suggest that OCT will be especially important in the diagnosis and management of three diseases in particular: macular holes, retinal edema, and glaucoma.[6,9–11]

Cardiovascular Optical Coherence Tomography Imaging

Nontransparent Tissue

In late 1995, we demonstrated the potential of OCT for identifying pathology in nontransparent tissue.[7,8] One of the most important ad-

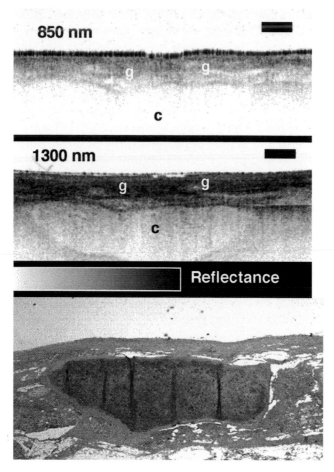

Figure 2. Wavelength dependency of optical coherence tomography (OCT) imaging. A major advance in OCT imaging was the identification of an "optical window" in the near infrared (1300 nm), which allowed significant penetration in nontransparent tissue. Here, we see OCT imaging performed at 850 nm and 1300 nm in an in vitro human epiglottis. The underlying cartilage can be seen at 1300 nm but not at 850 nm. The corresponding histology has been included. Bar represents 500 μm. Reproduced from Reference 7.

vances which allowed imaging to be performed in nontransparent tissue was an increase in the incident wavelength from 850 nm to 1300 nm that substantially increased the penetration.[7] This is demonstrated in Figure 2, in which a human epiglottis is imaged at the two wavelengths but the same incident power (100 μW). The underlying cartilage is seen at 1300 nm but not at 850 nm. The 1300-nm wavelength was chosen because it is well above the high scattering and absorption present in the visible region but below the relatively large absorption peak of water at 1500 nm.[16] Therefore, this wavelength takes advantage of the relatively low absorption and scattering that occurred in this optical window.

Early In Vitro Imaging

Initial in vitro imaging of human aorta demonstrated a strong correlation between data attained from atherosclerotic plaque and the corresponding histopathology. This imaging, which was performed at $16 \pm 1 \mu$m, delineated thin intimal caps and fissures at unprecedented resolution.[17] In addition, both high contrast between lipid and nonlipid tissue, and an ability to image through heavily calcified tissue were demonstrated.[7] Examples follow.

Data that demonstrate the potential of OCT for identifying high-risk coronary plaques are shown in Figure 3.[7] The top is an OCT image of an atherosclerotic plaque (p) abutting grossly normal intima. The most significant feature is the thin intimal layer overlying the plaque (arrow), which is less than 30 μm in diameter in some regions. An imaging technology capable of identifying fine microstructural detail, such as thin intimal walls, will likely be a powerful tool for patient risk stratification.

In addition to thin intimal walls, another characteristic of plaque instability is fissuring. Figure 4 demonstrates the ability of OCT to define fissuring within an aortic plaque.[7] A fissure extends from the vessel lumen into a large underlying plaque (p). The presence of the fissure and plaque are confirmed by histopathology.

An ability to generate high contrast between lipid and nonlipid tissue is important for the identification of high-risk coronary plaques. The ability of OCT to identify lipid collections within the wall of atherosclerotic plaques is shown in Figure 5.[7] In this heavily calcified plaque, a region of lipid (arrow) is noted over 500 μm below the tissue surface.

Of note, the ability of OCT to identify pathology in other organ systems, including the gastrointestinal tract, nervous system, reproductive tract, skin, and urinary tract, has been confirmed.[18-21]

Comparison with High-Frequency Ultrasound

Both catheter-based and linear OCT imaging have been directly compared with high-frequency ultrasound (IVUS), the current clinical technology with the highest resolution. These technologies were assessed both qualitatively and quantitatively. The axial resolution of both OCT and IVUS (30 MHz) were measured directly from the point-spread function off the surface of a mirror. The axial resolution of OCT was 16 ± 1 μm compared with 110 ± 7 μm for IVUS.[17]

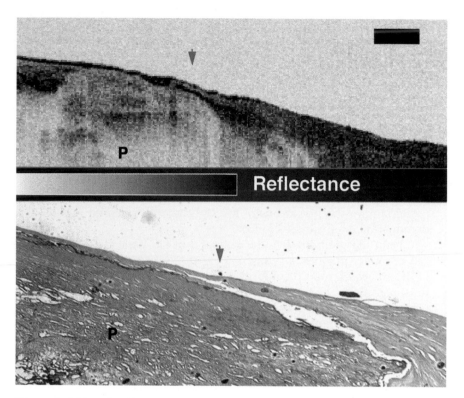

Figure 3. Thin intimal layer. The ability to identify thin intimal caps is important in patient risk stratification. An OCT image of an in vitro aortic plaque is shown here. The thin intimal cap (arrow) can be clearly identified above the plaque, which is less than 30 μm in diameter in some locations. Bar represents 500 μm. Reproduced from Reference 7.

When OCT and IVUS were compared qualitatively, OCT consistently demonstrated superior delineation of structural detail. In Figure 6, an aortic plaque was imaged in vitro with OCT and IVUS. In the IVUS image (top), though the presence of the plaque is suggested, no other structural detail is apparent.[17] In the OCT image, in addition to a plaque, a highly backscattered layer is seen within the intima, which appeared normal by ultrasound. This layer is confirmed by histopathology (bottom) to represent smooth muscle proliferation.

Once again, in the upper IVUS image (Fig. 7) a plaque can be identified but other structural information is minimal.[17] In the OCT image, not only is the plaque identified, but other localized areas of lipid are also detected within the wall of the plaque. Furthermore, the wall thickness of overlying intima, as assessed with OCT, strongly correlates with histopathology.

In Figure 8, an image of an in vitro human coronary artery, generated with a 2.9-French OCT catheter, is compared with that of a 2.9-French, 30-MHz IVUS catheter. Structural detail is superior with the OCT catheter when compared with the IVUS transducer.[22]

Advances Toward In Vivo Imaging

To develop OCT for in vivo intravascular imaging, the construction of a high-speed, catheter- based system is required. The OCT system

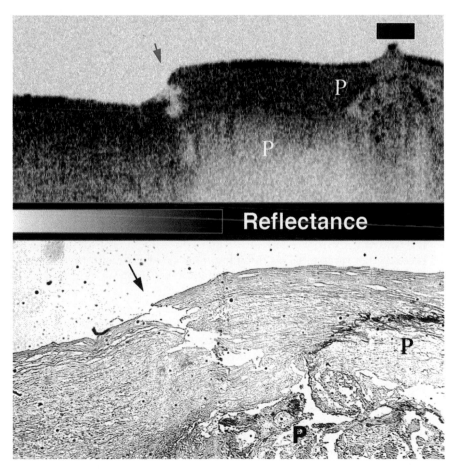

Figure 4. Fissure. Identification of signs of structural instability, such as fissures, is also critical for imaging technology. A fissure (arrow) in an in vitro aortic plaque is shown here. The fissures extends into a large underlying plaque. The corresponding histology has been included. The bar represents 500 μm. Reproduced from Reference 7.

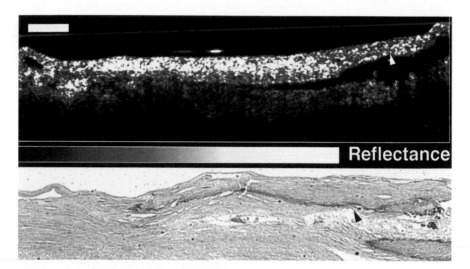

Figure 5. Lipid-filled plaque. The ability to distinquish between lipid and nonlipid tissue is important in the identification of high-risk plaques. Here, a lipid collection is noted on the left side of the image (arrow), embedded within this heavily calcified aorta. Bar represents 500 μm. Reproduced from Reference 7.

used to generate original in vitro images—which changed the optical pathlength in the reference arm with a linearly translating galvanometer (moving mirror)—had an acquisition rate of approximately 40 seconds per image.[8] This imaging rate is insufficient to eliminate the motion artifacts associated with in vivo imaging. Furthermore, commercial galvanometers do not generate sufficient mechanical translation rates to allow imaging in real time. An alternative method recently developed involves keeping the mirror stationary while stretching the fiber in the reference arm.[15] The fiber is wrapped around a piezoelectric crystal, which expands when voltage is passed across it. Acquisition rates of 4 frames per second have been achieved with this method. However, although piezoelectric fiber stretchers allow rapid scanning, they have very high power requirements, which may be dangerous in the clinical environment. In addition, it is difficult to increase acquisition rates above 10 frames per second with this method because of nonlinear fringe modulation due to hysteresis, uncompensated polarization dispersion matches, and poor temperature stability. For this reason, other methods are currently being aggressively pursed.

As stated above, a 2.9-French OCT imaging catheter that contains no transducer within the frame has been developed.[14] The catheter consists of an optical fiber, grin lens, light directing prism, speedome-

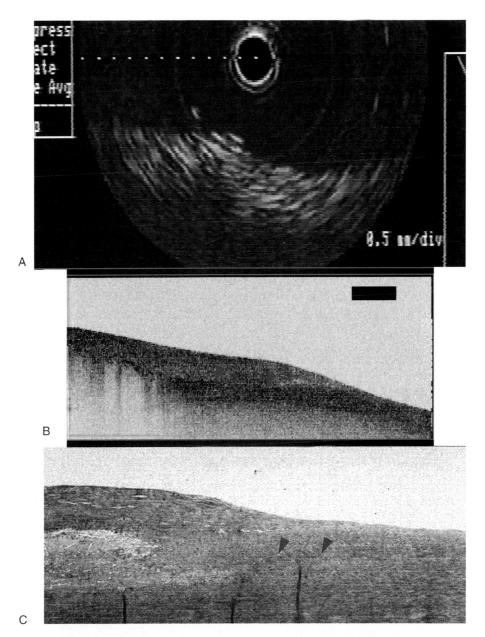

Figure 6. Comparison of optical coherence tomography (OCT) and high-frequency ultrasound (IVUS). **A.** Image of in vitro aortic plaque generated with a 30-MHz IVUS transducer. **B.** Image generated with OCT. OCT identified not only the plaque, but a layer of smooth muscle proliferation within the plaque. Bar and grid separations represent 500 microns. Reproduced from Reference 17.

ter cable, and external casing. Catheters are currently being constructed with smaller external diameters.

In vivo imaging of the rabbit esophagus, respiratory tract, and aorta has recently been performed.[23]

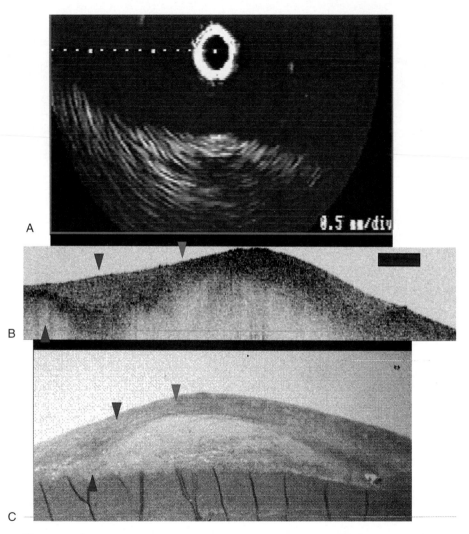

Figure 7. Comparison of optical coherence tomography (OCT) and high-frequency ultrasound (IVUS) **A.** Image of in vitro aortic plaque generated with a 30-Mhz IVUS transducer. **B.** Image generated with OCT. OCT identified both the plaque and localized lipid collections within the wall of the plaque. Bar and grid separations represent 500 µm. Reproduced from Reference 17.

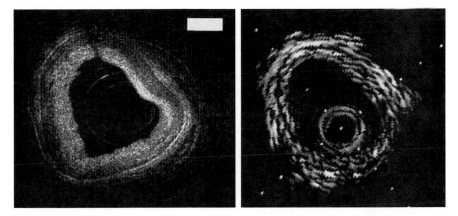

Figure 8. Comparison of optical coherence tomography (OCT) and high-frequency ultrasound (IVUS) catheter-based imaging. The image on the left is an OCT image of an in vitro coronary artery, compared with an IVUS image (right). The superior resolution of the OCT image is evident. Bar and grids represent 1 mm. Reproduced from Reference 22.

Limitations

The potential limitations of OCT for in vivo intravascular imaging are the possible reductions of image quality when imaging through blood or large volumes of tissue, the relatively slow current data acquisition rates, the current lack of a portable source for in vivo imaging, and multiple scattering.

Unlike most other tissue, blood is a dynamic scatter of light whose properties change with not only cell concentration, but also such factors as blood velocity, oxygenation state, and cell shape.[24] However, based on transmission data, it can be assumed that blood will lead to substantially higher scattering when compared with saline. This has been confirmed with preliminary data, which suggest that OCT imaging will be significantly altered in the presence of blood (Fujimoto et al, 1997; unpublished data). Therefore, for in vivo intravascular imaging, blood must be displaced by methods such as saline injections or balloon occlusion.

The ability of OCT to image through the width of a normal coronary artery has been demonstrated.[25] However, it is not known whether penetration through the various morphologies of atherosclerotic plaque will be as complete. This remains the subject of future investigation.

The current image acquisition rates of OCT at 4 frames per second are insufficient for vascular imaging. It is likely to be necessary for rates to exceed 10 frames per second in order to reliably measure luminal diameter. High-speed data acquisition is currently under investigation, and acquisition rates in this range appear probable.

The light source used for in vitro imaging was a diode similar in some ways to the ones used in laser pointers and CD players. However, a mode-locked laser was used to generate in vivo imaging,[23] due to the higher power requirements of imaging at faster acquisition rates (ie, the faster the acquisition rate, the less time spent on a given axial plane and, therefore, less power per plane). The mode-locked lasers are complex and expensive, making them unattractive for widespread clinical use. Clinically viable sources with similar wavelength and power profiles to these lasers are under investigation.

The relatively complex phenomenon of multiple scattering can potentially reduce the resolution of OCT under certain circumstances.[12] In general, OCT is designed to detect specific photons. These photons are ones which are single backscattered and have not had significant alterations of their mean wavelength, wavelength distribution (band width), or polarization state. If the number of scattering events is high in a given tissue, the system may become "overwhelmed" and begin detecting photons that are multiply scattered. This results in a reduction in resolution. In general, though, this represents an important theoretical problem; we have not observed it to be limiting in the interpretation of atherosclerotic plaque images.

Technical Appendix

Low Coherence Interferometry and Resolution

The heart of the OCT system is a Michelson interferometer.[26,27] If the illuminating source generates light with a broad bandwidth, then the autocorrelation function or AC-coupled photon current representing the interference is then proportional to:

$$I(\Delta l) \; \alpha \; r_s r_r Re[F\{S(\omega)\}]\cos(\omega_0 \tau_p) \tag{1}$$

where $I(\Delta l)$ is the intensity at the detector, $r_s r_r$ is the product of the reflections off the sample and mirror, $Re[F\{S(\omega)\}]$ is the real component of the Fourier transform of the power spectrum of the source, ω_0 is the center frequency of the source, and τ_p is the phase delay. The width of the spectrum and the width of the autocorrelation function (coherence length) are inversely related via the Fourier transform. Therefore, the resolution increases (shorter coherence length) with increasing source band width.[28]

If the source has a Gaussian spectrum with a FWHM (full width half maximum) bandwidth, $\Delta\lambda$, and a center λ_0, then the coherence length (Δl) or axial resolution is

$$\Delta l = (2\ln(2)/\pi)(\lambda^2/\Delta\lambda). \tag{2}$$

The lateral resolution is determined essentially by the focusing power of the system or the lens chosen. It is described by the formula:

$$d = (2b\lambda/\pi)^{.5} \tag{3}$$

where d is the spot size or FWHM of the Gaussian spatial distribution, and b is the confocal parameter, which is twice the Rayleigh parameter.

System Dynamic Range

OCT has been designed near the shot-noise limit by choosing a Doppler frequency (signal shift from moving mirror) above 10 KHz to avoid 1/f noise, and a proper transimpedance amplifier resistance and reference arm voltage to overcome thermal noise.[26,27] For shot-noise detection, the theoretical maximum signal-to-noise ratio (SNR) that can be achieved with OCT under the assumption of infinite linearity of electronics and infinite dynamic range of the digitization electronics can be expressed:

$$\text{SNR} = 10\log \{\eta P_s/2hv\text{NEB}) \tag{4}$$

where $\eta P_s/2hv$ is the number of electrons per unit time generated by the detector due to returning light and 1/NEB band pass filter band width. The measured SNR for the system was measured to be 109 dB and was determined from the maximum signal measured off a mirror, divided by the noise.

Conclusions

OCT has been shown to identify plaque microstructure at unprecedented resolutions with in vitro aorta and coronary arteries segments. OCT has also been directly compared with IVUS, where OCT demonstrated a superior qualitative and quantitative performance. High speed, catheter-based systems have now been developed that are ready to be applied to in vivo imaging. In summary, OCT represents a promising new technology for high-resolution intravascular imaging and the identification of high-risk coronary lesions.

References

1. Richardson PD, Davies MJ, Born GVR. Influence of plaque configuration and stress distribution on fissuring of coronary atherosclerotic plaques. *Lancet* 1989;i:941–944.

2. Falk E. Plaque rupture with severe pre-existing stenosis precipitating coronary thrombosis: Characteristics of coronary atherosclerotic plaques underlying fatal occlusive thrombi. *Br Heart J* 1983;50:127–134.
3. Davies MJ, Thomas AC. Plaque fissuring = mthe cause of acute myocardial infarction, sudden ischemic death, and crescendo angina. *Br Heart J* 1983; 53:363–373.
4. Fuster V, Badimon L, Badimon JJ, Chesebro JH. The pathogenesis of coronary artery disease and the acute coronary syndromes. *N Engl J Med* 1992; 326:242–250.
5. Badimon L, Badimon JJ, Gold HK, Fuster V. Coronary atherosclerosis: Morphology and characteristics to identify by evolving imaging technology. *Am J Card Imaging* 1992;6:278–288.
6. Huang D, Swanson EA, Lin CP, et al. Optical coherence tomography. *Science* 1991;254:1178–1181.
7. Brezinski ME, Tearney GJ, Bouma BE, et al. Optical coherence tomography for optical biopsy: Properties and demonstration of vascular pathology. *Circulation* 1996;93:1206–1213.
8. Fujimoto JG, Brezinski ME, Tearney GJ, et al. Optical biopsy and imaging using optical coherence tomography. *Nature Med* 1994;1:970–972.
9. Swanson EA, Izatt JA, Hee MR, et al. In vivo retinal imaging by optical coherence tomography. *Opt Lett* 1993;18:1864–1866.
10. Hee MR, Izatt JA, Swanson EA, et al. Optical coherence tomography of the human retina. *Arch Ophthalmol* 1995;113:325–332.
11. Puliafito CA, Hee MR, Lin CP, et al. Imaging of macular diseases with optical coherence tomography. *Ophthalmology* 1995;102:217–229.
12. Schmitt J, Knuttel A, Yadlowsky M, Eckhaus MA. Optical-coherence tomography of a dense tissue: Statistics of attenuation and backscattering. *Phys Med Biol* 1994;39:1705–1720.
13. Bouma BE, Tearney GJ, Boppart SA, et al. High resolution optical coherence tomographic imaging using a modelocked Ti:Al_2O_3 laser. *Opt Lett* 1995;20: 1486–1488.
14. Tearney GJ, Boppart SB, Bouma BE, et al. Scanning single mode fiber optic catheter- endoscope for optical coherence tomography. *Opt Lett* 1996; 21: 543–545.
15. Tearney GJ, Bouma BE, Boppart SB, et al. High speed optical coherence tomography. *Opt Lett* 1996;21:1408–1411.
16. Parsa P, Jacques SL, Nishioka NS. Optical properties of rat liver between 350 nm and 2200 nm. *Appl Opt* 1989; 28:2325–2330.
17. Brezinski ME, Tearney GJ, Weissman NJ, et al. Assessing atherosclerotic plaque morphology: Comparison of optical coherence tomography and high frequency intravascular ultrasound. *Heart* 1997;77:166–178.
18. Schmitt JM, Yadlowsky MJ, Bonner RF. Subsurface imaging of living skin with optical coherence microscopy. *Dermatology* 1995;191:93–98.
19. Brezinski ME, Tearney GJ, Boppart SA, et al. Optical biopsy with optical coherence tomography—feasibility for surgical diagnostics. *J Surg Res* 1997; 71:32.
20. Tearney GJ, Brezinski ME, Southern JF, et al. Optical biopsy in human urologic tissue using optical coherence tomography. *J Urol* 1997;157: 1913–1919.
21. Tearney GJ, Brezinski ME, Southern JF, et al. Optical biopsy in human gastrointestinal tissue using optical coherence tomography *Am J Gastroenterol* 1997;92:1800–1804.

22. Tearney GJ, Brezinski ME, Boppart SA, et al. Catheter based optical imaging of a human coronary artery. *Circulation* 1996;94:3013.
23. Tearney GJ, Brezinski ME, Bouma SA, et al. In vivo endoscopic optical biopsy with optical coherence tomography. *Science* 1997;276:2037–2039.
24. Lindberg LG, Oberg PA. Optical properties of blood in motion. *Opt Engin* 1993;32:253–257.
25. Brezinski, ME, Tearney GJ, Bouma BE, et al. Imaging of coronary artery microstructure with optical coherence tomography. *Am J Cardiol* 1996;77: 92–93.
26. Swanson EA, Huang D, Hee MR, et al. High-speed optical coherence domain reflectometry. *Opt Lett* 1992;17:151–153.
27. Hee MR, Izatt JA, Jacobson JM, et al. Femtosecond transillumination optical coherence tomography. *Opt Lett* 1993;18:950–952.
28. Haus HA. *Waves and Fields in Optoelectroncs.* Englewood Cliffs, NJ: Prentice Hall; 1984.

Panel Discussion III

Overview of Imaging:

Characterization of the Vulnerable Plaque with Emphasis on Other Atherosclerotic Regions and Imaging Modalities

Dr. Fuster: First let's summarize the second session of this morning which was about imaging. We learned that intravascular ultrasound is moving along with enthusiasm, and still we have questions about sensitivity and the specificity of the images. Then we learned from angioscopy, in possibly the first prospective of study, that it was actually quite impressive. I'm not entirely sure how this technique can be mastered by interventionalists to really understand what you see and what it represents. Questions for the future are, will it be a technique of general importance, or, as it appears now, is it going to be a technique of importance only in the hands of the people with the best experience? Then we discussed evaluating calcification by EBT scanning, a noninvasive ultrafast scan for the identification of calcium as a marker and as a risk factor for coronary artery disease.

Now about magnetic resonance, I want to be very sure that I understand where we stand with it. Dr. Pohost, in 1990, 7 years ago, you said magnetic resonance just needs a year, and it will be a "one-stop shop." Now we're now in 1997 and those predictions of 1990 don't look too good. I'd also like to go to Dr. Edelman because at that time he was talking about detection of coronary stenosis. What in the world has happened with you guys all these years?

Dr. Edelman: I'd like Dr. Pohost to come up and answer to that. But first, MR's had a lot of progress outside of the heart. For instance, we are now seeing that carotid MRI angiography has become a very

259

routine clinical tool similar to angiography for peripheral and abdominal thoracic studies. I remember back about the same time people saying carotid MRI angiography would never be useful. I think the problem is that we perhaps underestimated the difficulty in getting a clinically useful result out of the MR. We can now image coronary arteries fairly reliably at least in the proximal portions, but to get something that is of sufficient value that eliminates the need for cardiac catheterization, or provides information that changes a patient's outcome, we haven't succeeded. So I think we have to lower our expectations a little bit.

Dr. Fuster: Okay! I go to Dr. Toussaint, who I know very well as an MR colleague for three years. I was really surprised you did not discus your own work assessing carotid plaques with external imaging. I think it's one of the most interesting advances made. My colleague Dr. Shinnar tomorrow also has a lot of data. What better imaging procedure do we have to look at the wall of the carotid artery?

Dr. Toussaint: Maybe that's not being shy, but being cautious. We have only preliminary data from this study. Now you have started much larger scale studies. From these studies we will get larger confirmation of those data. Certainly this is one of the first and most important applications of MR to tissue characterization of atherosclerotic plaques in a large superficial vessel. This vessel can be imaged quite easily with surface coils. These technologies have improved very much. They provide higher resolution and promise to enable doing tissue characterization.

Dr. Fuster: Well it's interesting because what you started with the first six patients we have continued trying to correlate pathology with magnetic resonance. This will be presented tomorrow. We now have 87 cases. This is one area which is very, very promising.

I'd like to move for a moment into what Dr. Amarenco presented. First of all, I said this morning that when the brain receives a little blood, it usually but not always reacts to it very symptomatically. And all your studies of the aortic arch which have provided a significant insight into its causation of many strokes. My question to Dr. Amarenco is about the plaque thickness being more than 4 mm thickness; what is the pathology? Is this the same plaque we were talking this morning with a high lipid core, is it ulcerated?

Dr. Amarenco: We don't have a clear correlation with pathology yet.

Dr. Fuster: Four years ago Michael Davies studied unstable plaques in the aortic arch. There were thick plaques with ulcerations and a large lipid pool, but he did not have any imaging for correlation. So this was purely a pathological study. The assumption is that what you described today are in fact the same plaques that we see in the coronary arteries. They are not huge, but have a very high lipid content. This is very, very interesting in that we are probably dealing with the same disease, with the brain being very sensitive to the emboli.

Discussant from the Audience: Does Dr. Davies make a distinction between an atherosclerotic emboli and a thromboemboli?

Dr. Fuster: No he didn't. Dr. Davies only quantified three components: the extracellular matrix, the lipid, and the macrophages. The plaques that were thickest had very high enrichments of macrophages and lipids. He didn't address the issue of thrombosis, although some of these plaques had thrombi. The question is, what is the nature of the emboli or the nature of the particle that is going into the brain? Dr. Amarenco, do you want to comment on that? Is it a thrombus or a microthrombus? Is it plaque gruel?

Dr. Amarenco: I think it's thrombus. There are two or three large trials being developed which use patients who have the plaques that you describe and have hypercholesterolemia. The studies will see whether plaques that you have initially visualized directly can be modified by treatment with lipid-lowering drugs or with antithrombotics using follow-up with these new imaging technologies. This is a clear example of how this imaging technique can provide the significant information and insight that we need.

Dr. Wagner: I'm interested in the panel's view about where we're going in imaging methods for characterizing vulnerability. As Dr. Falk stressed this morning, plaque vulnerability is very complex and multifactorial. Is any one imaging method likely to become a clinically useful method, or are we going to need a combination of these methods? Or can we answer that question today?

Dr. Toussaint: For sure the absolutely noninvasive techniques will have attraction for the superficial vessel. We can address the progression of the disease, for example, both from ultrasound, possibly high-frequency ultrasound, and certainly from MRI. But progression of coronary lesions will come initially most probably from the angioscopy and the intravascular ultrasound. However, I heard of two things today that indirectly told me something. One was Dr. Amarenco's comment that his last prospective study showed a correlation between the thickness of the plaque of more than 4 mm and the risk of cardiovascular events including myocardial infarction. That's very important because you are really imaging an individual who you know already has active disease in one system, and that is imageable. It might tell you that atherosclerosis is "traveling" to another system, the coronary arteries. Second, this morning, Dr. Larry Hollier presented a study correlating pathology in different areas. Atherosclerotic disease in the legs means activity in the coronary artery. I think we have to begin to think in this way. Thus, we need an imaging technology that can go to the aortic arch or can go to the carotid arteries and tell us if the patient's coronaries are in trouble. In the meantime, let's develop technology to get into the coronary arteries. That is how I see the next 5 years or so.

Dr. Fuster: I suspect that the answer to this question won't be really clear until we have a great many more prospective studies such as that Dr. Uchida presented this morning. We simply don't know enough about the natural history of the vulnerable plaque. Dr. Brezinski, do you have any comments as you look at your own optical coherence tomography technique, and can you tell us an unbiased comment?

Dr. Brezinski: I can definitely tell you a biased comment. With any of the intravascular imaging techniques we first need a second terminology, noninvasive, to stratify patients by risk in order to identify the patients appropriate for intracoronary imaging. We're talking about a very large number of patients as any intracoronary technique is going to need a large patient group. Intracoronary techniques have, or appear to have, the resolution needed. Thus from my perspective you need two complementary imaging technologies for successfully selecting and examining patients.

Dr. Fuster: I tend to agree. As per Dr. Toussaint, I think we are going to need techniques for other regions that will identify prospectively the patient whose coronaries are in trouble.

Dr. Insull: I'd like to make a comment about imaging techniques that can be used efficiently only by selecting a proper study population. The best population is a high risk group, as exemplified by Greg Brown's FATS Trial *Circulation* 1993;87:1781–1791. He studied 146 men, with 94 under aggressive lipid-lowering treatments, and 53 in control with conventional treatment. He had a very dramatic reduction in coronary events immediately after starting aggressive treatment and this was sustained throughout the 4-year trial period. His diagrams show the number of lesions detected by pretreatment angiography. The control group's data provide an estimate of the probable maximum incidence of vulnerable lesions converted to culprit lesions in 4 years. These incidences demonstrate the numbers of lesions that have to be examined to detect highly vulnerable plaques. Brown observed four coronary events in 313 lesions with stenosis 10 percent to 40 percent, four events in 101 lesions with stenosis of 40 percent to 70 percent, and one event in 16 lesions with stenosis greater than 70 percent. The respective incidence rates of events per 4 years were 1.3 percent, 3.9 percent, and 6.3 percent. none of the 53 lesions with less than 10 percent stenosis developed culprit plaques causing coronary events. To find these highly vulnerable lesions with relatively low incidences would require extensive searching. We have seen how potentially that can be done in Dr. Nissen's IVUS study where he does a controlled rapid pullback followed by a computerized image reconstruction, and in Dr. Uchida's angioscopy study in which he can visually scan lesions. I think all this means that the very advanced technology described here today should be applied initially where a few high-risk patients can be studied extensively. That was the design principal of Brown's study.

Dr. Fuster: I think that this is an excellent point. It reminds me when we talk about secondary prevention versus primary prevention. If you have a high risk population, which is the one to develop disease readily, that's the population to look at in contrast to the population that has a lower risk of evolving clinical disease for the first time.

Dr. Shankar, from your radionuclear imaging, do you think that the macrophage is active?

Dr. Shankar: I believe so.

Dr. Fuster: Does the uptake of the glucose mean that the other functions of the macrophage remain intact?

Dr. Shankar: Glucose is essential for many cells. The only question is that in the atherosclerotic lesion it needs to be documented whether the glucose uptake is seen only in macrophages, or also in the smooth muscle cells or endothelial cells. But from what I understand about the vulnerable plaque, its content in macrophage cells is higher than in smooth muscle cells. If the macrophages are indeed a marker for vulnerable plaque, I believe that PET would be able to detect it.

Dr. Fuster: The reason that I'm asking this question is obviously a very important issue because if you really have a model, as you have, then you can detect an active macrophage, thereby getting the study into the vessel wall. And you can image and use pharmacological techniques. We have that in the rabbit model. In following the tissue changes using PET imaging, we might end up with a very interesting new pharmacological tool to assay for the activity of a cell that is critical in the arterial atherosclerotic process.

Dr. Insull: I suggest a very interesting experimental model for validating tissue characterization and the effect of treatment. Subcutaneous injection of extracts derived from seaweed causes a fibrous reaction. In the presence of hypercholesterolemia, this becomes laden with macrophage foam cells rich in cholesterol esters. The size of a fibroma can be manipulated to the size you want. The fibroma can be followed serially so it can be treated, for example, with statins. This provides an assay system that is easy to follow noninvasively and by serial biopsy since it's close to the skin surface because of the subcutaneous injection. This would be an easy pilot technique.

Dr. Fuster: Panel members, what do you expect for your technique for the next year, and what do you expect in the next 5 years?

Dr. Toussaint: First, for the next year there are a few things for MRI in vivo imaging that must be checked. What is the magnetic resonance nature of the tissue characteristics to detect, such as lipid infiltration and collagen? In the next 5 to 10 years at least, I believe we might get some answer about the low profile plaques inside the proximal coronary arteries.

Dr. Fuster: I think that one can safely expect that in 5 years MR angiography quality will be as good as what we expect from DSA today. So we will see MR replacing a number of angiographic studies. By 5 years from now we will have enough resolution to do reasonable plaque characterization.

Dr. Amarenco: From the neurological point of view, I think that we need a noninvasive imaging tool. It would be very important if the MRA and MRI techniques would be developed for the aortic arch plaques. We need them to evaluate therapy and to determine which treatment is the most effective for the plaques we described today.

Dr. Shankar: From my point of view, where I would be 5 years from now depends on funding, the bias of the funding agency, and the provision of adequate funds to do good work. A modest transfer of principles of these methodologies has a lot of potential, but unfortunately it requires funding. Carefully done studies can address the issue of identifying specific molecules that are responsible for plaque vulnerability. A key question is whether this kind of work will be funded by the National Institutes of Health. I think this is also research for industry support.

Dr. Fuster: I recently chaired a panel in New Orleans addressing clinical investigation, yesterday, today, and tomorrow. Funding is getting more and more difficult. However, I believe that if you have a good idea, it will go on, with the best qualified people working together. The initial collaboration between Dr. Toussaint and I on MRI of the coronary arteries started without funding. We have been able to get our ideas moving and not get stuck. Despite difficulties in funding, we all have to work creatively.

Dr. Insull: I'm looking back to a meeting and a book sponsored by the Vascular Lesions Committee 15 years ago, eds: Bonds MG, et al. *Clinical Diagnosis of Atherosclerosis, Quantitative Methods of Evaluation*, where I authored a chapter titled "Universal Reference Standards for Measuring Atherosclerotic Lesions: The Quest for the Gold Standard," which described criteria for standards. At that time we did not have standards for lesions. We knew there were a lot of different lesions, but we didn't know quite how they all fitted into the plaques' evolutionary sequence. Since 1982, we've learned that the most important lesion is the vulnerable lesion. The culprit lesion is important, but by definition that's the vulnerable lesion already after the fact of rupture causing clinical disease. We want to know what is the vulnerable lesion that becomes the culprit lesion. In 1983 we had a pathological description of lesions, and we've had that again today, only more sophisticated. I think we've had a reasonable start on a definition of the vulnerable lesion based on the culprit lesion, but it is still a retrospective description. What we need, and what we're looking for, is a prospective description so that we can identify the most vulnerable lesions before people become stricken by a culprit lesion. We lack a clear and comprehensive description of the vulnerable lesion that describes all the major characteristics and that is commonly accepted by all investigators, ie, a gold standard. Without this definition it is difficult for the new imaging technology to focus on the target of identifying these vulnerable lesions. I think the power of the technology that has been described today is very sophisticated and has great promise, as looking at lesions with the naked eye by angioscopy and being able to get measurements of tissue function, as described for radioisotope technology. To achieve these promises we need a definition of the vulnerable lesion that will be commonly accepted, and that can then be used as a common guide for applying the various imaging techniques that have been described today.

Dr. Fuster: This is a good summary. It's time to adjourn.

Chapter 15

De Novo Atherosclerotic Geometric Remodeling and Plaque Vulnerability

Gerard Pasterkamp, MD, PhD

Introduction

Until recently, plaque formation was considered to be the only determinant of atherosclerotic luminal narrowing. Recent postmortem and intravascular ultrasound studies, however, revealed that arterial remodeling is another important determinant of luminal narrowing in de novo atherosclerosis. *Arterial remodeling* refers to various changes in the geometry and structure of the artery.[1,2] The change in total arterial circumference ranges from excessive enlargement, with an actual increase in lumen, to arterial shrinkage that contributes to lumen narrowing. The mechanisms responsible for this spectrum of remodeling are unknown, but their identification will be important for the potential development of therapeutic strategies to promote favorable remodeling.

This chapter focuses on the two modes of remodeling of the artery in de novo atherosclerosis: compensatory enlargement, which decelerates, and shrinkage, which accelerates luminal narrowing by atherosclerotic plaque formation. The possible relationship between vascular geometry and markers for plaque instability is subsequently discussed.

Compensatory Enlargement

In experimental primate atherosclerosis, the artery adapts to lesion formation by enlargement, resulting in a long prestenotic phase of ath-

From: Fuster, V (ed). *The Vulnerable Atherosclerotic Plaque: Understanding, Identification, and Modification*. Armonk, NY: Futura Publishing Company, Inc.; © 1999.

erosclerosis.[3] Glagov et al[4] studied atherosclerotic enlargement in histologic cross sections of left main coronary arteries obtained from 136 human hearts. They found that coronary arteries enlarge proportionally to the increase in plaque area, and that the formation of a functionally important lumen stenosis is delayed until the lesion occupies approximately 40% of the area within the internal elastic lamina. Even overcompensatory enlargement of the coronary artery with increase of the luminal cross-sectional area may be observed.[4] At a certain limit the artery is maximally enlarged and additional plaque formation then encroaches on the lumen. These findings on (over)compensatory enlargement are supported by several in vivo studies in which geometric remodeling was studied by use of epicardial[5] and intravascular ultrasound.[6-10] Presently, intravascular ultrasound is the best diagnostic imaging modality, which allows the arterial geometry, and thereby arterial remodeling, to be studied in vivo. The conclusion that the artery initially enlarges in response to plaque accumulation was primarily based on a positive correlation between plaque area and the area encompassed by the internal elastic lamina. In most studies this positive correlation between the plaque area and the vessel size had been inferred from data pooled from many patients.[4,8,9,11,12] Pooling data from all subjects, however, may mask an individual variation in the susceptibility of the artery to undergo compensatory enlargement. We recently demonstrated that individual variation in the compensatory enlargement response may occur in the femoral artery.[13] It appeared that some arterial segments were well capable of enlargement in response to plaque formation, whereas other arterial segments were not. Compensatory enlargement has been demonstrated, so far, in atherosclerotic coronary arteries,[4,5,8,9,11,12] femoral arteries,[6,7,13] iliac arteries,[10] and carotid arteries.[14]

Shrinkage

During intravascular ultrasound studies of the atherosclerotic femoral artery, we observed that variation in plaque mass over the length of the arterial segment was not always accompanied by equal changes in luminal area. Moreover, the location with the smallest lumen area rarely contained the largest plaque mass, indicating that the decrease in lumen area could not be attributed to plaque increase alone.[6] Compared to a reference site that contained the least amount of plaque, we found that shrinkage of the artery was responsible for part of the decrease in lumen area (Fig. 1). In addition, less luminal narrowing was observed in compensatory enlarged arterial segments compared to shrunken arterial segments. From that study,[6] it was concluded that in

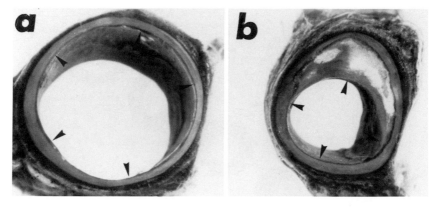

Figure 1. Impact of remodeling on percentage luminal narrowing. Two cross sections obtained from the identical femoral artery are shown. **a.** The reference cross section that contained the least amount of plaque: lumen area = 22.0 mm^2, vessel area = 22.3 mm^2, plaque area = 0.3 mm^2. **b.** The lesion site that is shrunken: lumen area = 8.1 mm^2, vessel area = 13.4 mm^2, plaque area = 5.3 mm^2. The black arrowheads indicate the luminal border. The illustrated cross sections are 0.5 cm in thickness. The dark areas behind the arrowheads represent the inner vascular wall. Difference in lumen area (13.9 mm^2) could not be fully explained by the increase in plaque area (5.0 mm^2). In this cross section, difference in vessel area (8.9 mm^2) accounted for 64% of the alteration in lumen area.

the femoral artery compensatory enlargement prevents, and shrinkage accelerates, luminal narrowing.

The contribution of arterial wall shrinkage to the development of critical arterial stenosis in the coronary artery has been reported by our group[15] and by others.[16–18] Nishioka et al[16] reported that in the group of enlarged arterial segments an average of 82% of plaque burden was compensated for, while reduction of the vessel area in the shrinkage group contributed 39% to the lumen area reduction. This percentage of vessel size reduction does not reflect the true impact of remodeling on percentage luminal stenosis, since had the artery been enlarged, the lumen would not have been narrowed at all. In addition to de novo atherosclerosis, the role of arterial remodeling in luminal narrowing has been recognized in restenosis after balloon angioplasty,[19,20] saphenous vein bypass grafts,[21] and transplanted hearts.[22] Thus, arterial remodeling, as well as intimal hyperplasia and plaque formation, may be considered an important determinant of luminal narrowing. In practice, an equal amount of plaque or intimal hyperplasia may lead to extreme differences in lumen area, varying from luminal enlargement to complete occlusion (Fig. 2).

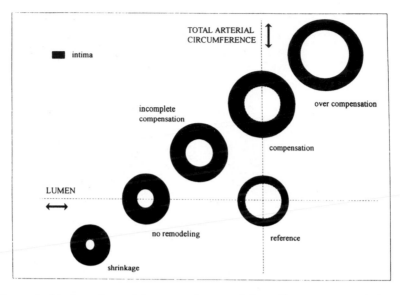

Figure 2. Modes of arterial geometric remodeling. Plaque accumulation or neointima formation in an artery may progress without reducing the lumen (compensation) or even with increasing lumen size (overcompensation) if the artery enlarges. If compensation is incomplete or if the artery does not remodel, plaque or intimal hyperplasia will narrow the lumen. A subset of arteries shrinks, thus aggravating lumen narrowing by plaque or intimal hyperplasia. In the model illustrated here, the cross-sectional area of the intima is held constant. (Reprinted from Post MJ, et al. *Atherosclerosis* 1995;118 (suppl):S115–S123, with kind permission from Elsevier Science Ireland Ltd., Ireland.)

Possible Mechanisms of De Novo Atherosclerotic Remodeling

The mechanisms that initiate the different remodeling responses in atherosclerosis are thus far unknown. It has been hypothesized that attenuation of the media that is frequently observed in atherosclerotic arteries[23] may explain the increase of the area encompassed by the internal elastic lamina. The extent of enlargement, however, mostly exceeds the medial area and can therefore not fully explain this phenomenon. It has been postulated that local increase in shear stress due to luminal narrowing may induce an endothelium compensatory dilatation of the artery.[4] Endothelial functions may be disturbed in atherosclerotic arteries[24] or in patients suffering from risk factors for cardiovascular disease.[25] Failure of the natural endothelial response to alterations in shear stress may lead to failure of the compensatory enlargement response or even to shrinkage of the artery.

Recent studies have shown that the prevalence of "inadequately enlarged" arterial segments is increased in smokers compared with nonsmokers,[26,27] which indicates that the increased risk for cardiovascular disease in smokers may be partly explained by a paradoxical shrinkage response.

Geometric Remodeling and Plaque Vulnerability

Lumen Area

Geometric variables such as lumen area, plaque area, and vessel area can easily be derived by use of histology and intravascular ultrasound, whereas angiography can only depict a silhouette of the luminal borders. Angiographic luminal diameter narrowing is not a predictive value for the onset of plaque rupture.[28–30] Angiographic studies of coronary arteries revealed that the preexisting, underlying lesion does not usually cause hemodynamically significant stenosis.[28,29] In fact, over 50% off all ruptured lesions are at sites with less than 50% luminal narrowing. In a pathological study, Mann and Davies[31] showed that determinants of plaque vulnerability, core size, and cap thickness were not related to the degree of luminal stenosis. This observation is often explained as a statistical phenomenon: the lesions with potential vulnerable plaques with minor luminal narrowing outnumber the lesions that are hemodynamically significantly narrowed.[30,32]

Plaque Area

Before the recognition of the concept of compensatory enlargement, plaque mass was thought to be the only determinant of luminal narrowing. Thus, it was assumed that the decrease in angiographic luminal diameter equalized the increase in plaque diameter. During the validation of intracoronary angiography as a diagnostic modality, several investigators reported that the angiogram underestimated the degree of luminal stenosis compared with histology.[33–35]

Marcus et al[35] hypothesized that the finding of an unobstructed coronary angiogram, despite moderate obstruction observed with histology, might be explained by outward displacement of the plaque. Thus, the definition of luminal stenosis used in histology (percentage of the area encompassed by the internal elastic lamina that is occupied by plaque) and in angiography (percentage luminal stenosis compared to a reference lumen) appeared not to be comparable. The type and degree of atherosclerotic remodeling explains this discrepancy.[36] Compensatory enlargement of the artery also explains why plaque rupture is mostly observed at lesions that are moderately stenosed on angiography[28-30] but severely narrowed in histology.[37,38]

The current consensus is that the propensity for plaques to rupture is independent of lumen size. Differences exist, however, in hypotheses on the relation between plaque vulnerability and plaque size. Mann et al[31] did not find a relation between the core size and plaque mass. The lack of a relation between plaque size and a marker for plaque vulnerability (core size) may be explained by the methodology used. In their study, Mann et al[31] used the absolute values of plaque area and core area for comparison. A high correlation between absolute plaque area and core area would be observed if, for instance, cross sections revealed plaque areas of 5.0 mm^2, 10.0 mm^2, and 20.0 mm^2 with corresponding core areas of 2.5 mm^2, 5.0 mm^2, and 10 mm^2, respectively, while no relation would be observed if the core area was expressed as percentage of total plaque area (in all cross sections 50%). Therefore, the hypothesis postulated by Fishbein and Siegel[38] may be valid: that not small but rather large plaques, which may not produce significant luminal stenosis, are the ones that undergo rupture with subsequent thrombosis.

Vessel Area, Remodeling

The relation between alterations in vessel area, ie, atherosclerotic arterial remodeling, and vulnerability of the plaque is unknown. The interpretations of the results of previous angiographic and postmortem studies may lead to the hypothesis that compensatory enlarged segments are more likely to be vulnerable to plaque rupture: (1) on angiography the preexisting lesions mostly show less than 50% luminal narrowing[28-30]; whereas (2) on histology most ruptures are observed at locations with more than 75% cross-sectional area narrowing.[37,38] Both observations can only be explained by the existence of compensatory enlargement prior to plaque rupture. It may be hypothesized that enlargement of the vessel area and fibrous cap rupture are initiated by identical mechanisms. Inflammatory responses may lead to the release of matrix-degrading enzymes, metalloproteinases. These enzymes may degrade matrix components beneath the fibrous cap as well as beneath the medial layer at the base of the plaque, leading to weakening of the fibrous cap and weakening of the arterial collagenous "skeleton," respectively. Subsequently, the first may initiate plaque rupture,[39] and the second may lead to compensatory enlargement or even aneurysm formation.[40]

Recently, Nishioka et al[41] demonstrated that unstable angina is more frequently observed at compensatory enlarged lesions in coronary artery lesions, as visualized with intravascular ultrasound. As with plaque rupture, unstable angina is found to be associated with the presence of inflammation in the vascular wall. The hypothesis that plaques in compensatory enlarged lesions are more prone to rupture may therefore be supported by the observations of Nishioka et al.[41]

Limitation in Atherosclerotic Remodeling Studies: The Reference

The limiting factor of research on de novo atherosclerotic remodeling is the choice of the reference site. In postmortem and single ultrasound observations only single static visualization on a dynamic process is obtained. Atherosclerotic remodeling is a process which is likely to occur over decades, in contrast to remodeling in restenosis, which occurs within 6 months.[19,20] The slow progression of de novo atherosclerosis virtually excludes serial intravascular ultrasound studies. Most investigators use a proximally or distally located "normal appearing" reference site to quantify the degree of atherosclerotic remodeling; but what is "normal appearing"? Most investigators who examine the intravascular ultrasound images still think in angiographic terms; in that case "normal appearing" equals "normal lumen." In investigations in remodeling, however, this equation should not be accepted; in the femoral artery, we have shown that most cross sections that showed a "normal" lumen were, in fact, compensatorily enlarged.[6] In those studies we considered the cross section with the least amount of plaque as the reference, assuming that it had been least affected by the atherosclerotic process. Still, this reference merits careful consideration. The artery may be generally affected by the atherosclerotic disease, which hampers the identification of a proper reference that contains the least amount of plaque. Secondly, tapering also influences arterial size. It may be difficult to correct for tapering if numerous side branches are present.

In summary, arterial remodeling is an important determinant of luminal stenosis: in the long term, compensatory enlargement prevents, and shrinkage accelerates, narrowing of the lumen. Future studies will reveal whether variation in vessel size is also related to the occurrence of acute arterial plaque rupture.

References

1. Gibbons GH, Dzau VJ. The emergent concept of vascular remodeling. *N Engl J Med* 1994;330:1431–1438.

2. Mulvany MJ. Determinants of vascular structure. *J Cardiovasc Pharmacol* 1992;19(suppl):S1–S6.
3. Armstrong ML, Heistad DD, Marcus ML, et al. Structural and hemodynamic responses of peripheral arteries of macaque monkeys to atherogenic diet. *Arteriosclerosis* 1985;5:336–346.
4. Glagov S, Weisenberg E, Zarins CK, et al. Compensatory enlargement of human atherosclerotic arteries. *N Engl J Med* 1987;316:1371–1375.
5. Mc Pherson DD, Sirna SJ, Hiratzka LF, et al. Coronary arterial remodeling studied by high frequency epicardial echocardiography: An early compensatory mechanism in patients with obstructive coronary atherosclerosis. *J Am Coll Cardiol* 1991;17:79–86.
6. Pasterkamp G, Wensing PJW, Post MJ, et al. Paradoxical arterial wall shrinkage contributes to luminal narrowing of human atherosclerotic femoral arteries. *Circulation* 1995;91:1444–1449.
7. Pasterkamp G, Borst C, Gussenhoven EJ, et al. Remodeling of de novo atherosclerotic lesions in femoral arteries: Impact on the mechanism of balloon angioplasty. *J Am Coll Cardiol* 1995;26:422–428.
8. Hermiller JB, Tenaglia AN, Kisslo KB, et al. In vivo validation of compensatory enlargement of atherosclerotic coronary arteries. *Am J Cardiol* 1993;71:665–668.
9. Ge J, Erbel R, Zamorano J, et al. Coronary artery remodeling in atherosclerotic disease: An intravascular ultrasonic study in vivo. *Coron Artery Dis* 1993;4:981–986.
10. Losordo DW, Rosenfield K, Kaufman J, et al. Focal compensatory enlargement of human arteries in response to progressive atherosclerosis. *Circulation* 1994;89:2570–2577.
11. Gerber TC, Erbel R, Görge G, et al. Extent of atherosclerosis and remodeling of the left main coronary artery determined by intravascular ultrasound. *Am J Cardiol* 1994;73:666–671.
12. Zarins CK, Weisenberg E, Kolettis G, et al. Differential enlargement of artery segments in response to enlarging atherosclerotic plaques. *J Vasc Surg* 1988;7:386–394.
13. Pasterkamp G, Borst C, Post MJ, et al. Atherosclerotic arterial remodeling in the superficial femoral artery: Individual variation in local compensatory enlargement response. *Circulation* 1996;93:1818–1825.
14. Steinke W, Els T, Hennerici M. Compensatory carotid artery dilatation in early atherosclerosis. *Circulation* 1994;89:2578–2581.
15. Clarijs JAGM, Pasterkamp G, Schoneveld AH, et al. Compensatory enlargement in coronary and femoral arteries is related neither to the extent of plaque free vessel wall nor to lesion eccentricity: A post mortem study. *Arterioscler ThrombVasc Biol* 1997. In press.
16. Nishioka T, Luo H, Eigler NL, et al. Contribution of inadequate compensatory enlargement to development of human coronary artery stenosis: An in vivo intravascular ultrasound study. *J Am Coll Cardiol* 1996;27:1571–1576.
17. Wong CB, Porter TR, Xie F, Deligonul U. Segmental analysis of coronary arteries with equivalent plaque burden by intravascular ultrasound in patients with and without angiographically significant coronary artery disease. *Am J Cardiol* 1995;76:598–601.
18. Mintz GS, Kent KM, Pichard AD, et al. Contribution of inadequate arterial remodeling to the development of focal coronary artery stenoses: An intravascular ultrasound study. *Circulation* 1997;95:1791–1798.
19. Post MJ, Borst C, Kuntz RE. The relative importance of arterial remodeling

compared with intimal hyperplasia in lumen renarrowing affer balloon angioplasty: A study in the normal rabbit and the hypercholesterolemic Yucatan micropig. *Circulation* 1994;89:2816–2821.

20. Kakuta T, Currier JW, Haudenschild CC, et al. Differences in compensatory enlargement, not intimal formation, account for restenosis after angioplasty in the hypercholesterolemic rabbit model. *Circulation* 1994;89:2809–2815.

21. Mendelsohn FO, Foster GP, Palacios IF, et al. In vivo assessment by intravascular ultrasound of enlargement in saphenous vein bypass grafts. *Am J Cardiol* 1995;76:1066–1069.

22. Lim TT, Liang DH, Botas J, et al. Role of compensatory enlargement and shrinkage in transplant coronary artery disease. Serial intravascular ultrasound study. *Circulation* 1997;95:855–859.

23. Isner JM, Donaldson RF, Fortin AH, et al. Attenuation of the media of coronary arteries in advanced atherosclerosis. *Am J Cardiol* 1986;58:937–939.

24. Zeiher AM, Schachinger V, Hohnloser SH, et al. Coronary atherosclerotic wall thickening and vascular wall reactivity in humans. *Circulation* 1994; 89:2525–2532.

25. Reddy KG, Nair RN, Sheenan HM, Hodgson JmcB. Evidence that selective endothelial dysfunction may occur in the absence of angiographic or ultrasound atherosclerosis in patients with risk factors for atherosclerosis. *J Am Coll Cardiol* 1994;23:833–843.

26. Tauth JG, Sullebarger JT, Swartz S, et al. Determinants of coronary arterial remodeling patterns: An intravascular ultrasound study. *J Am Coll Cardiol* 1997(suppl);29:391A.

27. Weissman NJ, Chari R, Mendelsohn FO, et al. Patient and plaque characteristics associated with coronary artery remodeling: An intravascular ultrasound analysis. *J Am Coll Cardiol* 1997(suppl);29:124A.

28. Ambrose JA, Tannenbaum, Alexopoulos D, et al. Angiographic progression of coronary artery disease and the development of myocardial infarction. *J Am Coll Cardiol* 1988;12:56–62.

29. Little WC, Constantinescu M, Applegate RJ, et al. Can coronary angiography predict the site of a subsequent myocardial infarction in patients with mild-to-moderate coronary artery disease? *Circulation* 1988;78:1157–1166.

30. Alderman EL, Corley SD, Fisher LD, et al, and CASS Participating investigators and staff. Five-year angiographic follow-up of factors associated with progression of coronary artery disease in the Coronary Artery Surgery Study (CASS). *J Am Coll Cardiol* 1993;22:1141–1154.

31. Mann JM, Davies MJ. Vulnerable plaque. Relation of characteristics to degree of stenosis in human coronary arteries. *Circulation* 1996;94:928–931.

32. Falk E, Shah PK, Fuster V. Coronary plaque disruption. *Circulation* 1995; 92:657–671.

33. Isner JM, Kishel J, Kent KM, et al. Accuracy of angiographic determination of left main coronary arterial narrowing. *Circulation* 1981;63:1056–1064.

34. Schwartz JN, Kong Y, Hackel DB, Bartel AG. Comparison of angiographic and post- mortem findings in patients with coronary artery disease. *Am J Cardiol* 1975;36:174–178.

35. Marcus ML, Armstrong ML, Heistad DD, et al. Comparison of three methods of evaluating coronary obstructive lesions: Post-mortem arteriography, pathologic examinations and measurements of regional myocardial perfusion during maximal vasodilation. *Am J Cardiol* 1982;49:1699–1706.

36. Pasterkamp G, Wensing PJW, Hillen B, et al. Impact of local atherosclerotic remodeling on the calculation of percent luminal narrowing. *Am J Cardiol* 1997;79:402–405.

37. Qiao J-H, Fishbein MC. The severity of coronary atherosclerosis at sites of plaque rupture with occlusive thrombosis. J Am Coll Cardiol 1991;17: 1138–1142.
38. Fishbein MC, Siegel RJ. How big are coronary atherosclerotic plaques that rupture? *Circulation* 1996;94:2662–2666.
39. Galis ZS, Sukhova GK, Lark MW, Libby P. Increased expression of matrix metalloproteinases and matrix degrading activity in vulnerable regions of human atherosclerotic plaques. *J Clin Invest* 1994;94:2493–2503.
40. Dobrin PB, Baker WH, Gley WC. Elastolytic and collagenolytic studies of arteries: Implications for the mechanical properties of aneurysms. *Arch Surg* 1984;119:405–409.
41. Nishioka T, Luo H, Nagai T, et al. Impact of coronary artery remodeling on clinical manifestations of patients with de novo coronary artery lesions. *J Am Coll Cardiol* 1997;(suppl)·:125A.

Chapter 16

Lipids in Atherosclerotic Lesion Progression

John R. Guyton, MD

Atherosclerosis represents a gross derangement of tissue lipid metabolism in a specific site—the arterial intima. In most body organs and tissues, lipoproteins admirably perform their various functions, which include regulating the cholesterol content of cells and helping to control lipid oxidation. In the arterial intima, lipoproteins fail to regulate cholesterol and to protect against oxidation. As a result, lipid chemistry in the arterial intima is dramatically altered, and the consequences for tissue viability and arterial function are severe.

A full review of the chemical and structural characteristics of lipids in atherosclerosis is well beyond the scope of this chapter. We focus here on major features considered critical to the initiation, progression, and development of propensity to rupture in atherosclerotic plaques. The reader is referred to worthwhile reviews by Smith,[1] Small,[2] Williams and Tabas,[3] and Guyton and Klemp[4] for consideration of other topics.

High Low-Density Lipoprotein Concentrations in Arterial Intima

The tissue concentration of low-density lipoproteins (LDL) in the arterial intima is very high compared to all other connective tissues in the body. By quantitative immunoassay, the concentration of LDL in the arterial intima is about equal to the plasma LDL concentration.[1,5] In contrast, the LDL concentration in the tunica media is very low,

Supported by NIH Grants HL29680, HL45619, and M01-RR-30.

From: Fuster, V (ed). *The Vulnerable Atherosclerotic Plaque: Understanding, Identification, and Modification.* Armonk, NY: Futura Publishing Company, Inc.; © 1999.

usually unmeasurable. What is the usual LDL concentration found in the interstitial space of other connective tissues? The best estimate comes from measurements in peripheral lymph, which yield approximately one tenth of the plasma concentration.[6] Therefore, the connective tissue in the arterial intima sees an LDL concentration that is approximately 10 times as high as that seen by any other connective tissue in the body.

Why is this so? Figure 1 shows that the arterial intima is a loosely organized tissue, whereas the arterial media is tightly organized. Particles the size of LDL appear to be sterically excluded from the arterial media. The arterial media possesses not only dense elastic lamellae, but also collagen fibers and proteoglycans that are packed tightly among the smooth muscle cells and elastic lamellae. Overall, the medial tissue layer represents a permeability barrier analogous to the endothe-

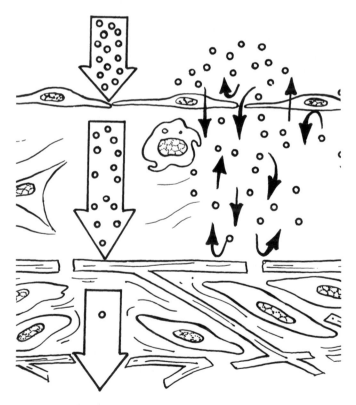

Figure 1. Lipoprotein transport in the arterial wall. Both endothelium (near top of figure) and internal elastic lamina are permeability barriers. Few LDL particles penetrate the tunica media. Both convection (left) and diffusion (right) of LDL are depicted.

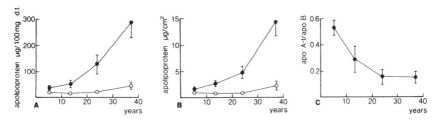

Figure 2. Age-related increases of apoB (closed circles) and apoA-1 (open circles) detected immunochemically in human aortic intima, expressed in two ways (**A** and **B**). ApoB, associated with LDL, can be considered atherogenic, while apoA-1, associated with HDL, might be antiatherogenic. The ratio of apoA-1 to apoB declines with age (**C**). Reproduced from Reference 7, with permission.

lial permeability barrier. Therefore, the intima resides between two permeability barriers. This observation suggests that LDL not only are present in the intima in high concentration, but also that the intimal LDL are stagnant. The half-life of LDL in the plasma is 2 to 3 days. Measurement of the half-life of LDL in arterial intima is one goal of current research. It may be as long as weeks or months, depending on the thickness of the intima.

Yla-Ierttuala et al[7] measured apolipoprotein concentrations in autopsied human aortas at varying ages, as shown in Figure 2. Apolipoprotein A-I intimal concentrations increase modestly with age, but apoB concentrations increase greatly as adult life is attained. By age 40, intimal apoB mass concentrations are fivefold greater than apoA-I concentrations, despite the fact that apoA-I mass in plasma is usually greater than apoB mass.[7] Since these apolipoproteins are found on LDL and HDL (high density lipoproteins), respectively, a corresponding increase in LDL relative to HDL in the arterial intima must occur.

To summarize, LDL are found in a much higher concentration in arterial intima than in any other connective tissue in the body. This is almost certainly the reason that cholesterol deposition regularly occurs with aging in the arterial intima but rarely occurs at all in other sites.

High Levels of Unesterified Cholesterol in the Early Atherosclerotic Core

A critical juncture in atherosclerotic lesion development is the transition from fatty streak to fibrous plaque. Fatty streaks are flat, harmless lesions, often found in teenagers, that have no propensity to rupture. Fibrous plaques are raised atherosclerotic lesions, which usually possess a lipid core. Those with marked core development are prone to rupture. In recent years it has become clear that most fibrous plaques arise from fatty streaks.[8]

Fibrous plaques differ from fatty streaks in two major ways: their fibroproliferative character and their possession of a necrotic lipid-rich core. We asked which of these differences occurs first, as fatty streaks progress toward becoming fibrous plaques. Is the initial change in the fatty streak a fibromuscular expansion, or does the development of the lipid core occur before major fibromuscular expansion? Evidence gathered from a number of human autopsy studies suggests a surprising answer: that initiation of the lipid core *precedes* major fibromuscular expansion as fatty streaks progress to become fibrous plaques. Moreover, particular kinds of lipid deposits—vesicles with a high content of unesterified cholesterol, sometimes accompanied by cholesterol crystals—are characteristic of the early atherosclerotic core.

The first evidence for this sequence came from a study by Katz et al.[9] By microscopic examination of saline minces of arterial intima, the authors found cholesterol crystals in a subset of flat human aortic lesions resembling fatty streaks. Lesions with cholesterol crystals also showed relatively high levels of unesterified cholesterol by chemical analysis. These lesions were termed *intermediate* (between fatty streaks and fibrous plaques), on the basis of their lipid composition.

To better understand lesion progression, we examined, by use of a combination of chemical and microscopic methods, the smallest distinct raised lesions we could find in human aorta. In histologic sections, approximately three fourths of these small lesions had lipid deposits in two distinct locations: foam cells near the luminal surface, and a deeper lying lipid core (Fig. 3). We have called these lesions *fibrolipid lesions*; by topology and features they may also be considered small or early fibrous plaques. The histology and chemistry of the foam cell cap in the fibrolipid lesion are indistinguishable from the features of a fatty streak. However, the lesions as a whole, and particularly the microdissected cores, show a marked increase in unesterified cholesterol, quite unlike fatty streaks. On average, 63% of total cholesterol in the early core is unesterified. Partial disappearance of cells from the core region in these early lesions is also observed.[10–12]

In the study of small raised lesions, whenever the lesion had foam cells, it also possessed a lipid core.[10] This finding led us to speculate that by the time a fatty streak begins a process of fibromuscular expansion, it may already possess a lipid core. If so, then some *flat* fatty lesions may also possess lipid cores at an earlier stage of development. We examined 31 flat human aortic fatty lesions and found deep intimal cholesterol clefts in 6 of them (cholesterol clefts correspond to the spaces left in fixed tissues when cholesterol monohydrate crystals are extracted by solvents use in histologic processing). In the deep intimal sublayer near the clefts, a significant decrease in overall cell volume was determined morphometrically. The combination of cholesterol clefts and cell disappearance demonstrates the origin of the atherosclerotic core in these lesions.[13] This study provides histologic confirmation of the intermediate lesion described almost two decades previously by Katz et al.[9] Importantly, the study demonstrates that the atherosclerotic core often originates before the onset of major fibromuscular thickening in lesion development.

Therefore, lesion transition from fatty streak to fibrous plaque is marked initially by deep intimal accumulation of unesterified cholesterol and simultaneously by evidence of cell toxicity (disappearance of cells). Somewhat later, fibromuscular expansion occurs. The mechanism for accumulation of unesterified cholesterol is unknown; potential mechanisms are discussed elsewhere.[4]

It has recently become clear that excessive cholesterol may itself be toxic to cells. When macrophages and other cells become overloaded with cholesterol, they ordinarily sequester it in a nontoxic form by esterifying it and forming cytoplasmic oily droplets of cholesteryl ester. If this did not occur, then cell membrane dysfunction and ultimately toxicity would be expected, as cell membranes develop unphysiological

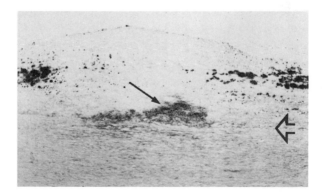

Figure 3. Early formation of the atherosclerotic core demonstrated in frozen section of a small fibrolipid lesion (lumen at top). The core, which has a hazy appearance by Oil Red O staining, is found in the musculoelastic, deeper sublayer of the intima (arrow). Foam cell infiltrates, staining more densely with Oil Red O, appear in the more superficial intimal sublayer at the shoulders of this lesion. The difference in staining characteristics reflects the differing compositions of core lipids— mostly cholesterol-rich vesicles—and foam cell lipids—mostly cholesteryl ester-rich oily droplets. The open arrow indicates location of the internal elastic lamina. Reproduced from Reference 4, with permission. ($\times$ 800.)

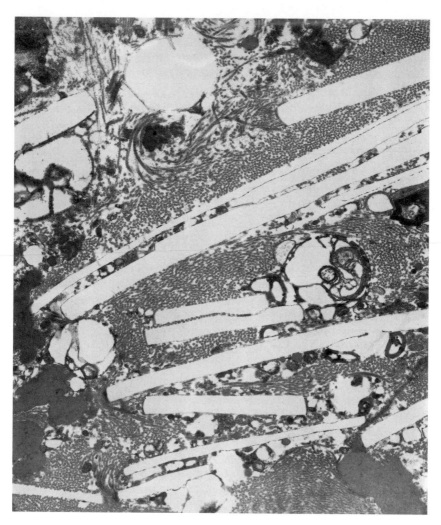

Figure 4. Cholesterol clefts inserted among collagen fibrils in the deep intima of a flat human aortic lesion resembling a fatty streak. Vesicular lipid structures are also present. Electron micrograph reproduced from Reference 13 with permission.

cholesterol-to-phospholipid ratios. With use of an inhibitor of the esterifying enzyme, acylCoA:cholesterol acyltransferase, Warner et al[14] demonstrated that cholesterol loading via unregulated uptake of modified lipoproteins was toxic to macrophages. Subsequently Tabas et al[15] demonstrated that a last line of defense for cells in this situation is an increase in phosphatidylcholine synthesis, presumably to keep cholesterol/phosphatidylcholine ratios nearly normal in cell membranes.[15]

These experiments demonstrate that modeling of cholesterol excess in cell culture is difficult. A critical difference between cell culture and the arterial wall may be the dramatically reduced diffusion and convection of lipoproteins, including HDL and LDL, in the arterial intima. The arterial intima lacks a microcirculation. This should profoundly limit reverse cholesterol transport within the intima. In order to function effectively in reverse cholesterol transport, HDL must be able to transfer cholesteryl ester along to larger lipoproteins such as LDL and very low density lipoproteins (VLDL).[16,17] However, VLDL are largely excluded from the intima, and LDL move in and out of the intima very slowly. Thus, one must suspect that reverse cholesterol transport in this tissue is impaired. This is especially true in comparison with cell culture, where typically a 3000-μm thick layer of freely mobile fluid (culture media) perfuses a layer of cells several micrometers thick. Formation of cholesterol crystals has been particularly difficult to model in cell culture, although formation of cholesterol crystals within lysosomes of cultured cells has recently been demonstrated.[18] However, in the arterial wall cholesterol crystals probably initiate and unquestionably enlarge in the extracellular space, especially in association with bundles of collagen fibrils (Fig. 4).[12] The difference between the in vivo and in vitro situations might be due mostly to the stagnant condition of lipoprotein movement in the arterial wall. More quantitative data are obviously needed in this area.

Lipid Oxidation

The third critical factor in lipid biochemistry of atherosclerosis is lipid oxidation. This is a vast topic, which is well covered elsewhere in this volume and in other reviews.[19-21] Ample evidence indicates a role for lipid oxidation in inflammatory responses in arterial cells, including recruitment of monocytes to lesions.[22] The cytotoxic effect of oxidized LDL on arterial cells in culture has been ascribed to oxysterols and to the potent cytotoxin, 7-β-hydroperoxycholesterol.[23-25]

Conclusive evidence for the presence of oxidized lipoproteins and lipids in atherosclerotic lesions has been presented.[26] However, some confusion exists regarding the quantitation of lipid oxidation in lesions. One recent article began with the statement that *most of the lipids in the atherosclerotic plaque are oxidized.* That is hardly true. Carpenter et al[27] addressed this question in a careful study using gas chromatography for quantitation of native and oxidized lipids in human atherosclerotic

Table 1

Extent of Oxidation of Atheromatous Lipids

	μg/100 μg chol.	Ratio of oxidized lipid to parent lipid	Ratio in copper-oxidized LDL
HODEs (primary products of 18:2 fatty acid oxidation)	0.77	6%	5–25%
7-β-OH cholesterol (from peroxidation)	0.14	0.14%	≈25%
26-OH cholesterol (from enzymatic oxidation)	0.61	0.61%	0

LDL = low-density lipoprotein.

plaques.[27] An abbreviated summary of results is shown in Table 1. All of the oxidized lipids detected amounted to approximately 2% of the mass of unoxidized cholesterol. Polyunsaturated fatty acids have the greatest susceptibility to oxidation. The primary oxidation products of linoleic acid (18:2) amounted to 6% of the mass of unoxidized linoleic acid. Cholesterol oxidation products include multiple products of non-enzymatic lipid peroxidation, most of which have oxygen attached to carbon 7 (in biologic systems), and a single product, 26-OH cholesterol, which is exclusively derived from the 26-hydroxylase enzyme (also termed 27-hydroxylase). In the analysis of Carpenter et al, 7-keto-cholesterol and 7-β-hydroperoxycholesterol were reduced with sodium borohydride and thus added to the total of 7-β-OH cholesterol measured chromatographically. Together these major lipid peroxidation products of cholesterol amounted to only 0.14% of the total mass of cholesterol. The enzymatic oxidation product was considerably more abundant, 0.61% of the mass of cholesterol. These findings are in contrast to measurements of oxysterols in LDL oxidized by copper ions in vitro, where levels of oxysterols are far greater (unpublished data from this laboratory). The measurements of accumulated oxysterols in atherosclerotic lesions underestimate their production, since oxysterols diffuse out of the tissue much more readily than cholesterol. Oxidized products of linoleic acid remain largely esterified (to cholesterol and phospholipids) and thus do not diffuse away. In any case, the low abundance of oxysterols in lesions raises questions as to whether some of their effects demonstrated in cell culture are relevant in vivo.

A crucial question to answer in understanding the development of the vulnerable atherosclerotic plaque is: what kills cells in the necrotic core region? Much attention has been given to the possibility that oxidized lipids are toxic to the cells. However, another strong possibility is that unesterified cholesterol itself is the culprit. Distinguishing between these possibilities has important therapeutic implications and should be a priority for future research.

References

1. Smith EB. The relationship between plasma and tissue lipids in human atherosclerosis. *Adv Lipid Res* 1974;12:1–49.
2. Small DM. Cellular mechanisms for lipid deposition in atherosclerosis. *N Engl J Med* 1977;297:873–877.
3. Williams KJ, Tabas I. The response-to-retention hypothesis of early atherogenesis. *Arterioscler Thromb Vasc Biol* 1995;15:551–561.
4. Guyton JR, Klemp KF. Development of the lipid-rich core in human atherosclerosis. *Arterioscler Thromb Vasc Biol* 1996;16:4–11.
5. Hoff HF, Heideman CL, Gaubatz JW, et al. Quantification of apolipoprotein B in grossly normal human aorta. *Circ Res* 1977;40:56–64.
6. Reichl D. Extravascular circulation of lipoproteins: Their role in reverse transport of cholesterol. *Atherosclerosis* 1994;105:117–129.
7. Yla-Herttuala S, Solakivi T, Hirvonen J, et al. Glycosaminoglycans and apolipoproteins B and A-1 in human aortas. *Arteriosclerosis* 1987;7:333–340.
8. Stary HC, Chandler AB, Glagov S, et al. Special report: A definition of initial, fatty streak, and intermediate lesions of atherosclerosis. *Arterioscler Thromb* 1994;14:840–856.
9. Katz SS, Shipley GG, Small DM. Physical chemistry of the lipids of human atherosclerotic lesions: Demonstration of a lesion intermediate between fatty streaks and advanced plaques. *J Clin Invest* 1976;58:200–211.
10. Bocan TM, Guyton JR. Human aortic fibrolipid lesions. Progenitor lesions for fibrous plaques, exhibiting early formation of the cholesterol-rich core. *Am J Pathol* 1985;120:193–206.
11. Bocan TM, Guyton JR. Ultrastructure of the human aortic fibrolipid lesion. Formation of the atherosclerotic lipid-rich core. *Am J Pathol* 1986;123:413–424.
12. Guyton JR, Klemp KF. Development of the atherosclerotic core region: Chemical and ultrastructural analysis of microdissected atherosclerotic lesions from human aorta. *Arterioscler Thromb* 1994;14:1305–1314.
13. Guyton JR, Klemp KF. Transitional features in human atherosclerosis: Intimal thickening, cholesterol clefts, and cell loss in human aortic fatty streaks. *Am J Pathol* 1993;143:1444–1457.
14. Warner GJ, Stoudt G, Bamberger M, et al. Cell toxicity induced by inhibition of acyl coenzyme A: Cholesterol acyltransferase and accumulation of unesterified cholesterol. *J Biol Chem* 1995;270:5772–5778.
15. Tabas I, Marathe S, Keesler GA, et al. Evidence that the initial up-regulation of phosphatidylcholine biosynthesis in free cholesterol-loaded macrophages is an adaptive response that prevents cholesterol-induced cellular necrosis. Proposed role of an eventual failure of this response in foam cell necrosis in advanced atherosclerosis. *J Biol Chem* 1996;271:22773–22781.
16. Reichl D, Miller NE. Pathophysiology of reverse cholesterol transport: Insights from inherited disorders of lipoprotein metabolism. *Arteriosclerosis* 1989;9:785–797.

17. Jonas A. Lecithin-cholesterol acyltransferase in the metabolism of high-density lipoproteins. *Biochim Biophys Acta* 1991;1084:205–220.
18. Tangirala RK, Jerome WG, Jones NL, et al. Formation of cholesterol mono-hydrate crystals in macrophage-derived foam cells. *J Lipid Res* 1994;35: 93–104.
19. Steinberg D, Parthasarathy S, Carew TE, et al. Beyond cholesterol. Modifications of low- density lipoprotein that increase its atherogenicity. *N Engl J Med* 1989;320:915–924.
20. Parthasarathy S, Rankin SM. Role of oxidized low density lipoprotein in atherogenesis. *Prog Lipid Res* 1992;31:127–143.
21. Steinbrecher UP, Zhang H, Lougheed M. Role of oxidatively modified LDL in atherosclerosis. *Free Radic Biol Med* 1990;9:155–168.
22. Berliner JA, Territo MC, Sevanian A, et al. Minimally modified low density lipoprotein stimulates monocyte endothelial interactions. *J Clin Invest* 1990; 85:1260–1266.
23. Hughes H, Mathews B, Lenz ML, Guyton JR. Cytotoxicity of oxidized low density lipoprotein to porcine aortic smooth muscle cells is associated with the oxysterols 7- ketocholesterol and 7-hydroxycholesterol. *Arterioscler Thromb* 1994;14:1177–1185.
24. Guyton JR, Lenz ML, Mathews B, et al. Toxicity of oxidized low density lipoproteins for vascular smooth muscle cells and partial protection by antioxidants. *Atherosclerosis* 1995;118:237–249.
25. Chisolm GM, Ma G, Irwin KC, et al. 7-Beta-hydroperoxycholest-5-en-3-beta-ol, a component of human atherosclerotic lesions, is the primary cyto-toxin of oxidized human low density lipoprotein. *Proc Natl Acad Sci U S A* 1994;91:11452–11455.
26. Yla-Herttuala S, Palinski W, Rosenfeld ME, et al. Evidence for the presence of oxidatively modified low density lipoprotein in atherosclerotic lesions of rabbit and man. *J Clin Invest* 1989;84:1086–1095.
27. Carpenter KLH, Taylor SE, Ballantine JA, et al. Lipids and oxidised lipids in human atheroma and normal aorta. *Biochim Biophys Acta* 1993;1167: 121–130.

Chapter 17

Extracellular Matrix of the Vulnerable Atherosclerotic Plaque

William D. Wagner, PhD

Introduction

Components of the extracellular matrix play a significant role in the development and potential transition of atherosclerotic lesions to vulnerable plaques. Major components of the extracellular matrix of the atherosclerotic lesion include collagen, elastic fibers, and glycoproteins. The normal function of the arterial wall depends on the extracellular matrix synthesized and secreted mainly by smooth muscle cells and endothelial cells of the intimal and medial layers, as well as by fibroblasts in the adventitia. Typically, type I collagen provides tensile strength to the artery wall and is significantly increased in the fibromuscular cap of atherosclerotic lesions. Reduced collagen levels at sites such as the growing edges of lesions result in compromised tissue strength. Elastic fibers normally provide the elastic recoil property of the arterial wall. Elastases present in specific regions of the atherosclerotic plaque degrade the elastin moiety of the elastic fiber, preventing a normal function as well as producing elastin peptides chemotactic for macrophages. A major fraction of the glycoprotein component of matrix includes several types of proteoglycans. Proteoglycans consist of a protein component, and possess covalently bound, linear, and pendant sulfated glycosaminoglycan chains as part of their carbohydrate complement. The oligosaccharide sequence of the glycosaminoglycan, as

Studies were supported by National Institutes of Health grants HL25161, HL45848, and HL45095.

From: Fuster, V (ed). *The Vulnerable Atherosclerotic Plaque: Understanding, Identification, and Modification.* Armonk, NY: Futura Publishing Company, Inc.; © 1999.

well as the extent and location of sulfate groups, results in specific functional properties which influence cell-matrix and matrix-matrix interaction, binding of growth factors and enzymes, binding of coagulation/anticoagulation factors, and regulation of cell proliferation. Structural and functional properties of versican, a chondroitin sulfate-containing proteoglycan; decorin and biglycan, two dermatan sulfate-containing proteoglycans; and the syndecans, cell surface heparan sulfate-containing proteoglycans, function in a variety of specific mechanisms that potentially lead to vulnerable atherosclerotic lesions. In this chapter, current and newly emerging data are presented to indicate that primary alterations in specific proteoglycans are key in the development of the vulnerable atherosclerotic plaque.

Proteoglycan Structure

The functional properties of proteoglycans depend on the structure of both the core protein and the glycosaminoglycan component. There are several types of glycosaminoglycan structures that tend to be associated with distinct proteins. Each of these proteins is a specific gene product. Glycosaminoglycans are classified as sulfated or nonsulfated. The sulfated glycosaminoglycans present in arteries are chondroitin sulfate, dermatan sulfate, and heparan sulfate.[1] Minor amounts of keratan sulfate and heparin are described in arteries. Chondroitin sulfate is a linear polysaccharide consisting of repeating disaccharide units of glucuronic acid and N-acetyl galactosamine. The sulfate groups are present on the hexosamine. Sulfation is usually at either the 4th or 6th position of galactosamine, although disulfated and trisulfated disaccharides can occur in the polysaccharide. The precise structure of chondroitin sulfate varies depending on the cell of origin. The variation may include differences in chain length and sulfation patterns. Presumably, sulfation pattern differences result from changes in the availability of precursors and/or activities of the glycosyl and sulfate transferases. Chondroitin sulfate synthesis[2] begins on an acceptor serine residue in the core protein initially by the transfer of a xylose residue, followed by two consecutive galactose residues and a glucuronic acid residue, and then repetitive addition of N-acetyl galactosamine and glucuronic acid. Sulfation of the N-acetyl galactosamine occurs during the chain elongation. Dermatan sulfate, although biosynthetically similar to chondroitin sulfate, differs by having the presence of iduronic acid instead of selective glucuronic acid residues. Iduronic acid residues are formed from glucuronic acid by the action of an epimerase. The presence of iduronic acid adds additional potential functional properties to the chain, because polysaccharides containing iduronic acid residues as opposed to glucuronic acid residues are relatively more electronegative and also, conformationally, more flexible. Heparan sulfate has the same linkage trisaccharide as chondroitin sulfate and dermatan sulfate.[2] This is also attached to a serine residue in the core protein. Synthesis of the repeating disaccharide structure in the heparan sulfate polysaccharide chain involves the sequential addition of glucuronic acid and N-acetyl glucosamine. Some of the glucosamine residues undergo a process of deacetylation and subsequent N-sulfation. This process is regulated by a specific enzyme, N- deacetylase N-sulfotransferase. The activity of this enzyme is unique to the synthesis of heparan sulfate and heparin. The factor that distinguishes heparan sulfate from heparin is that in contrast with heparan sulfate, the majority of the glucosamine residues in the polysaccharide chain of heparin are deacetylated and subsequently N-sulfated. In the synthesis of heparan sulfate, a variable proportion of the glucuronic acid residues can undergo epimerization to iduronic acid. This is followed by O-sulfation at both the 6th position of glucosamine and the 2nd position of iduronic acid residues. In some cases, the 3rd position of glucosamine residues may also undergo sulfation. This variation in the extent of the events that occur during the biosynthesis of heparan sulfate makes heparan sulfate heterogeneous in structure, depending upon the activities of the specific enzymes in synthesis. Keratan sulfate has been described as a minor component in arteries.[3] Keratan sulfate does not contain hexuronic acid; instead it is composed of a repeating disaccharide of galactose and N-acetyl glucosamine. The hexosamine residue is typically sulfated at the 6th position, but sulfation can also occur at the 6th position of galactose. Hyaluronic acid is a nonsulfated glycosaminoglycan present in artery wall. Hyaluronic acid does not require a protein acceptor to initiate synthesis. Synthesis occurs at the plasma membrane of the cell by consecutive addition of glucuronic acid and N-acetyl glucosamine, elongating the polysaccharide chain. The precursors are added at the internal surface of the cell membrane and the growing polysaccharide chain is extruded directly into the extracellular space. Hyaluronic acid differs from the sulfated glycosaminoglycans in that it has an extremely long length, where the molecular weights can approach 1 million daltons. It also does not contain any polymer modifications. One specific function of hyaluronic acid is to interact with the proteoglycans that contain a hyaluronic acid-binding region on their core protein, and thus produce a supermolecular weight aggregate of proteoglycans in the extracellular space.

Proteoglycan Classification

There are several ways to classify proteoglycans of arteries. One method is to put proteoglycans in families based on the type of glycosaminoglycan chain covalently linked to the core protein.[4] This creates a chondroitin sulfate proteoglycan family, a dermatan sulfate proteoglycan family, and a heparan sulfate proteoglycan family. Another way to classify the protein is based on the actual gene trivial name; for example, versican is the major member of the chondroitin sulfate proteoglycan family. Decorin and biglycan are two major family members of the dermatan sulfate proteoglycan family, and specific syndecans are members of the heparan sulfate family. In this chapter the trivial names of the proteoglycans are used in order to indicate that specific functional properties of these molecules depend on either the core protein or the polysaccharide chain and that modification occurs in the atherosclerotic lesion.

Versican

Versican has been cloned and sequenced.[5] This proteoglycan has the unique property of interacting ionically with hyaluronic acid to form a supermolecular weight aggregate. This is the major extracellular proteoglycan of arteries (50% to 60% of total proteoglycan).[6] One specific function of versican is derived primarily from its ability to occupy a large space within the extracellular domain. One important function, therefore, is to provide a viscoelasticity property to the arterial wall. This is dependent on an ionic association with hyaluronic acid and the maintenance of a supermolecular weight aggregate. Alterations in artery versican in the human atherosclerotic lesion primarily include reductions in the hyaluronic acid-binding region, resulting in a reduced size of aggregate. Consequences include enhanced permeability to plasma components such as low-density lipoprotein.[6]

Decorin and Biglycan

The structure and function of dermatan sulfate proteoglycans (15% to 20% of total artery proteoglycan) have recently been characterized in a number of different tissues. There are two types of dermatan sulfate proteoglycans, decorin and biglycan, which have similar core protein molecular weights of approximately 45 to 50 kDa but differ in degree of substitution with glycosaminoglycan or oligosaccharide.[7] The decorin and biglycan genes have been cloned and sequenced from human bone.[8,9] Studies have demonstrated that within a tissue there are specific types of dermatan sulfate proteoglycans,[10] and the distribution of dermatan sulfate proteoglycan type may vary depending upon age.[11]

A number of functional roles for decorin have been reported.[12–18]

Although most of these studies were not conducted with decorin from artery or from cells derived from arteries, similar functions may operate in the artery wall and in atherosclerosis. Decorin has been reported to interact by way of the core protein with several components of the extracellular matrix. A role in collagen fibrillogenesis has been suggested[12] as a result of the interaction with collagen types I, II, and VI.[13,14] Alterations in the collagen types in human atherosclerotic plaque have been reviewed.[15,16] Decorin could potentially either impair healing of the atherosclerotic plaque through slowing of type I collagen fiber formation, or facilitate healing by orienting collagen molecules into functional molecules. A role for decorin in the reduction of cell proliferation by use of transfected Chinese hamster ovary (CHO) cells has been reported[17] to result from its binding to transforming growth factor-β (TGFβ).[18] It is unclear whether the effect of TGFβ on the artery wall results in smooth muscle cell inhibition or proliferation. In vitro TGFβ may inhibit or stimulate smooth muscle cell proliferation, depending on concentration of TGFβ, cell age, density, the line of cells, or the presence of other cellular factors.

Syndecans

A variety of biological functions has been described for syndecans which reflects a highly variable heparan sulfate structure.[19–21] The glycosaminoglycan chains located on the ectodomain of heparan sulfate proteoglycans can serve to mediate communication between the cell and its environment via their interaction with cell adhesion molecules such as fibronectin and thrombospondin, matrix molecules such as collagen and laminin, or with growth factors such as fibroblast growth factor (FGF) or platelet-derived growth factor (PDGF). In addition, the heparan sulfate proteoglycans core protein can provide a transmembrane link between the cytoskeleton and the extracellular environment.[22,23] The specificity of function of heparan sulfate proteoglycans resides in the heparan sulfate chains. The binding of syndecan to several matrix proteins (types I, III, V collagen, fibronectin, thrombospondin, and tenascin), as well as to basic FGF, is also mediated through the heparan sulfate chain.[24] The structure of the heparan sulfate chain on syndecan varies according to the cell of origin, and the variation affects the potential interaction and strength of binding.

The structural properties and sequence of the core proteins of the integral membrane heparan sulfate proteoglycans on cells has been reviewed.[19,24,25] Major types found on smooth muscle cells are syndecan 2 and syndecan 4. Syndecan 2 obtained its trivial name, *fibroglycan*, based on the isolation initially from fibroblasts. Syndecan 2 is the major heparan sulfate proteoglycan of mesodermal cells but is hardly detectable in epithelial cells. It is a type I integral membrane protein of 201 amino acids that carries three or four heparan sulfate chains. It contains a transmembrane domain of 25 amino acid residues and a short C-terminal domain of 32 amino acids.[26] It has been cloned and sequenced in human skin fibroblasts[26] and rat smooth muscle cells.[27] Syndecan 4, also termed *ryudocan* or *amphiglycan*, has been cloned and sequenced in two independent laboratories.[28,29] The other heparan sulfate proteoglycans belonging to the family of type I integral membrane proteoglycans are syndecan 1 and syndecan 3. Syndecan 1 was originally identified in mouse mammary epithelial cells as a hybrid molecule carrying both heparan sulfate and chondroitin sulfate chains.[30] Syndecan 1 is abundant and is expressed in epithelial cells rather than in mesenchymal cells.[24] Very low levels of syndecan expression have been reported in rat artery smooth muscle cells.[31,32] All of the syndecans show limited but significant structural similarities.

Proteoglycan–Low-Density Lipoprotein Interaction

Complexes of low-density lipoprotein and arterial wall proteoglycans occur, and cholesteryl ester accumulation in macrophages is promoted by these complexes in vitro.[33–35] Lipoprotein-proteoglycan complexes in vivo have been demonstrated, and have been isolated from atherosclerotic lesion in humans.[36] We have, based on immunohistochemical studies of human atherosclerotic lesions, demonstrated that decorin specifically is colocalized with low-density lipoprotein, and further identified an accessory molecule, lipoprotein lipase (LpL), that participates in the interaction. Lipoprotein-proteoglycan complexes isolated from human atherosclerotic lesions stimulate cholesteryl ester synthesis in foam cells isolated from rabbit lesions by a dose-dependent, receptor- mediated process, and result in intracellular accumulation of cholesteryl ester.[35] In this study, the stimulation of cholesteryl ester synthesis was inhibited 32% to 37% by polyinosinic acid, 50% by acetyl low-density lipoprotein, only 6% by cytochalasine D, and not at all by native low-density lipoprotein, suggesting that complexes were taken up primarily by the scavenger receptor.

LpL, a key enzyme in regulation of blood lipoproteins, interacts with heparan sulfate proteoglycan on the surface of endothelial cells[37] and in the subendothelial matrix. Normally, LpL hydrolyzes triglycerides of low-density lipoprotein and chylomicrons, but the enzyme has been demonstrated to be involved in atherosclerosis through binding to low-density lipoprotein in the arterial wall. This interaction with low-density lipoprotein is independent of LpL enzymatic activity.

Studies in smooth muscle cells[38] have demonstrated augmented cellular binding properties of low-density lipoprotein by way of heparan sulfate proteoglycans. Low-density lipoprotein uptake mechanisms may be mediated by the turnover of the heparan sulfate proteoglycan or may facilitate the positioning of low-density lipoprotein in proximity to receptors such as the low-density lipoprotein receptor-like protein. In recent studies[39] we have observed that LpL not only interacts with heparan sulfate on cells but also with dermatan sulfate proteoglycans isolated from arterial tissue. Both heparan sulfate and dermatan sulfate contain similar carbohydrate structural features but are two distinct glycosaminoglycans that may play independent roles in LpL binding. Dermatan sulfate proteoglycans in contrast to versican showed enhanced potential to bind low-density lipoprotein when LpL was present.[39] Therefore, since it is significantly increased in the developing atherosclerotic lesion and can be found widespread throughout the intercellular matrix, LpL can be a mechanism to enhance low-density lipoprotein accumulation in the atherosclerotic plaque. The molecular interactions of LpL with dermatan sulfate proteoglycans and low-density lipoprotein may represent a significant mechanism leading to cellular uptake as well as to interference in low-density lipoprotein efflux from the vessel wall.

Proteoglycan-Heparin Cofactor II Interaction

In addition to generating fibrin, thrombin may also promote early cellular inflammatory and proliferative events in atherosclerosis.[40] Thrombin is a smooth muscle cell mitogen and monocyte chemoattractant. These cellular effects are mediated by a specific thrombin receptor that has been detected on several cell types. In human atherosclerotic lesions, high levels of thrombin receptor expression have been identified in areas that are rich in macrophages or proliferating smooth muscle cells. In early lesions such as fatty streaks, thrombin receptor expression is observed in the intima. The underlying media does not typically show expression of receptor activity.[41] These findings suggest that thrombin receptors are important during early stages of the development of the atherosclerotic lesion and that modulation of the thrombin activation of the receptor may be important for inhibition of thrombin action. Mechanisms that could be targeted in atherosclerosis include the regulation of thrombin binding to the thrombin receptor rather than modulation of thrombin receptor expression; regulation of the thrombin receptor is poorly understood and studies investigating this mechanism may in fact be difficult because it is regulated by multiple inflammatory mediators. The approach therefore would be to modify thrombin activity in the lesion. One potential manner is to modify thrombin activity through regulation of heparin cofactor II activity.

Heparin cofactor II and antithrombin III (ATIII) are protease inhibitors that both form inactive covalent complexes with target proteases. While ATIII inhibits all proteases of the intrinsic coagulation pathway,[42] heparin cofactor II only inhibits thrombin.[43] In the presence of heparin, the thrombin inhibitory activity of both ATIII and heparin cofactor II is significantly enhanced (up to 1000 times).[42,44] Dermatan sulfate also accelerates the inhibition of thrombin by heparin cofactor II but has no effect on ATIII. ATIII activates in vivo by binding to heparan sulfate on endothelial cells.[45,46] It is unclear how and by what mechanism thrombin is inhibited at sites below the endothelium and within the intimal lesion. It has been postulated that heparin cofactor II inhibits thrombin in vivo in tissue where cells produce significant amounts of dermatan sulfate.[47] Studies with cultured fibroblasts[47] and purified decorin and biglycan[48] have demonstrated that dermatan sulfate proteoglycans accelerate the rate of thrombin inhibition by heparin cofactor II. Our recent findings indicate that artery smooth muscle cells produce syndecans and dermatan sulfate proteoglycans, which significantly upregulate heparin cofactor II inhibitory activity of thrombin.[49]

These findings suggest a model wherein intramural thrombin activity can be inhibited by heparin cofactor II at two different sites. One site comprises dermatan sulfate proteoglycans in the vicinity of collagen-rich interstitial extracellular matrix. A second line of defense is heparan sulfate proteoglycans at or near the smooth muscle cell surface. Because of heparan sulfate distribution, heparan sulfate proteoglycan interaction would provide regulation of thrombin activity near thrombin receptors on the smooth muscle cell surface. Heparan sulfate proteoglycan content in the atherosclerotic lesion is reduced compared to normal arterial tissue; therefore, the progression of atherosclerosis may be associated with increased thrombin generation at a time when one of the potential thrombin regulatory mechanisms is downregulated.

In another study[50] we examined whether dermatan sulfate proteoglycans from advanced stages of atherosclerosis were capable of stimulating heparin cofactor II inhibition of thrombin. In this study decorin and biglycan were purified from human aorta and tested for their ability to upregulate heparin cofactor II. The results of these studies indicate that as atherosclerosis advances, the decorin present in the lesion has reduced ability to upregulate the inhibitory activity of heparin cofactor II. The precise mechanism whereby the dermatan sulfate chain influences heparin cofactor II activity is not fully understood. In preparations of commercial dermatan sulfate, specific oversulfated oligosaccharide sequences responsible for upregulation of heparin cofactor II activity have been identified.[51] We hypothesize that the dermatan sulfate present in advanced atherosclerotic lesions is defective in the content of these specific oligosaccharides.

Conclusion

It is clear that proteoglycans participate in a variety of mechanisms important to our understanding of the vulnerable atherosclerotic plaque. Mass increases of proteoglycans in atherosclerotic lesions provide a mechanism for increased binding capacity for insudated plasma low-density lipoprotein. Studies on the qualitative nature of the glycosaminoglycan and alterations in atherosclerotic plaques have provided new mechanisms to consider in the resolution of the atherosclerotic lesion. One such mechanism involves an impaired regulation of thrombin through heparin cofactor II.

Acknowledgement The author expresses gratitude to all collaborators who participated in the studies described and to Sharon Ireland and Lisa Gotow, who contributed to the manuscript preparation.

References

1. Stevens RL, Colombo M, Gonzales JJ, et al. The glycosaminoglycans of the human artery and their changes in atherosclerosis. *J Clin Invest* 1976;58: 470–481.
2. Silbert JE. Structure and metabolism of proteoglycans and glycosaminoglycans. *J Invest Dermat* 1982;79(suppl 1):131–137.
3. Robbins RA, Wagner WD, Register TC, et al. Demonstration of a keratan sulfate-containing proteoglycan in atherosclerotic aorta. *Arterioscl Thromb* 1992;12:83–91.
4. Poole AR. Proteoglycans in health and disease: Structures and functions. *Biochem J* 1986;236(1):1–14.
5. Zimmermann DR, Ruoslahti E. Multiple domains of the large fibroblast proteoglycan, versican. *EMBO J* 1989;8(10):2975–2981.
6. Wagner WD. Proteoglycan structure and function as related to atherosclerosis. *Ann N Y Acad Sci* 1985;454:52–68.
7. Kresse H, Hausser H, Schönherr E, Bittner K. Biosynthesis and interactions of small chondroitin/dermatan sulphate proteoglycans. *Eur J Clin Chem Clin Biochem* 1994;32:259–264.
8. Fisher LW, Termine JD, Young MF. Deduced protein sequence of bone small proteoglycan I (biglycan) shows homology with proteoglycan II (decorin) and several nonconnective tissue proteins in a variety of species. *J Biol Chem* 1989;264:4571–4576.
9. Fisher LW, Heegaard AM, Vetter U, et al. Human biglycan gene: Putative promoter, intron-exon junctions, and chromosomal localization. *J Biol Chem* 1991;266:14371–14377.
10. Bianco P, Fisher LW, Young MF, et al. Expression and localization of the

two small proteoglycans biglycan and decorin in developing human skeletal and non-skeletal tissues. *J Histochem Cytochem* 1990;38:1549–1563.

11. Melching LI, Roughley J. The synthesis of dermatan sulphate proteoglycans by fetal and adult human articular cartilage. *Biochem J* 1989;261:501–508.

12. Vogel KG, Paulsson M, Heinegard D. Specific inhibition of type 1 and type II collagen fibrillogenesis by the small proteoglycan of tendon. *Biochem J* 1984;223:587–597.

13. Scott PG, Winterbottom N, Dodd CM, et al. A role for disulphide bridges in the protein core in the interaction of proteodermatan sulphate and collagen. *Biochem Biophy Res Comm* 1986;138:1348–1354.

14. Bidanset DJ, Guidry C, Rosenberg LC, et al. Binding of the proteoglycan decorin to collagen type VI. *J Biol Chem* 1992;267:5250–5256.

15. Wagner WD. Modification of collagen and elastin in the human atherosclerotic plaque. *Pathobiol Human Atheroscler Plaque* 1989;167–188.

16. Stary HC, Blankenhorn DH, Chandler AB, et al. A definition of the intima of human arteries and of its atherosclerosis-prone regions. *Circulation* 1992; 85:391–405.

17. Yamaguchi Y, Ruoslahti E. Expression of human proteoglycan in chinese hamster ovary cell inhibits cell proliferation. *Nature* 1988;336:244–246.

18. Yamaguchi Y, Mann DM, Ruoslahti E. Negative regulation of transforming growth factor-β by the proteoglycan decorin. *Nature* 1990;346:281–284.

19. Rosenberg RD, Shworak NW, Liu J, et al. Heparan sulfate proteoglycans of the cardiovascular system. *J Clin Invest* 1997;99:2062–2070.

20. Gallagher JT, Lyon M, Steward WP. Structure and function of heparan sulphate proteoglycans. *Biochem J* 1986;236:313–325.

21. David G. Structural and function diversity of the heparan sulfate proteoglycans. In: Lane DA, et al eds: *Heparin and Related Polysaccharides*. New York: Plenum Press; 1992:69–78.

22. Woods A, Couchman JR, Höök M. Heparan sulfate proteoglycans of rat embryo fibroblasts. *J Biol Chem* 1985;260:10872–10879.

23. Rapraeger A, Jalkanen M, Bernfield M. Cell surface proteoglycan associates with the cytoskeleton at the basolateral cell surface of mouse mammary epithelial cells. *J Cell Biol* 1986;103:2683–2696.

24. Bernfield M, Kokenyesi R, Kato M, et al. Biology of the syndecans: A family of transmembrane heparan sulfate proteoglycans. *Ann Rev Cell Biol* 1992; 8:365–393.

25. David G. Integral membrane heparan sulfate proteoglycans. *FASEB J* 1993; 7:1023–1030.

26. Marynen P, Zhang J, Cassiman J-J, et al. Partial primary structure of the 48- and 90-kilodalton core proteins of cell surface-associated heparan sulfate proteoglycans of lung fibroblasts. *J Biol Chem* 1989;264:7017–7024.

37. Cizmeci-Smith G, Stahl RC, Showalter LJ, Carey DJ. Differential expression of transmembrane proteoglycans in vascular smooth muscle cells. *J Biol Chem* 1993;268:18740–18747.

28. Kojima T, Shworak NW, Rosenberg RD. Molecular cloning and expression of two distinct cDNA-encoding heparan sulfate proteoglycan core proteins from a rat endothelial cell line. *J Biol Chem* 1992;267:4870–4877.

29. David G, van der Schueren B, Marynen P, et al. Molecular cloning of amphiglycan, a novel integram membrane heparan sulfate proteoglycan expressed by epithelial and fibroblastic cells. *J Cell Biol* 1992;118:961–969.

30. Rapraeger A, Jalkanen M, Endo E, et al. The cell surface proteoglycan from mouse mammary epithelial cells bears chondroitin sulfate and heparan sulfate glycosaminoglycans. *J Biol Chem* 1985;260:11046–11052.

31. Cizmeci-Smith G, Asundi V, Stahl RC, et al. Regulation expression of syndecan in vascular smooth muscle cells and cloning of rat syndecan core protein cDNA. *J Biol Chem* 1992;267:15729–15736.
32. Cizmeci-Smith G, Langan E, Youkey J, et al. Syndecan 4 is a primary-response gene induced by basic fibroblast growth factor and arterial injury in vascular smooth muscle cells. *Arterioscler Thromb Vasc Biol* 1997;17: 172–180.
33. Wagner WD, Edwards IJ, St. Clair RW, Barakat H. Low density lipoprotein interaction with artery derived proteoglycan: The influence of LDL particle size and the relationship to atherosclerosis susceptibility. *Atherosclerosis* 1989;75:49–59.
34. Vijayagopal P, Srinivasan SR, Xu JH, et al. Lipoprotein-proteoglycan complexes induce continued cholesteryl ester accumulation in foam cells from rabbit atherosclerotic lesions. *J Clin Invest* 1993;91:1011–1018.
35. Vijayagopal P. Regulation of the metabolism of lipoprotein-proteoglycan complexes in human nonocyte-derived macrophages. *Biochem J* 1994;301: 675–681.
36. Srinivasan SR, Dolan P, Radhakrishnamurthy B, et al. Lipoprotein-acid mucopolysaccharide complexes of human atherosclerotic lesions. *Biochim Biophys Acta* 1975;388:58–70.
37. Parthasarathy N, Goldberg IJ, Sivaram P, et al. Oligosaccharide sequences of endothelial cell surface heparan sulfate proteoglycan with affinity for lipoprotein lipase. *J Biol Chem* 1994;269:22391–22396.
38. Mulder M, Lombardi P, Jansen H, van Berkel TJC, et al. Low density lipoprotein receptor internalizes low density and very low density lipoproteins that are bound to heparan sulfate proteoglycans via lipoprotein lipase. *J Biol Chem* 1993;268:9369–9375.
39. Edwards IJ, Goldberg IJ, Parks JS, et al. Lipoprotein lipase enhances the interaction of low density lipoproteins with artery-derived extracellular matrix proteoglycans. *J Lipid Research* 1993;34:1155–1163.
40. Baykal D, Schmedtje JF Jr., Runge MS. Role of the thrombin receptor in restenosis and atherosclerosis. *Am J Cardiol* 1995;75:82B–87B.
41. Nelken NA, Soifer SJ, O'Keefe J, et al. Thrombin receptor expression in normal and atherosclerotic human arteries. *J Clin Invest* 1992;90:1614–1621.
42. Rosenberg RD. Biologic actions of heparin. *Semin Hematol* 1977;14:427–440.
43. Parker KA, Tollefssen DM. The protease specificity of heparin cofactor II. *J Biol Chem* 1985;260:3501–3505.
44. Tollefsen DM, Majeru DW, Blank MK. Heparin Cofactor II: Purification and properties of a heparin-dependent inhibitor of thrombin in human plasma. *J Biol Chem* 1982;257:2162–2169.
45. Busch C, Owen WG. Identification in vitro of an endothelial cell surface cofactor for antithrombin III: Parallel studies with isolated perfused rat heart and microcarrier cultures of bovine endothelium. *J Clin Invest* 1982; 69:726–729.
46. Marcum JA, Fritze L, Galli SJ, et al. Microvascular heparinlike species with anticoagulant activity. *Am Physiol Soc* 1983;83:H725–H733.
47. McGuire EA, Tollefsen DM. Activation of heparin cofactor II by fibroblasts and vascular smooth muscle cells. *J Biol Chem* 1987;262:169–175.
48. Whinna HC, Choi HU, Roenberg LC, Church FC. Interaction of heparin cofactor II with biglycan and decorin. *J Biol Chem* 1993;268:3920–3924.
49. Shirk RA, Church FC, Wagner WD. Arterial smooth muscle cell heparan sulfate proteoglycans accelerate thrombin inhibition by heparin cofactor II. *Arterioscler Thromb Vasc Biol* 1996;16(9):1138–1146.

50. Wagner WD, Shirk RA, Church FC. Biglycan is increased in the human atherosclerotic plaque, and is defective in regulation of thrombin via heparin cofactor II activation. *FASEB J* 1997;11(3):A317.
51. Mascellani G, Liverani L, Prete A, et al. Active sites of dermatan sulfate for heparin cofactor II. *J Carbo Chem* 1995;14(8):1165–1177.

Structural and Cellular Components of the Vulnerable Plaque

Dr. Fuster: I would like the inflammation people to be on that side and the mechanically oriented people on this side. The session this morning was oriented toward the two probably most important mechanisms leading to the vulnerability of a plaque: inflammatory forces, and mechanical forces, stress and so forth. So I would like to begin by asking a question to the first panel and actually, specifically, to Dr. Pasterkamp. I must say that I had a completely different idea of remodeling until I listened to you this morning. I will tell you what my idea was and then you tell me how wrong I was. Basically, my understanding of how a plaque develops and the lumen changes is that as the plaque begins to develop, as Dr. Glagov describes, the lumen gets larger. But as the plaque keeps growing, at the very end you end up with a very stenotic lesion and a small lumen. It never occurred to me that when the stenosis is very severe, the mass is the same as when the lumen is large. This is not what I heard you say.

Dr. Pasterkamp: No, that's correct. You point out the importance of our methods. With respect to all the important work Dr. Glagov has performed in the past, and is performing right now, from our point of view, that concept is not correct. It happens in part of the arterial segments. We think that if plaque accumulates, that the artery will not always enlarge and adapt to the plaque formation, but that you're very lucky if that happens. In some locations, something totally different will happen and that is that the artery will not adapt, will not enlarge, but will shrink and at those locations the stenotic problem will occur. So the concept of the very famous graph or plot of Dr. Glagov from initial enlargement is true, but only for part of the cross sections.

Dr. Fuster: Yes, except that when you presented the curves, I was very impressed by the fact that you were not talking about the exception, you were talking about the rule.

299

About a different issue, you said that the vulnerable components are more predominant, when there is an increase in the mass of the atherosclerotic plaque. I just have a problem with this. This means that the very beginning of the lesion formation is the stable period, which in fact it's not. The stable period is at the very end, when the disease is very stenotic and is very fibrotic. So I have a problem there.

Dr. Pasterkamp: We didn't study the initial lesions here. What I didn't mention is, that the femoral arteries we studied for plaque instability came from people from 90 years old on average. So these people were very old, with very advanced lesions and I think we only looked at lesions of type 4, 5 and 6. But coming back to your question of the amount of plaque, as it relates to plaque instability, I think we used a methodology which no one else has used. We took two cross sections from one artery, from one individual, and compared those cross sections with the extremes in geometry within the same individual. In this way, you avoid individual differences in plaque morphology. I totally agree with you that it may be conflicting with other results, but we use different methodology and I can't explain all the differences at this point.

Dr. Fuster: Well I think you contributed significantly this morning to point out that whatever lumen we see, we don't know what is going on underneath in terms of mass and remodeling. I think that's very important. You really changed our way of understanding how the plaque and the lumen change over time and I think that's part of what we try in this meeting is to break from old concepts and go into forward.

Dr. Libby: In the context of Dr. Pasterkamp's presentation, I'd like to suggest that you focus your attention on the adventitia instead of thinking about the fibrous cap. I'd like you to look on the other side of the vessel, and consider the inflammation and enzymes that may be important in the expansion of the artery. It must enlarge through the peri-adventitial connective tissue. Inflammation in the adventitia may be crucial in producing that compensatory enlargement. In the context of restenosis, we know we have a risk of adventitial inflammation, which most people have ignored over the years. Now that we're focused as we were yesterday by Steve Nissen's presentation on the failure of positive remodeling or actual active constriction at the level at the adventitia, I think we have to be refocusing our attention on the adventitia. For example, when we have a predominance of TGFβ in the adventitial inflammatory response, we may have a heightened production of collagen which might cause wound shrinkage and constriction. Whereas, we may have an increase in metalloproteinase activity, a decrease in matrix synthesis, and that will allow the adaptive remodeling. So I think, we have to refocus on the adventitia and I suggest that in your experiments, you probe the adventitia as well.

Discussant from the Audience: I look at post mortem specimens, and I would like to address my questions to the inflammatory group. Dr. Ross and Dr. Fuster have both emphasized that atherosclerosis is an active inflammatory fibroproliferative disease process. When I see adventitial inflammatory cells, am I safe in saying that the patient has active atherosclerotic disease regardless of whether the lumen is narrowed or whether I can see anything at the innermost surface? Can I ask you how often do you see these? Have you quantified? Can you give us a sense?

Dr. Falk: Yes I've studied the whole coronary tree histologically and I see it very often. Perhaps 60 percent of the time, and it doesn't seem to be related to the degree of stenosis, it does seem to be related to ulceration.

Dr. Fuster: I think this is a critical question today and I'm glad you mentioned it. Actually Peter already eluded briefly to the importance of the adventitia. Frankly we know very little and we are now beginning to talk about failing angioplasty and the issue of remodeling and constriction making the adventitia partially responsible. Certainly in my own development of the understanding of this disease, the adventitia didn't play a role in my thinking until very recently so it's very hard for me to make any comments except I am learning. So maybe other people could make comments.

Dr. Rosenfeld: I found in a knockout mouse model, rampant adventitial inflammation especially at those sites that were most stenotic. We also found that in each case where it had occurred, there was also deposition of cholesterol clefts both at the interface, at the internal elastic lamina, and in the media. These were highly correlated with extensive thinning of the media. So I think there's something to Peter's suggestion that there are inflammatory mediators coming from the adventitial surface and that the attraction of those inflammatory cells to the adventitia may be in response to the deposition of cholesterol deep within the lesion.

Dr. Fuster: I'd like to ask a question to Dr. Libby and then to Dr. Guyton. Do you think the cholesterol always comes from the lumen or maybe the part of the cholesterol may come through the vasa vasorum in some way? I'm just asking the question because the cholesterol plaque is very close to the adventitia, and you begin to wonder how it got there.

Dr. Libby: I think it's a possibility, I don't know how likely it is. The only way that I can address that is based on the studies we did on oxidation. When we used antibodies that allowed us to see where there were lipid oxidation products, you always see them very strongly on the adventitial surface. I don't know whether this is due to the presence of lipoproteins that have been oxidized or whether there's a very high oxygen tension in the adventitia and endogenous lipids cause the oxidation. That's the only evidence that lipid mediators may be coming from the adventitial surface.

Dr. Guyton: In answer to your question about causality, I think in ordinary atherosclerosis, the pathway for inflammation goes from inside out, from intimal inflammation through to the adventitia. But as for the question whether it's possible to have outside in, I think we've learned a lot from the transplantation models. About a third of my lab works on transplantation arteriosclerosis where you have an acute rejection of brisk response, inflammatory response in the myocardium with perivascular cuffing as one of the hallmarks of acute rejection. Sometimes when there's eccentric perivascular cuffing with a lymphocyte cluster on the adventitial side, we would see an intimal reaction that was at the same position radially. So that was a strong suggestion that you can have outside/in signaling. Since then we've done experimental studies where we've looked at this symptomatically where we've induced myocardial rejection by withdrawing cyclosporin cyclically and been able to document outside/in signaling in the vessels. So that's an example, an experimental example, which I think illustrates the possibility of this outside/in pathway

Discussant from the Audience: Of course, I find Dr. Rosenfeld's observations extremely intriguing, particularly with regard to the role of free cholesterol in that inflammatory process or the oxidation. But I want to go back to the previously mentioned observation that the ulcerated lesions had more inflammation. And that may be possibly related to an increase convection of fluid at the point where you disrupt the endothelium. One of the things that may be happening is that you're convecting more fluids from the arterial wall and sweeping those inflammatory mediators from the intimal layer into the adventitia. This may be coupled, once you've denuded the endothelium, with an edema and a swelling of the media so that the permeability properties of the media may also change when you change the endothelial permeability.

Discussant from the Audience: I would just like to support the concept of the effect of early disease on, not only on the intima, but also in the whole vessel wall. I would like to share with you some of our data in the hypercholesterolemic pig. This is a model that Dr. Fuster was developing earlier. The pig was fed with cholesterol for 10 or 12 weeks and this pig is characterized by very early lesion, if any lesion at all. We actually demonstrated that some of the major effect is actually localized to the adventitia and what we are able to see is that at the same time, we have an apotopic process, mildly, in the intima. The media was spared, but most of the process was actually in the adventitia. This is a concept that is not new. I think it's a pretty old concept. Also, we were able to demonstrate that there is increased density of vasa vasorum in this model, while the intima proliferation was very, very mild. So I think that the concept that early atherosclerosis affects only the intima, we probably have to look at the whole vessel wall including the vasa vasorum, adventitia, and external elastic membrane. I would like to challenge the panel after all this interesting 2 days. All our data is from autopsies or after death events. What kind of animal model should we use now to follow this disease? Which plaque is vulnerable? How do we define the plaque rupture in an animal model?

Dr. Taubman: Regarding this issue of the adventitia. About a year ago David Gertz came to Mount Sinai to do a sabbatical and brought with him two different rabbit models. One in which the animal was initially injured and then cholesterol fed for a month, the other in which he was essentially cholesterol fed first after a mild denudation and then injured. And what he found, and I don't know if a lot of other investigators have found this, is in the animal which was initially not cholesterol fed, but rather was injured and then cholesterol fed, most of the macrophages appeared to line up at the medial adventitial border; they all expressed tissue factor. On the other hand, the animal which originally was cholesterol fed and then injured, most of the macrophages appeared to be in the intima. I'd like you to comment on what you think about that. That was my other issue. Both MCP1 and tissue factor are obviously constitutively expressed in the adventitia. When you injure, you tend to see an increase in both MRNA and protein in the adventitia. You now see it in the media as well as where you didn't before. But one could argue that in the absence of severe injury, that the gradient may absolutely be coming from the adventitia and may be most important at the level of the vasa vasorum. If you do a severe injury in an animal that's already cholesterol fed, it is already essentially in an activated state, then you get these agents induced in the media, and your gradient then extends to the lumen.

Dr. Fuster: Thank you. The mechanical people are getting very anxious.

Chapter 18

Mechanical Stress and Strain and the Vulnerable Atherosclerotic Lesion

*Luis Rohde, MD, MSc and
Richard T. Lee, MD*

Acute catastrophic vascular events are frequently due to a structural failure of a component of a diseased vessel. Thus, it is not surprising that mechanical features of the atherosclerotic lesion significantly influence its probability of rupture. Recognition of specific features that increase vulnerability to disruption may allow prediction of plaques that are most likely to cause acute events in the future. This chapter introduces basic principles of vascular mechanics, focusing on topics related to stress and strain, in order to provide the appropriate background for understanding the mechanical catastrophe of plaque rupture. Evidence is reviewed that suggests that increased circumferential stress is a major pathophysiological factor involved in plaque rupture. The chapter concludes with a discussion of the critical concept that a loss of atherosclerotic matrix integrity at specific locations in the atherosclerotic lesion is a major determinant of plaque stability.

Vascular Mechanics: Important Basic Principles

The general purpose of studying the mechanics of materials is to ensure that a structure will be safe when confronted with the combined effect of applied forces. By understanding the behavior of different

Supported in part by a Grant-in-Aid from the American Heart Association and a grant from the National Heart Lung and Blood Institute (HL-54759). Dr. Rohde is sponsored by Capes/Brazil.

From: Fuster, V (ed). *The Vulnerable Atherosclerotic Plaque: Understanding, Identification, and Modification.* Armonk, NY: Futura Publishing Company, Inc.; © 1999.

materials under different conditions, we can estimate the probability that a structure can withstand the stresses it will see in the future. It is important to realize that with all materials, including biological materials, fracture is a probability distribution determined by the nature of the imposed stress and the strength of the material.

How do we characterize the mechanical properties of a structure as complex as the diseased artery? If we apply an external force to an object, it will tend to deform in the direction of the applied force, depending on the material properties and geometry of the structure. The resistance to deformation is an important mechanical property of biological tissues that is usually described qualitatively as "stiffness." We need more quantitative measures of material behavior, and therefore we must understand the meaning of stress and strain. Here we introduce some of these concepts to provide us with a common-ground vocabulary for the discussion of the mechanics of the vulnerable lesion; more in-depth overviews can be found in a number of texts and reviews.[1-3]

Stress

Stress is defined as a force acting on a surface and is expressed in units of force divided by the area of the surface. Because force is a vector (that is, it has a direction), stress is also a vector. When the force is applied perpendicular to the surface, such as the stress that blood pressure applies to the lumen of the vessels, it is called a *normal* stress. Normal stresses may be compressive (when the structure tends to shrink) or tensile (when the structure tends to elongate). Stress can also be applied parallel to a surface; this is called *shear* or *tangential* stress. Shear stress causes an angular deformation of a material (Fig. 1).

One type of stress on an object can lead to another. When a cylinder is pressurized, the radial stress of the pressure must be balanced by a circumferential tensile stress in the vessel wall. Under the assumption that the wall of the cylinder is thin relative to the diameter of the vessel, it can be shown that:

$$\sigma = P\,r\,/\,h \qquad (1)$$

where σ is the tensile wall stress, P is the pressure in the vessel, r is the radius of the vessel, and h is the thickness of the vessel (Fig. 2). In this case, the dominant stress component is a tensile stress oriented in the circumferential direction. This is a well-known relationship known as Laplace's law. This concept explains, for example, why the probability of rupture of aortic aneurysms is closely related to the maximal size of the aneurysm. As the radius of the aneurysm enlarges, the circumfer-

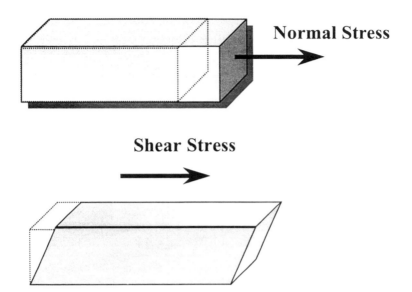

Normal Stress

Shear Stress

Figure 1. Normal versus shear stress. On a given block of a material stress can be applied perpendicular or normal to one of the faces on the block. A shear stress or tangential stress is applied parallel to a face. On any given face of the block there may be two shear stresses and one normal stress.

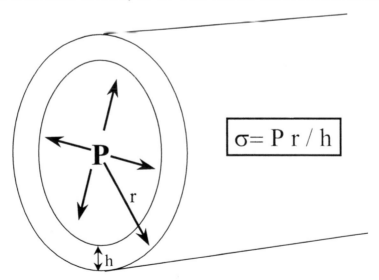

$$\sigma = P\,r\,/\,h$$

Figure 2. Laplace's law. When pressure is applied to the inner lumen of a cylinder or vessel, the force must be balanced by tension or circumferential stress in the vessel wall. If the cylinder is thin relative to the radius, a simple calculation derives the well-known Laplace relation. This explains why thin and large vessels such as aortic aneurysms are much more prone to rupture.

ential wall stress increases; this increase in wall stress is amplified by the thinning of the wall that often accompanies aneurysm expansion.

Strain and the Stress-Strain Relation

When a surface is subject to an externally applied force, the ensuing deformation is the strain. As strain is related to changes in length of a material, it is usually expressed as a fraction or percentage, without units (Fig. 3). Strains can also be tensile (positive strain) or compressive (negative strain) and can be angular, as in strain in response to shear stress. For the same amount of stress (force on a surface) acting on two materials with different mechanical properties, the strains will be

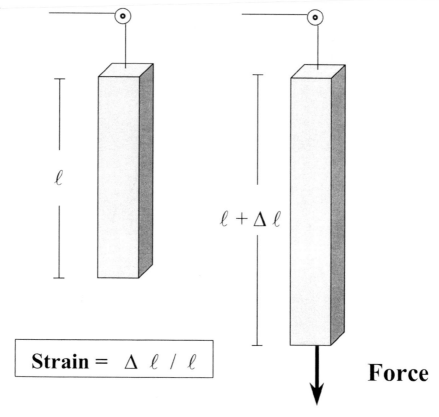

Figure 3. Strain. Strain occurs as a result of stress, but the two terms should not be used interchangeably. In its simplest form, strain in one dimension can be expressed as the percentage of its initial length that a structure increases in length when the stress is applied.

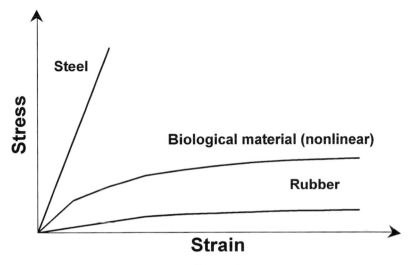

Figure 4. One way to express the stiffness of a material is to plot stress against strain. Stiff materials, such as steel, will have very little strain for a given stress, while materials like rubber have large strains for small stresses. Note that a biological material will have a nonlinear stress- strain relation, typically getting stiffer with increasing strain. In reality, the differences between steel and rubber would be even more marked.

distinct. So, the stress-strain diagrams of two or more materials can be compared to define which one is stiffer (Figure 4). *E* is the ratio of stress to strain and is called *the elastic modulus* or *the Young's modulus*:

$$E = \text{stress/strain} \qquad (2)$$

Nonlinear Elasticity

In many nonbiological materials, the relation between stress and strain is constant over the range of stresses imposed on that structure. When this relation is constant we can say that the material has a linear elastic behavior, and Young's modulus can describe much of the material's behavior. Biological materials, however, rarely behave as linear elastic materials. As the stress on a biological material is increased, the increment of strain for each increment of stress decreases, so that the material actually becomes stiffer; hence we say that these materials have nonlinear elasticity (see Figure 4).

Anisotropy

A block of steel or plastic has material properties that are the same in every direction, a property called *isotropy*. Most biological materials respond differently to the force applied in different directions; this asymmetric behavior is called *anisotropy*. The artery, with layers of smooth muscle cells, extracellular matrix, and other components, is a markedly anisotropic structure. The anisotropic nature of the biological materials makes it more difficult to describe their mechanical behavior through simple parameters.

The Atherosclerotic Plaque: Biomechanical Considerations

Most of the stress load of the normal arterial wall is probably carried by the medial layer. The media comprises concentric layers of smooth muscle cells, collagen, and elastin with extracellular matrix proteoglycans. Elastin is an important contributor to the normal pulsatile behavior of the vessels and behaves mechanically close to a linear elastic material (that is, it has a constant Young's modulus and returns to its initial shape when the stress is removed). Although elastin can be stretched to many times its initial length at rest without rupturing, it will fracture at relatively low stresses. Collagen, in contrast, is an extremely stiff protein: the tensile modulus of individual collagen fibers is approximately 5000 times that of elastin. Analysis of mechanical properties of individual collagen fibers from rat tendon tail shows very high tensile strength, with rupture only at stresses equivalent to 250,000 mm Hg.

While many other factors help to determine how the artery responds to stress, it is useful to consider the network of elastin and collagen in the concept of nonlinear stiffness. At low stresses and strains, the collagen fibers are relaxed and the "rubber-band–like" behavior of the elastin fibers dominates the mechanical behavior of the artery. At higher stresses and strains, the elastin fibers are stretched to their limit, and the collagen fibers become progressively "recruited" so that the vessel becomes stiff and more resistant to rupture. Stress and strain measurements in human arteries have confirmed this nonlinear elastic behavior. Because the normal artery is relatively symmetric, useful analyses of material properties can be made with noninvasive techniques, considering the artery as relatively homogeneous.[4]

Mechanical Stress in Complex Atherosclerotic Lesions

In contrast with the normal artery, the materials and geometries of the atherosclerotic lesion are too complex to be analyzed with simple formulas such as the Laplace equation. Atherosclerotic lesions have stiff fibrous materials, focal calcifications, and very soft necrotic lipid pools. Investigators have used a technique called *finite element analysis* to approach the mechanical properties of the vulnerable lesion. Finite element analysis is a widely used engineering technique used to study complex three-dimensional structures. The distribution of stress within the original complex structure can be calculated by subdividing the structures into much smaller sections and assigning specific mechanical properties for each element. Airplanes and bridges are examples of tremendously complex structures that bear enormous amounts of stress and that can be designed through finite element analysis. For example, the current Boeing 777 aircraft was designed completely by finite element analysis.

Because the atherosclerotic plaque is such a complex structure, it would be unrealistic to attempt to simulate all of its biomechanical behavior. Instead, one may take the approach of identifying the most critical or dominant parameters, measuring these whenever possible, and designing a finite element approach that can be realistically applied to individual coronary artery lesions (Fig. 5). As described below, this

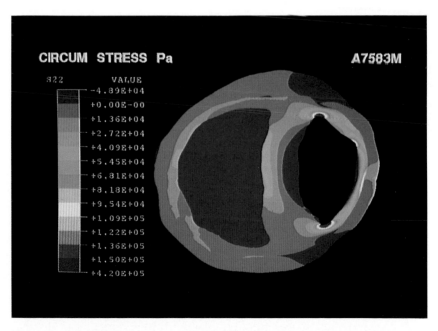

Figure 5. Stress in a human atherosclerotic lesion. This is a finite element model of stress in a human atherosclerotic lesion. The deep blue lipid pool has almost no stress. The red locations are very–high-stress regions (the color scale at the left is in pascals, a unit of stress measurement).

approach has provided insight into the nature of the vulnerable lesion and the approach is supported by postmortem findings as well as clinical data.

In 1989, Richardson et al[5] presented landmark data on finite element analysis and the association of the pathology of the vulnerable lesion with plaque rupture. In this study of coronary plaque fissures, the investigators suggested that the particularly common configuration of a fissure through the edge or center of a fibrous cap was due to high circumferential tensile stress in the fibrous cap. This increased stress was caused by the inability of the soft lipid core of the atheroma to bear stress. We extended these observations in a study of coronary artery models based on biomechanical measurements in hundreds of actual aortic atherosclerotic lesions.[6] We speculated that stenosis severity was not a major indicator of lesion stability, while lipid content and fibrous cap thickness were the dominant factors. Our studies indicated that lesion area reduction is, in fact, a negligible factor in determining stress in the fibrous cap. In fact, very severe stenoses tend to have slightly lower stresses, because the radius of curvature of the lumen is small. This may be one reason that very severe stenoses, as detected by angiography, tend to cause asymptomatic occlusion rather than massive infarctions.

In contrast, the thickness of a fibrous cap overlying a lipid pool is a critical factor in determining lesion stress. When fibrous cap thickness falls below 200 μm, stress in the fibrous cap can skyrocket to many thousands of mm Hg, the level of stress necessary to fracture human atherosclerotic tissue. It is interesting to note that most plaques that rupture have fibrous cap thicknesses of 50 to 180 μm postmortem. Unfortunately, with our current routine clinical tools, there is no method for measuring fibrous cap thickness in vivo, particularly in the submillimeter range. These data suggest, however, that imaging modalities such as intravascular ultrasound and optical coherence tomography may have the resolution to identify vulnerable lesions.

What is the role of calcification in plaque rupture? Occasionally, thrombi in coronary arteries can be found at locations where a nodule of calcium has apparently "eroded" through the fibrous cap, causing the disruption. Overall, however, most plaques that rupture are not heavily calcified, and focal calcifications are not as important as fibrous cap thickness in causing high-stress locations. In contrast, calcification of lesions has a significant impact on the outcome of balloon angioplasty, where calcium deposits may accentuate the dissection that generally accompanies successful angioplasty.[7] It may appear paradoxical that calcification has a major influence on balloon angioplasty but perhaps less on spontaneous plaque rupture. However, balloon angioplasty in most cases is successful due in part to shear between layers of the artery as the balloon expands to diameters that the artery does not experience under normal conditions. In this circumstance, tearing of tissue past the stiff calcification is more likely to occur. In addition, some complex atherosclerotic lesions with heavy calcification have sub-intimal fibrillar collagen bands with an appearance that suggests that plaque rupture has already occurred and has healed. This raises the intriguing possibility that calcification may accompany asymptomatic plaque rupture and healing that relieves high-stress regions. This scenario would explain why ruptured lesions often are not heavily calcified.

Computational biomechanical modeling of any phenomenon is interesting but subject to criticism without support and validation from the actual biology. We have evaluated the concept that increased circumferential stress is associated with plaque fracture sites by studying actual patient lesions in detail.[8] In reconstructions of ruptured and non-ruptured lesions, stresses in plaques that ruptured were significantly higher than in unruptured plaques (4091 versus 1444 mm Hg, $P<0.0001$). In most lesions, the actual plaque ruptures occurred in high-stress locations, defined as regions with stresses greater than 2250 mm Hg. These data support the hypothesis that high circumferential stress regions are also the vulnerable rupture locations.

However, plaques do not always rupture at the absolute highest stress region; often the rupture occurs at the second or even third highest region. One simple and trivial explanation for this is error in our methods, but these data also suggest an important biological explanation. It is clear when one handles human atherosclerotic tissue that the tissue is very heterogeneous, with some tough regions and other friable regions. This heterogeneity probably explains why plaque rupture does not always occur at the highest stress region in a given lesion. At the highest stress location, the tissue may be more resistant to fracture, while the tissue may be weaker at the second or third highest stress region. This heterogeneity in tissue strength, which has been confirmed with careful biomechanical experiments with human tissue,[9] suggests that strategies to improve lesion strength could modestly lead to major improvements in plaque stability.

High-Stress Regions and the Dynamic Atheroma Matrix

Tissue structure requires a balance between synthesis, organization, and degradation of extracellular matrix. Even in normal tissues this process is ongoing at a very slow rate. In atherosclerotic lesions, enzymes that degrade extracellular matrix proteins may play an impor-

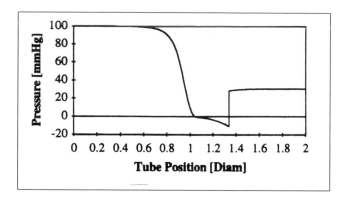

Figure 4. Area versus distance along stenosis, showing compression just downstream of the throat.

dilate, the distal pressure falls. The blood flow increases, and the throat pressure falls even more. The stenosis eventually stops any more flow through the throat, limiting the hemodynamic "flow reserve," a phenomenon called *flow choking* by fluid mechanicians.[7] Flow choking occurs even when there is no viscosity, and is the main limit to flow in a dynamic stenosis.[8,9] The stenosis may even "collapse" when the throat pressure falls too low.

Several factors can influence flow choking, including degree of stenosis, distal pressure, external pressure, and plaque stiffness. Severity of stenosis is the dominant of these factors.[10] Low distal pressures seen during ischemia/hyperemia can induce choking. High external pressures, as during a Valsalva maneuver, compress the plaque. A calcific plaque may stent the artery open.

When the pressure in the throat of the stenosis falls below the external pressure, the plaque cap undergoes compression loading instead of tension loading (Fig. 4).[11] The cap may cycle between compression during the high flow phase of a cardiac cycle and tension during the slow flow phase. This is a loading condition that arteries typically never experience; thus, arteries probably are not built to withstand intermittent compression.

A diseased carotid artery was modeled with elastic materials shaped in the form of a stenosis.[6a] These models allowed for variations in stenosis severity, wall thickness, and stiffness. Two elastic materials were used to form the tubes: a silicone rubber material (Sylgard 184, Dow Corning Corp., Midland, MI), and a latex rubber dipping compound. Each of these compounds had different stiffness and application properties. The silicone rubber was applied uniformly on the outer surface of the mandrel with a stiff brush. The mandrel was continuously rotated to ensure uniform thickness of the liquid layer. Wall thickness could be controlled by the amount of material applied and the rate of rotation. The polymer was exposed to gentle heating to accelerate the curing process. The latex stenoses were made by first dipping the clean mandrel in a calcium nitrate solution, then dipping the coated mandrel in the liquid latex compound. Latex wall thickness was governed by the dipping time.

The pressure-area relationship was slightly different for the proximal, throat, and distal portions of the model, due to manufacturing variations. The values for a silicone tube are shown in Figure 5. Curves for a fresh bovine carotid artery and a latex Penrose tube-law are also shown in this figure for comparison. The silicone model behaved similarly to the latex rubber tube. However, the models were much stiffer than the bovine artery for high positive pressures. Likewise, for highly negative pressures, the silicone model was much stiffer. Around small negative pressures, all of the tubes collapsed at similar magnitudes. Thus, the buckling point of the silicone tube appears to be a reasonable model for experiments that focus on the initial collapse of an artery. Additionally, it is likely that diseased stenotic arteries would be much stiffer than normal arteries or tubes of constant diameter.

The various parameters of stenosis severity, proximal pressure, stiffness, and axial strain can be compared in order to gain insight into the relative importance of these factors on collapse. A factorial design analysis at two levels was performed on the results of these experi-

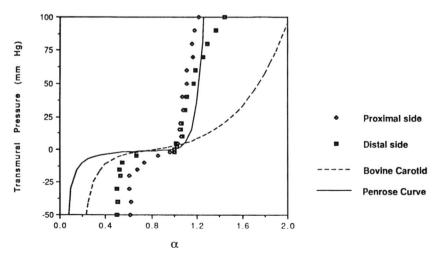

Figure 5. Pressure versus area for an artery, and models made of silicone and latex rubber for negative and positive pressures.

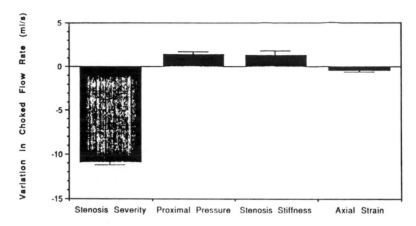

Figure 6. Relative strength of various parameters in producing flow choking and compression. Note that severity of stenosis is most influential.

ments.[6a] Figure 6 illustrates the relative influence of these parameters on the choked flow rate. By far, the most important parameter was the severity of stenosis, as a change in severity from 71% to 78% reduced the choked flow by almost 11 mL/s. An increase in perfusion pressure by 30 mm Hg or an increase in tube stiffness by 25 Pa increased the choked flow rate by approximately 1.5 mL/s. The axial strain differences yielded a small decrease in choked flow rate of about 1 mL/s.

A multiple regression analysis was also performed on the results of 60 independent experiments.[6a] A 95% confidence interval can be plotted for choked flow rate as a function of stenosis severity. Likewise, a plot of the coefficient of multiple determination r^2 as a function of the variables in the model can be made. This analysis shows that stenosis severity accounts for 89.9% of the choked flow, whereas the addition of inlet pressure or axial strain only increases the coefficient of multiple determination by 0.5%.

There is now an unusual loading condition in this artery, which is built like a composite material. In engineering, the typical use of the term *composite material* refers to polymers with fibers made from petroleum products formed under high pressure. However, a true composite is any material composed of fibers and a matrix used for a structure. Thus, an artery is a natural composite structure made by the body. We then asked the question: how would a plaque cap respond to such a cyclic compressive load?

Materials engineers have a great deal of experience with composite materials and their failure modes. In general, cyclic loads can cause failure of a material even when a single load of this magnitude is not detrimental. The worst type of repetitive loading happens when the loads cycle between tension and compression—commonly seen when one breaks a paper clip by bending it back and forth. Similarly, old airplane bolts can fail catastrophically after years of cyclic loading. When an artery is subjected to compression, it initially shrinks, but then it buckles and bends into a new shape. Stress concentrations can reach very high levels in the cap. Our hypothesis is that the strength of the plaque cap is weakened by the cyclic compressive loading (Fig. 7).[11]

We have subjected a series of human arteries with atherosclerotic plaque caps to cyclic loading between tension and compression. The intimal surface exhibited a high frequency of rupture at the point of maximal compression in comparison with control arteries loaded only in tension (n = 24, $P<0.01$).[12] Thus, we concluded that the cyclic compression of high-grade arterial stenoses can contribute to localized plaque cap weakness and can increase the propensity to plaque cap rupture.

We have further explored the physiological likelihood of this scenario.[13] During high flow conditions, the stenosis severity can increase, ie, a dynamic stenosis.[9] The throat diameter decreases from the low pressures there, and the upstream diameter tends to increase from the higher resistance. Compression is highly likely for arterial stenoses greater than 70% by diameter. It is interesting to note that this amount of stenosis appears to be a common clinical criterion for hemodynamically significant stenosis. Soft lipid-laden plaques should be more likely to compress than stiff calcific plaques. In one ultrasound study of carotid disease, echo-lucent lipid plaques were much more likely to become symptomatic than echo-dense or calcific plaques in the greater than 70% category.[14]

General pressures are strongly increased with heavy lifting, and severe exercise might be expected to produce sudden increases in pressure, leading to collapse of the stenosis. The distal pressure past a stenosis is a difficult quantity to measure. An approximate value can be obtained by measuring the stump pressure of the internal carotid artery during an endarterectomy operation in which the flow in the artery is stopped. Approximately 25% of stump pressures are lower than 20 mm Hg, which can put this population at greater risk for plaque compression.

Arterial spasm near a stenosis may be precipitated by local wall compression, which may be exacerbated by pharmacological interventions designed to decrease the downstream resistance. If opposing endothelial cells should touch during a collapse, denudation of endothelial cells and exposure of collagen is possible. When the plaque cap ruptures, we have found that platelets adhere and accumulate most

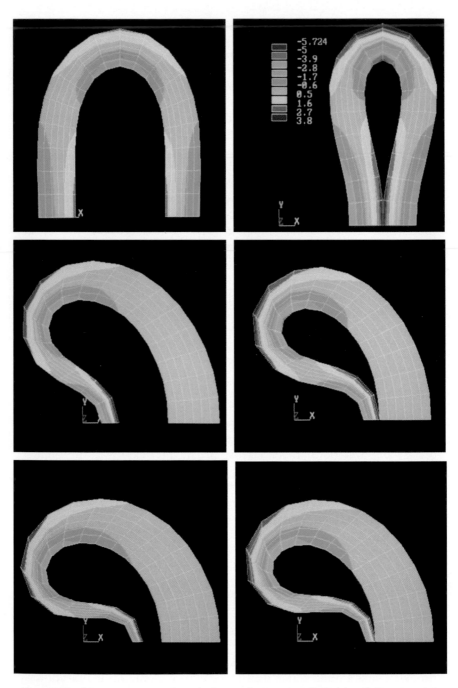

Figure 7. Artery cross section during collapse, predicted by finite element modeling.

strongly at the throat of a collagen-coated stenosis, where the shear stresses are greatest.[15]

In conclusion, the hemodynamic forces surrounding high-grade stenosis are complex but may be analyzed in fluid mechanical terms. The stenosis causes high velocities in the throat, which in turn lower the intraluminal pressure. The low pressure at the throat increases the severity of the stenosis and causes compression of the plaque cap with each cardiac cycle. The cyclic compression on the plaque cap can produce a localized mechanical weakening, which combined with local accumulations of matrix metalloproteinases, may produce focal plaque rupture of a catastrophic nature. An understanding of the combination of local mechanical forces and biochemical factors may be important to the prediction and treatment of the terminal events in atherosclerosis.

References

1. North American Symptomatic Carotid Endarterectomy Trial (NASCET) Collaborators. Beneficial effect of carotid endarterectomy in symptomatic patients with high-grade carotid stenosis. *N Engl J Med* 1991;325:445–453.
2. Young B, Moore WS, Robertson JT, et al. An analysis of perioperative surgical mortality and morbidity in the asymptomatic carotid atherosclerosis study. Asymptomatic Carotid Atherosclerosis Study (ACAS) Investigators. *Stroke* 1996;27(12):2216–2224.
3. Alderman EL, Fisher L, Maynard C, et al. Determinants of coronary surgery in a consecutive patient series from geographically dispersed medical centers. Coronary Artery Surgery Study (CASS). *Circulation* 1982;66(2 pt 2): I6–I15.
4. Davies MJ, Thomas AC. Plaque fissuring–The cause of acute myocardial infarction, sudden ischemic death, and crescendo angina. *Br Heart J* 1985; 53:363–373.
5. Clark JM, Glagov S. Transmural organization of the arterial media–the lamellar unit revisited. *Arteriosclerosis* 1985;5:19–34.
6. Binns RL, Ku DN. The effect of stenosis on wall motion: a possible mechanisms of stroke and transient ischemic attack. *Arteriosclerosis* 1989;9: 842–847.
6a. Biz S. *Flow in Collapsable Stenosis: An Experimental Study*. Atlanta, GA: Georgia Institute of Technology; 1993. Thesis.
7. Shapiro HH. Steady flow in collapsible tubes. *J Biomech Eng* 1977;9:126–147.
8. Ku DN, Zeigler MN, Downing JM. One-dimensional steady inviscid flow through a stenotic collapsible tube. *ASME J Biomech Eng* 1990;112:444–450.
9. Gould KL. Pressure-flow characteristics of coronary stenoses in unsedated dogs at rest and during coronary vasodilation. *Circ Res* 1978;43(2);2–253.
10. Downing JM, Ku DN. Effects of frictional losses and pulsatile flow in the collapse of stenotic arteries. *J Biomech Eng* 1997;119(3):317–324.
11. Aoki T, Ku DN. Collapse of diseased arteries with eccentric cross section. *J Biomech Eng* 1993;26(2):133–142.
12. Ku DN, McCord BN. Cyclic stress causes rupture of the atherosclerotic plaque cap. *Circulation* 1993;88(4 pt 2, suppl):1362.

13. Ku DN. Blood flow in arteries. *Ann Rev Fluid Mech* 1997;29:399–434.
14. Johnson J, Kennelly MM, Decesare D, et al. Natural history of asymptomatic carotid plaque. *Arch Surg* 1985;120:1010.
15. Markou CP, Hanson SR, Siegel JM, et al. The role of high wall shear rate of thrombus formation in stenoses. *Adv Bioeng ASME BED* 1993;26:555–558.

Chapter 20

Effect of Rheology on Thrombosis

Juan Jose Badimon, PhD, Lina Badimon, PhD, and Valentin Fuster, MD, PhD

The causative role of coronary thrombotic occlusion in acute myocardial infarction was postulated at the turn of the century. Only recently have clinical and pathological observations and experimental investigation led to a better understanding of platelet-vessel wall interaction and thrombus formation and its implication in the onset of coronary ischemic events.

Pathological studies of patients who died suddenly or shortly after a coronary event have shown that the existence of an acute thrombus on a disrupted atherosclerotic plaque is fundamental in the onset of the acute ischemic events. Emerging evidence also suggests that plaque rupture, subsequent thrombus formation, and fibrous organization of thrombus are important in the progression of atherosclerosis in asymptomatic patients and those with stable angina. In addition, within the past few years it has become apparent that coronary atherosclerotic lesions with less severe angiographic disease are associated with rapid progression to severe stenosis or total occlusion and that these lesions may account for unstable angina or acute myocardial infarction in up to two thirds of patients who develop these conditions. Studies on atherosclerotic plaques from stable angina patients have revealed old, organized thrombi that were difficult to differentiate from atherosclerotic changes seen in the arterial wall. Therefore, it is clear that plaque disruption with mural thrombus formation, its subsequent fibrotic organization, significantly contributes to the fast progression of atherosclerotic plaques seen in some cases.

From: Fuster, V (ed). *The Vulnerable Atherosclerotic Plaque: Understanding, Identification, and Modification.* Armonk, NY: Futura Publishing Company, Inc.; © 1999.

Pathophysiology of Thrombus Formation

The major role of normal endothelium is to maintain the fluidity of the blood within the blood vessels. Disruption of the integrity of the blood vessels results in a cascade of events leading to normal hemostasis or thrombosis. Platelets have long been considered to play a primary role in the events associated with hemostasis and thrombosis. Circulating platelets rapidly become activated by the exposure to collagen from the arterial wall and thrombin generated by the activation of the coagulation cascade, as well as to circulating agonists.

In the initial stages of endothelial injury, with functional alterations but without major morphological changes, no significant platelet deposition or thrombus formation can be demonstrated. A few scattered platelets may interact with such subtly injured endothelium and contribute, by the release of growth factors, to very mild intimal injury, form a monolayer to a few layers of platelets, which may deposit on the lesion, with or without mural thrombus formation. In severe injury, with exposure of components of deeper layers of the vessels, as in spontaneous plaque rupture or in angioplasty, marked platelet aggregation with mural thrombus formation follows. Vascular injury of this magnitude also stimulates thrombin formation through both the intrinsic (surface-activated) and extrinsic (tissue factor-dependent) coagulation pathways, in which the platelet membrane facilitates interactions between clotting factors. This concept for vascular injury as a trigger of the platelet coagulation response is important in understanding the pathogenesis of various vascular diseases associated with atherosclerosis and coronary artery disease.[1,2]

Platelet Activation

Exposed matrix from the vessel wall, thrombin generated by the activation of the coagulation cascade, and circulating epinephrine are all powerful platelet agonists. Adenosine diphosphate (ADP) is a platelet agonist that may be released from hemolyzed red cells in the area of vessel injury. Most platelet aggregation agonists seem to act through the hydrolysis of platelet membrane phosphatidylinositol by phospholipase C, which causes the mobilization of free calcium from the platelet-dense tubular system. Calcium mobilization promotes the contraction of the platelet, with the subsequent release of the content of its various storage organelles. Platelet-released ADP and serotonin stimulate adjacent platelets, further enhancing the process of platelet activation. Arachidonate, which is released from the platelet membrane by the stimulatory effect of collagen, thrombin, adenosine diphosphate, and serotonin, is another platelet agonist. Arachidonate is converted to thromboxane A_2, and not only promotes further aggregation, but is also a potent vasoconstrictor (Fig. 1).

The initial recognition of a damaged vessel wall by platelets involves: (1) adhesion, activation, and adherence to recognition sites on the thromboactive substrate (extracellular matrix proteins; eg, von Willebrand factor (vWF), collagen, fibronectin, vitronectin, laminin); (2) spreading of the platelet on the surface; and (3) aggregation with each other to form a platelet plug or white thrombus. The efficiency of the platelet recruitment depends on the underlying substrate and local geometry. A final step of recruitment of other blood cells also occurs; erythrocytes, neutrophils, and occasionally monocytes are found on evolving mixed thrombi (Fig. 2).

Platelet function depends on adhesive interactions, and most of the glycoproteins on the platelet membrane surface are receptors for adhesive proteins. Many of these receptors have been identified, cloned, se-

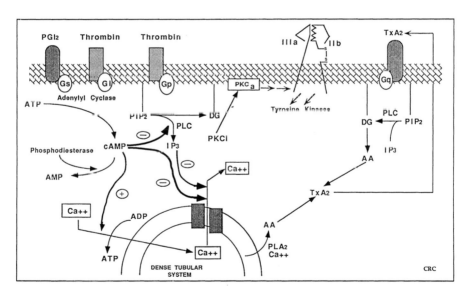

Figure 1. Signal transduction mechanisms initiated upon binding of agonists to platelet membrane receptors. Binding activates G-proteins and triggers intracellular second messengers (IP^3, DG). The final outcome is the activation of platelet secretion, IIb/IIIa receptor exposure, and aggregation. PGI^2, = prostacyclin; TxA^2 = thromboxane A^2; PIP^2 = phosphoinositol diphosphate; PLC = phospholipase C; PKC and PKCa = protein kinase C inactivated and activated, respectively; DG = diacylglycerol; IP^3 = inositol 1,4,5-triphosphate; AA = arachidonic acid; PLA^2 = phospholipase A^2; Gs, Gi, Gp, Gq = guanine nucleotide-binding regulatory proteins; IIb/IIIa = glycoprotein receptor for adhesive ligands, which supports platelet aggregation.

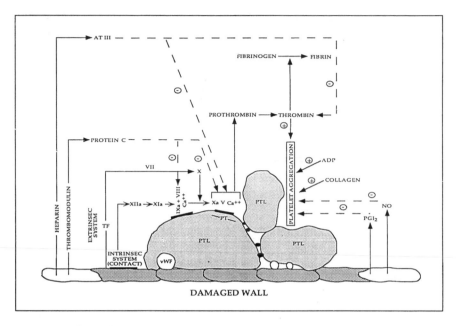

Figure 2. Simplified diagram of platelet-vessel wall, platelet-platelet interaction and coagulation enzymes. Platelet adhesion to recognition sites occurs in lesioned areas of the endothelium. Adhesion spreading and aggregation of newly arriving platelets contributes to mural thrombosis. Aggregation is enhanced by agonists present in the microenvironment (arrows with (+) signs), while there are spontaneous pathways of inhibition (arrows with (-) signs) derived from neighboring normal endothelium. TF = tissue factor; AT III = antithrombin III; NO = nitric oxide; PT = prothrombinase complex; vWF = von Willebrand factor.

quenced, and classified within large gene families that mediate a variety of cellular interactions (Table 1).[3,4] The most abundant is the integrin family, which includes GPIIb-IIIa, GPIa-IIa, GPIc-IIa, the fibronectin receptor, and the vitronectin receptor, in decreasing order of magnitude. Another gene family present in the platelet membrane glycocalyx is the leucine-rich glycoprotein family, represented by the GPIb-IX complex, receptor for vWF on unstimulated platelets, that mediates adhesion to subendothelium and GPV. Other gene families include the selectins (such as GMP-140) and the immunoglobulin domain protein (HLA class I antigen and cell adhesion molecule-related PECAM-1). Unrelated to any other gene family is the GPIV (IIIa) (Table 1).[3]

Therefore, platelet activation triggers intracellular signaling and expression of platelet membrane receptors for adhesion and initiation of cell contractile processes that will induce shape changes of platelets and secretion of the granular contents. The expression of the integrin

Table 1

Platelet Membrane Glycoprotein Receptors

Glycoprotein receptor	Ligand[1]	Function
GPIIb-IIIa (αIIb β_3)	Fg, vWF, Fn, Ts, Vn	Aggregation, adhesion at HSR[2]
Receptor Vn ($\alpha_v\beta_3$)	Vn, vWF, Fn, Fg, Ts	Adhesion
GP Ia-IIa (VLA-2, α_2 β_1)	C	Adhesion
GP Ic-IIa (VLA-5, α_5 β_1)	Fn	Adhesion
GP Ic'-IIa (VLA-6, α_6 β_1)	Ln	Adhesion
GP Ib-IX	vWF, T	Adhesion
GP V	substrate T	Unknown
GP IV (GP IIIb)	Ts, C	Adhesion
GMP-140 (PADGEM)	unknown	Interaction with leucocytes
PECAM-1 (GP IIa)	unknown	Unknown

[1]Fg = fibrinogen; vWF = von Willebrand factor; Fn = fibronectin; Ts = thrombospondin; Vn = vitronectin; C = collagen; L = laminin; T = thrombin. [2]HSR = high shear rate.

IIb/IIa (aIIb b$_3$) receptors for adhesive glycoprotein ligands (mainly fibrinogen and vWF) in the circulation initiate platelet-platelet interaction. The process is perpetuated by the arrival of passing-by platelets. Most of the glycoproteins in the platelet membrane surface are receptors for adhesive proteins or mediate cellular interactions.

Regulation of Thrombus Formation

Platelet arterial wall interactions and thrombus formation are modulated by the local fluid dynamics, the nature of the exposed substrate, and by systemic factors.

An investigation into the local fluid dynamic conditions is essential for an understanding of events occurring at the blood-surface interface. Blood flow determines the rate of transport of cells to and away from the substrate, and imposes fluid forces that affect the removal of material deposited at the surface. These forces may also lead to physical activation of secretory processes.[5,6]

Fluid Dynamics

From the rheologic point of view, blood is essentially incompressible and viscous. Because it is incompressible, it is insensitive to the pressure to which it is subjected, responding only to differences among neighboring points.[7,8] Therefore, the mechanical forces produced in blood vessels may result from (1) luminal pressure changes that cause blood flow (which yields shear stress); or (2) transmural pressure changes that cause circumferential deformation of the layers of the vessel wall during the cardiac cycle (caused by tensile stress). Fluid shear stress is the force per unit area generated by flow of a viscous liquid. Tensile stress produces strain, which is a measure of the percent change in vessel circumference generated by the expansion and contraction of the vascular lumen. Strain is the force which would tear a cell, or layer, from its normal position within the vessel wall.

The term *shear* has the precise physical meaning of a sliding motion between two adjacent planes. Blood flow can be described as an infinite number of laminae sliding one across another, each lamina suffering some frictional interference with the other laminae. Blood flow in a tubular chamber generates a parabolic flow profile. This results in maximal velocity and minimal shear at the center of the blood flow stream, and minimal velocity and maximal shear rate at the vessel wall. Shearing forces are generated by the different velocities between the laminae of the blood flow.

The shear rate, according to its definition for one-dimensional flow, is the velocity gradient in the direction perpendicular to the flow. The magnitude of the shear rate at the wall (wall shear rate) is particularly important in that it reflects the movement near the wall where most of the mass transport and reaction processes occur. In tubular vessels, wall shear stress of newtonian fluid can be calculated as a function of the volumetric flow rate: $\tau = 4\mu Q/\Pi r^3$, where μ is viscosity, Q is the volumetric flow, and r is the radius of the tubular chamber. Shear rate decreases with increasing vessel diameter for the same flow rate. Shear stress, which is mathematically the product of the fluid viscosity and the shear rate, is another basic parameter. In accordance with this for-

---

Table 2

Typical Ranges of Wall Shear Rates and Wall Shear Stresses in Human Blood Vessels

Blood vessel	Wall shear rate	Wall shear stress
Larges arteries	300–800	11.4–30.4
Arterioles	500–1,600	19.0–60.8
Veins	20–200	0.76–7.6
Stenotic vessels	800–10,000	30.4–380

Assuming a blood viscosity of 0.038 Poise. Wall shear rates expressed as seconds^{-1}, and shear stress as dynes/cm^2. Modified from Reference 43.

mula, Table 2 presents the typical ranges of wall shear rate and wall shear stresses.

The value of wall shear rate represents the force per unit area applied by the fluid on the vascular wall. Although these two parameters differ only in magnitude by a coefficient of viscosity [shear stress $\tau = -\mu \, (dv_z/dr)$; where μ is viscosity and (dv_z/dr) is shear rate], from a physical point of view, they have different functions in the event at the wall. It is the shear stress that directly exerts a force on substances, tending to strip them from the wall, while the shear rate contributes to the convective transport of material to the area and the removal of detached (soluble) material from the area.

Effect of Flow on Thrombus Formation in a Tubular Perfusion Chamber

Platelet-vessel wall interactions and thrombus formation in vivo take place under flow conditions. Several in vitro systems capable of modeling the different flow conditions developing in the blood vessels have been developed to investigate the mechanisms by which mechanical forces affect platelet-thrombus formation. Table 3 presents a summary of different flow systems used by other investigators.

Table 3

Different Flow Systems for Studying the Effects of Flow on Blood Cells-Surfaces Interactions

Type	Shear stress	Surface
Cone viscosimeter[44]	<1 to >200	None, cells, proteins, ECM
Annular chamber[45]	<10 to 800	Everted rabbit aorta
Parallel plate chamber[46]	<10 to >500	None, cells, protein, ECM, biomaterials
Tubular chamber[9]	<10 to >250	Aortic tissue, proteins, cells, biomaterials, ECM
Flow viscosimeter[47]	>1000	None
Filter aggregation[48]	?	Glass fiber
Flow column[49]	15 to 52	Proteins
Filtragometry[50]	?	Siliconized nickel filter
Stenotic Chambers		
Tubular chamber[51]	<10 to >500	Aortic tissue, proteins, biomaterials, ECM
Parallel plate chamber[52]	<10 to >500	None, cells, protein, ECM, biomaterials

ECM = extracellular mass.

To investigate the dynamics of platelet deposition and thrombus formation following vascular damage and to study the influence of various biochemical and physical factors, we developed a tubular perfusion chamber that retains the cylindrical shape of the vascular system and permits ex vivo exposure of such surfaces to blood under controlled flow conditions (Fig. 3). The description and rheologic characterization of the chamber has been described.[12]

To allow for the evaluation of platelet-thrombus formation on the exposed substrate to flowing blood, autologous platelets were labeled with 111 Indium. Platelet deposition was assessed from the ration between the platelet count and blood radioactivity in the animal and the radioactivity deposited in the exposed substrate. Dual labeling of fibrinogen allowed us to study the deposition of both platelet and fibrin(ogen).[9]

Exposure of de-endothelialized vessel wall (thus mimicking mild vascular injury) to blood demonstrated the shear dependence of platelet

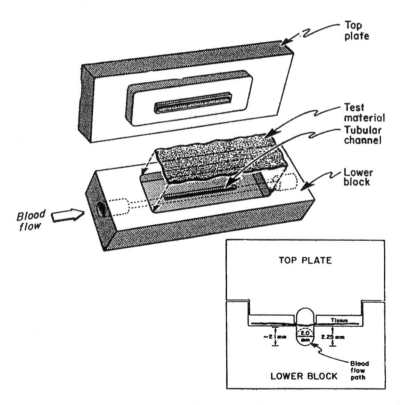

Figure 3. Sketch of the Badimon perfusion chamber used to expose material to flowing blood. From Reference 9.

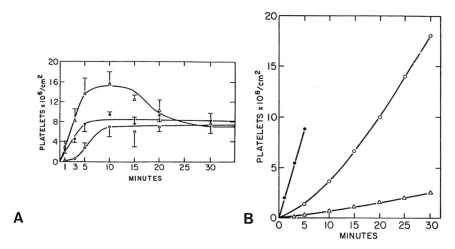

Figure 4. Platelet deposition on subendothelium (**A**) and on collagen (**B**) at different wall shear rates. Wall shear rates expressed as sec^{-1}. ○ = 1690; ● = 212, and Δ = 106. From Reference 10.

deposition (Fig 4., Panel A). At low shear rates, platelet deposition reached a maximum within 5 to 10 minutes of exposure, after which platelet deposition remained relatively constant. At high wall shear rate (1690/s), initial platelet deposition rate was higher that at the lower shear rates. Maximum platelet deposition was also observed at 5 to 10 minutes of exposure. However, the thrombi could be dislodged from the substrate by the flowing blood, suggesting that the thrombus was labile. At longer periods of perfusion, platelet deposition decreased to values not significantly different from those seen at the lower shear rate levels.

Exposure of fibrillar collagen (thus mimicking a deeper injury into the vessel wall) to blood produced platelet deposition of more than two orders of magnitude greater than on subendothelium (Fig. 4, panel B).[10] Even at high shear rate, platelet thrombus that formed was not dislodged, but remained adherent to the surface. These observations emphasize not only the importance of the shear rate but also the influence of the degree of injury on platelet deposition and thrombus formation. Overall, it is likely that when injury to the vessel wall is mild, the thrombogenic stimulus is relatively limited and the resulting thrombotic occlusion is transient, as occurs in unstable angina. On the other hand, deep vessel injury secondary to plaque rupture or ulceration results in exposure of collagen, tissue factor, and other elements of the vessel matrix, leading to relatively persistent thrombotic occlusion and myocardial infarction.[12]

The majority of flow studies have been performed in laminar flow conditions. Laminar flow conditions are not maintained in atherosclerotic vessels, since stenotic narrowings induce flow disturbances that modify cell-cell and cell-vessel wall interactions as well as the local concentrations of fluid-phase chemical mediators necessary for cell interaction. Using a modification of our perfusion chamber that allowed us to study the effects of varying degrees of stenosis on acute platelet deposition,[11] we found that platelet deposition on the damaged artery

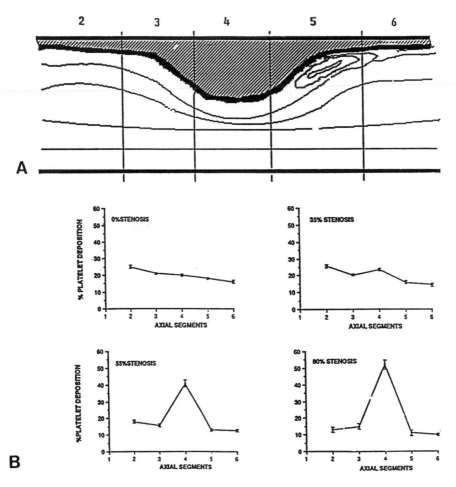

Figure 5. Axial distribution of platelet deposition on no-parallel stream lines. **A.** Scheme of the stream lines developing on an eccentric stenosis. **B.** Axial dependence of platelet depsition following perfusion at different degrees of stenosis. Blood flow was from left to right. Results are expressed as percentage of platelet deposition on the whole segment. From Reference 11.

increased with increasing stenosis. In addition, the axial distribution of platelet deposition clearly indicated that platelet thrombi grew preferentially at the apex of the stenosis, where the highest shear rate develops, even though similar damaged vessels were exposed in the segments with different flow profiles (Fig. 5).

Vessel characteristics also regulate fibrin(ogen) deposition kinetics; a significantly different outcome in fibrin(ogen) deposition (^{125}I-fibrinogen) kinetics is observed on mildly and severely damaged vessel wall.[12] Fibrin(ogen) deposition to damaged vascular wall was studied at a constant laminar flow typical of unobstructed medium size arteries. Mildly damaged (subendothelial) and severely damaged (below internal elastic lamina) vascular wall were studied as triggers of thrombosis. Fibrin deposition per surface area, as well as longitudinal axial dependence of fibrin deposition and its relationship to platelet deposition, were studied by segmental analysis of the substrates exposed in the flow chamber placed in an extracorporeal shunt. Fibrin(ogen) deposition was similar in nonanticoagulated and heparinized bloods in acute perfusions, and significantly higher on severely damaged vessels than on mildly damaged vessels. Segmental dependence analysis showed a significant decrease in fibrin deposition with distal location on both types of lesions. The ratio of fibrin(ogen) to platelet deposition was similar at all perfusion times on mild injury, while on severe injury a higher ratio was found at short perfusion times. That is, fibrin deposition is higher in the thrombus layers closest to the vessel wall on severe injury. Even under low shear conditions of arterial thrombosis, fibrin deposition and fibrin-to-platelet ratio are highly dependent on the degree of vascular damage.[12]

Overall, it is likely that when injury to the vessel wall is mild, the thrombogenic stimulus is relatively limited and the resulting thrombotic occlusion is transient, as occurs in unstable angina.

Effects of Shear Rate on Vessel Wall

Fluid dynamics also affect the interface between blood and the vascular wall; endothelial cells are capable of responding to local hemodynamic forces. These forces include shear stress and shear strain. Flow forces induce endothelial cells to modulate the synthesis and release of a variety of vasoactive and antithrombotic substances. Flow-induced vasoadaptation is mediated by the release of two vasoactive products, Prostacyclin PGI2 and endothelium-derived relaxing factor (EDRF/NO), from shear-exposed endothelial cells.[13–16] In addition to having vasoactive properties, these products are also powerful antiplatelet agents. PGI2 acts by raising intracellular levels of cyclic adenosine monophosphate (cAMP) in vascular smooth muscle cells and platelets.

Nitric oxide (NO) is also a potent vasodilator and antiplatelet agent. Its effects are mediated by elevation of the intracellular levels of cyclic guanine monophosphate (cGMP) in smooth muscle cells and platelets. The release of EDRF by endothelial cells is activated by both shear stress and cyclic strain.[17] The release of NO in response to increased shear rates seems to be mediated by upregulation of cyclic nitric oxide synthase messenger ribonucleic acid (cNOS mRNA).[18]

Another indirect mechanism of the inhibition of platelet activation and deposition is an increase in the levels of tissue plasminogen activator (tPA). It has been reported that tPA and plasmin inhibit shear-induced platelet aggregation.[19] High levels of shear stress stimulate secretion of tPA without modification of the plasminogen activator inhibitor-1 (PAI-1) levels.[20]

All of these actions are mediated by the shear rate stimulation of the shear-stress–responsive element (SSRE) regions on the promoter of shear-responsive genes. The transcriptional factor NF-KB, which accumulates in the nuclei of endothelial cells exposed to shear stress, binds to the SSRE and has been implicated in the rheologic activation of endothelial cells.[21]

A recent report of the induction of the tissue factor gene by shear stress indicates that it is not only the genes that contain SSRE in their promoter regions that could be induced by shear stress.[22] Shear-stress induction of tissue factor is mediated through and increased Sp1 transcriptional activity with a concomitant hyperphosphorilation of Sp1.

Effect of the Substrate on Platelet Deposition

It is likely that the nature of the substrate exposed after spontaneous or intervention-related plaque rupture would help to determine whether an unstable plaque proceeds rapidly to an occlusive thrombus or persists as nonocclusive mural thrombus. Although observational data show that plaque rupture is a potent stimulus for thrombosis, and although exposed collagen is suggested to have a predominant role in thrombosis, the relative thrombogenicity of different components of human atherosclerotic plaques is not well established. We have studied the relative contribution of different components of human atherosclerotic plaques to acute thrombus formation after 5-minute blood perfusions. Foam-cell–rich matrix (obtained from fatty streaks), collagen-rich matrix (from sclerotic plaques), collagen-poor matrix without cholesterol crystals (from fibrolipid plaques), atheromatous core with abundant cholesterol crystals (from atheromatous plaques), highly cel-

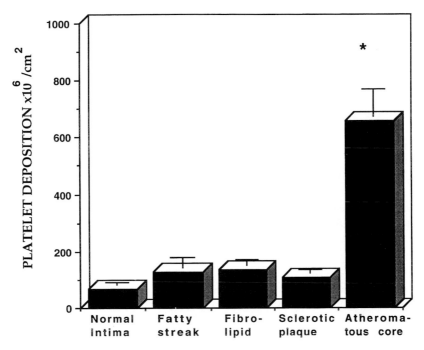

Figure 6. Platelet deposition on different types of human atherosclerotic plaques. Human plaques were perfused for 5 minutes in the Badimon perfusion system at high shear rate conditions. From Reference 23.

lular plaque (hyperplastic), and segments of normal intima derived from human aortas at necropsy were comparatively studied (Fig. 6). Specimens were mounted in the Badimon chamber, placed within an ex vivo extracorporeal perfusion system, and exposed to flowing blood for 5 minutes at high shear rate conditions mimicking medium-grade stenosis. Thrombus formation on atheromatous core was up to sixfold greater than on other substrates, including collagen-rich matrix. The atheromatous core is the most thrombogenic component of human atherosclerotic plaques and, therefore, plaques with large atheromatous core contents are at high risk to lead to thrombosis after spontaneous or mechanically induced rupture, due to the increased thrombogenicity of their content.[23] Human atherosclerotic plaque thrombogenicity seems to be related to tissue factor content.[24]

Systemic Thrombogenic Risk Factors

Focal thrombosis may lead to a local hypercoagulable or thrombogenic state of the circulation that may favor progression or recurrence of the thrombi. In addition, there is increasing experimental and clinical evidence that a primary hypercoagulable or thrombogenic state of the circulation exists, that can favor focal thrombosis. Thus, experimentally, platelet aggregation and the generation of thrombin may be activated by circulating catecholamines[25]; this interrelationship could be of importance in humans because it may be a link between conditions of emotional stress or circadian variation (early morning hours)[26] with catecholamine effects[27,28] and the development of myocardial infarction. Of importance is the increasing evidence of enhanced platelet reactivity in cigarette smokers,[29,30] which may or may not be related to catecholamine stimulus[31]; indeed, in agreement with the thrombogenic role of cigarette smoking, it has been observed that after discontinuation of smoking there is a sharp decrease in acute vascular events most often associated with thrombosis.[32]

Of no less importance is the increasing clinical and experimental evidence of hypercoagulability (fibrinogen, factor VII, vWF, poor fibrinolysis) in patients with progressive coronary disease[33] and of enhanced platelet reactivity at the site of vascular damage in experimental hypercholesterolemia[34] and in humans,[35] which supports previous clinical observation.[36] Within this context of metabolic abnormalities in young patients with coronary disease, high plasma levels of homocysteine after methionine loading and of lipoprotein(a) are also beginning to be identified as powerful thrombogenic risk factors. Homocystinemia in its heterozygous trait is now being identified as an important risk factor for atherosclerotic disease in young individuals with a strong family history of coronary disease.[37] Lipoprotein(a), which is very similar to low-density lipoproteins (LDL) in its configuration,[38,39] has been shown to be an important risk factor for ischemic heart disease, presumably for thrombotic occlusion and particularly in familial hypercholesterolemia.[40]

A deficient fibrinolysis may also be considered as a thrombogenic risk factor in coronary disease patients. One of the parameters of the fibrinolytic system is PAI-1; some studies suggest that high levels of PAI-1 are a risk factor for ischemic heart disease[41] and myocardial infarction.[42] Finally, aside from the possibility that true defective fibrinolysis with high PAI-1 levels is a thrombogenic risk factor, other hemostatic parameters, specifically fibrinogen, vWF, and factor VII levels, have also clearly been involved.[43,44]

References

1. Fuster V, Badimon L, Badimon JJ, Chesebro JH. The pathogenesis of coronary artery disease and the acute coronary syndromes. (Part I and II) *N Eng J Med* 1992;326:242–250.

2. Badimon JJ, Fuster V, Chesebro JH, Badimon L. Coronary atherosclerosis. *Circulation* 1993;87(suppl II):3–16.
3. Kieffer N, Phillips DR. Platelet membrane glycoproteins: Functions in cellular interactions. *Annu Rev Biol* 1990;6:329–357.
4. Kunicki T. Organization of glycoproteins within the platelet plasma membrane. In: George JN, Nurden AT, Philips DR eds: *Platelet Membrane Glycoproteins*. New York: Plenum Press; 1985:87–101.
5. Merril EW. Rheology of the blood. *Physiol Rev* 1969;49:863–888.
6. Goldsmith HL, Turitto VT. Rheological aspects of thrombosis and haemostasis: Basic principles and applications. *Thromb Haemost* 1986;55:415–435.
7. Brown CH, Leverett LB, Lewis CW. Morphological, biochemical, and functional changes in human platelets subjected to shear stress. *J Lab Invest* 1975;85:462–468.
8. Leonard E. Rheology of thrombosis. In: Colman R, Hirsh J, Marder V, Salzman E eds: *Haemostasis and Thrombosis. 2nd Edition.* New York: J.B. Lippincott Co; 1994:1211–1223.
9. Badimon L, Turitto V, Rosemark J, et al. Characterization of a tubular flow chamber for studying platelet interaction with biologic and prosthetic materials. *J Lab Clin Med* 1987;110:706–718.
10. Badimon L, Badimon JJ, Galvez A, et al. Influence of arterial damage and wall shear rate on platelet deposition. *Arteriosclerosis* 1986;6:312–320.
11. Badimon L, Badimon JJ. Mechanisms of arterial thrombosis in non-parallel streamlines: Platelet thrombi grow on the apex of stenotic severely injured vessel wall. *J Clin Invest* 1989;84:1134–1144.
12. Mailhac A, Badimon JJ, Fallon JT, et al. Effect of an eccentric severe stenosis on fibrin(ogen) deposition on severely damaged vessel wall in arterial thrombosis. Relative contribution of fibrin(ogen) and platelets. *Circulation* 1994;90:988–996.
13. Alshihabi SN, Chang YS, Frangos JA, Tarbell JM. Shear stress-induced release of PGE2 and PGI2 by vascular smooth muscle cells. *Biochem Biophys Res Commum* 1996;224:808–814.
14. Ando J, Kamiya A. Flow-dependent regulation of gene expression in vascular endothelial cells. *Jpn Heart J* 1996;37:19–32.
15. Malek AM, Izumo S. Control of endothelial cell gene expression by flow. *J Biochem* 1995;28:1515–1528.
16. Rubanyi G, Romero J, Vanhoutte P. Flow-induced release of endothelium-derived relaxing factor. *Am J Physiol* 1986:250⊥145.
17. Awolesi MA, Sessa WC, Sumpio BE. Cyclic-strain upregulates NO-synthase in cultured bovine aortic endothelial cells. *J Clin Invest* 1995;96:1449–1456.
18. Nishida K, Harrison DG, Navas JP, Fisher AA, et al. Molecular cloning and characterization of the constitutive bovine endothelial cell nitric oxide synthase. *J Clin Invest* 1992;90:2092–2097.
19. Coller B. Platelets and thrombolytic therapy. *N Engl J Med* 1990;33:322–328.
20. Diamond SL, Eskin SG, McIntire LV. Fluid flow stimulates tissue plasminogen activator secretion by cultured human endothelial cell. *Science* 1989;243:1483–1486.
21. Khachigian L, Resnick N, Gimbrone M, Collins T. Nuclear factor-kb interacts functionally with the PDGF B-chain shear stress response element in vascular endothelial cells exposed to fluid flow. *J Clin Invest* 1995;96:1169–1175.
22. Lin MC, Almus-Jacons F, Chen HH, et al. Shear stress induction of tissue factor gene. *J Clin Invest* 1997;99:737–744.

23. Fernandez-Ortiz A, Badimon JJ, Falk E, et al. Characterization of the relative thrombogenicity of atherosclerotic plaque components: Implications for consequences of plaque rupture. *J Am Coll Cardiol* 1994;23:1562–1569.
24. Toschi V, Gallo R, Lettino M, et al. Tissue factor modulates the thrombogenicity of human atherosclerotic plaques. *Circulation* 1997;95:594–599.
25. Rowsell HC, Hegardt B, Downie HG, et al. Adrenalin and experimental thrombosis. *Br J Haematol* 1966;12:66–73.
26. Mueller JE, Stone PH, Turi ZG, et al. The MILIS Study Group. Circadian variation in the frequency of onset of acute myocardial infarction. *N Engl J Med* 1985;313:1315–1322.
27. Willich SN, Linderer T, Wegscheider K, et al. Increased morning incidence of myocardial infarction in the ISAM study: Absence with prior beta-adrenergic blockade. *Circulation* 1989;80:853–858.
28. Tofler GH, Brezinski D, Schafer AL, et al. Morning increase in platelet response to ADP and epinephrine: Association with the time of increased risk of myocardial infarction and sudden cardiac death. *N Engl J Med* 1987; 316:1514–1518.
29. Fuster V, Chesebro JH, Frye RL, Elveback L. Platelet survival and the development of coronary artery disease in the young adult: Effects of cigarette smoking, strong family history and medical therapy. *Circulation* 1981;63: 546–551.
30. Winniford MD, Wheelan KR, Kremers MS, et al. Smoking-induced coronary vasoconstriction in patients with atherosclerotic coronary artery disease: Evidence for adrenergically mediated alterations in coronary artery tone. *Circulation* 1986;73:662–667.
31. Buhler FR, Vesanen K, Watters JT. Impact of smoking on heart attacks, strokes, blood pressure control, drug dose, and quality of life aspects in the International Prospective Primary Prevention Study in Hypertension. *Am Heart J* 1988;115:282–288.
32. Paul O. Background of the prevention of cardiovascular disease. II. Arteriosclerosis, hypertension and selected risk factors. *Circulation* 1989;80: 206–214.
33. Thompson SG, Kienast J, Pyke SDM, et al, for the European Concerted Action on Thrombosis and Disabilities Angina Pectoris Study Group. Hemostatic factor and the risk of myocardial infarction or sudden death in patients with angina pectoris. *N Engl J Med* 1995;332(10):635–641.
34. Hunt BJ. The relation between abnormal hemostatic function and the progression of coronary disease. *Curr Opin Cardiol* 1990;5:758–765.
35. Badimon JJ, Badimon L, Turitto VT, Fuster V. Platelet deposition at high shear rates is enhanced by high plasma cholesterol levels. In vivo study in the rabbit model. *Arteriosclerosis* 1991;11:395–402.
36. Lacoste L, La JY, Hung J, et al. Hyperlipidemia and coronary disease. Correction of the increased thrombogenic potential with cholesterol reduction. *Circulation* 1995;92:3172–3177
37. Carvalho ACA, Colman RW, Lees RS. Platelet function in hyperlipoproteinemia. *N Engl J Med* 1974;290:434–438.
38. Boers GHJ, Smals AGH, Trijbels FJM, et al. Heterozygosity for homocystinuria in premature peripheral and cerebral occlusive arterial disease. *N Engl J Med* 1985;313:709–715.
39. Dahlen GH, Guyton JR, Attar M, et al. Association of levels of lipoprotein Lp(a), plasma lipids, and other lipoproteins with coronary artery disease documented by angiography. *Circulation* 1986;74:758–765.

40. Seed M, Hoppichler F, Reaveley D, et al. Relation of serum lipoprotein(a) concentration and apolipoprotein(a) phenotype to CHD patients with familial hypercholesterolemia. *N Engl J Med* 1990;332:1494–1499.
41. Olofsson BO, Dahlen G, Nilsson TK. Evidence for increased levels of plasminogen activator inhibitor and tissue plasminogen activator in plasma of patients with angiographically verified coronary artery disease. *Eur Heart J* 1989;10:77–82.
42. Hamsten A, Wilman B, de Faire U, Blomback M. Increased plasma levels of a rapid inhibitor of tissue plasminogen activator in young survivors of myocardial infarction. *N Engl J Med* 1980;303:897–902.
43. Alevriadou BR, McIntire L. Rheology. In: Loscalzo J, Schaffer A eds: *Thrombosis and Haemorrhage*. Blackwell Science 1995:369–383.
44. Joist JH, Zeffren DI, Bauman JE. A programmable, computer-controlled cone-plate viscosimeter for the application of pulsatile shear stress to platelet suspensions. *Biorheology* 1988:25:449–456.
45. Weiss H, Baumgartner H, Tschopp TB, et al. Correction by factor VII of the impaired adhesion to subendothelium in von Willebrand's disease. *Blood* 1978:51:267–275.
46. Sakariassen KS, Aarts P, De Groot PG, et al. A perfusion chamber developed to investigate platelet interaction in flowing blood with human vesssel wall cells, their extracellular matrix, and purified components. *J Lab Clin Med* 1983:102:522–531.
47. Wurzinger LJ, Opiz R, Blasberg P, Schnid-Schonbein H. Platelet and coagulation parameters following milliseconds exposure to laminar shear stress. *Thromb Haemost* 1985:54:381–395.
48. O'Brien JR, Salmon GP. Shear stress activation of platelet GP IIb/IIIa plus von Willebrand factor causes aggregation: Filter blockage and the long bleeding time in von Willebrand's disease. *Blood* 1987:70:1354–1360.
49. Polanoiwska-Grabowska R, Gear ARL. High-speed platelet adhesion under conditions of high shear rate. *Proc Natl Acad Sci U S A* 1992;89:5754–5761.
50. Hornstra G, ten Hoor F. The filtragometer: A new device for measuring platelet aggregation in venous blood of man. *Thromb Diath Haemorr* 1975; 34:531–544.
51. Badimon L, Badimon JJ. Mechanisms of arterial thrombosis in non-parallel streamlines. Platelet thrombi grow on the apex of stenotic severely injured vessel wall. *J Clin Invest* 1989;84:1134–1144.
52. Barstard RM, Kierulf P, Sakariassen K. Collagen-induced thrombus formation at the apex of eccentric stenoses. A time-course study with non-anticoagulated human blood. *Thromb Haemost* 1996;75:685–692.

Chapter 21

The Potential Role of Endothelium in Acute Coronary Syndromes:
Vasomotion, Inflammation, Thrombosis

Scott Kinlay, MBBS, PhD,
Andrew P. Selwyn, MD, and Peter Ganz, MD

Introduction

The acute coronary syndromes of myocardial infarction, unstable angina, and sudden cardiac death are typically associated with disruption of the plaque and coronary artery thrombosis.[1-5] Atherosclerotic plaques that are prone to rupture characteristically have a thin fibrous cap, a large necrotic lipid pool core, prominent macrophages, and activated vascular smooth muscle cells and T-lymphocytes.[6] Increasing evidence implicates functional abnormalities of the endothelium in the development of the vulnerable plaque, plaque disruption, and thromboses that lead to the acute coronary syndromes.[7]

The possible mechanisms that relate the endothelium to the destabilization of atherosclerotic plaques and the acute coronary syndromes include the following:

1. By regulating vascular tone and compliance, the endothelium could mediate extrinsic events that trigger plaque rupture. However, the possibility that vasoconstriction provides the mechanical stimulus to plaque disruption seems unlikely, as acute coronary syndromes are typically not ob-

From: Fuster, V (ed). *The Vulnerable Atherosclerotic Plaque: Understanding, Identification, and Modification.* Armonk, NY: Futura Publishing Company, Inc.; © 1999.

served as results of provocative studies of vasoconstriction with acetylcholine, ergonovine, or other vasoconstrictor compounds.

2. The endothelium is an intrinsic determinant of plaque stability; it regulates inflammation within the intima, mediated by changes in the expression of cellular adhesion molecules and chemoattractants.

3. The endothelium modulates the consequences of plaque disruption through its control of vascular tone and its antithrombotic and antiplatelet functions.

The evidence for the last two roles of the endothelium on the development of acute coronary syndromes is discussed below.

Intimal Inflammation and the Endothelium

Atherosclerotic plaques that are vulnerable to rupture exhibit several inflammatory features that arise from the oxidation of low-density lipoproteins (LDL) within the intima and from the reduced availability of endothelium-derived nitric oxide.

Progressive oxidation of LDL within the arterial wall leads to a loss of its intrinsic antioxidants and the conversion of fatty acids on the outer surface to reactive hydroxyl forms (minimally oxidized LDL).[8,9] This is followed by greater structural changes, including modification of the apo B protein moiety and the formation of lysophosphatidylcholine.[10-12] In vitro studies have shown that these molecules can induce inflammatory gene products in endothelial cells. Minimally oxidized LDL increases the expression of monocyte chemoattractant protein-1 (MCP-1) and macrophage colony stimulating factor,[13-15] and activates NF-κB transcriptional regulatory factors[16,17] that lead to increased expression of adhesion molecules including vascular cell adhesion molecule-1 (VCAM-1).[18,19] Oxidized LDL and lysophosphatidylcholine also increase the expression of cellular adhesion molecules on the surface of endothelial cells.[20,21] The increased expression of cellular adhesion molecules and chemoattractants allows the endothelial cells to capture leucocytes and assist in their migration into the arterial wall. Macrophage colony stimulating factor also plays an important role in the conversion of recently trapped monocytes to macrophage (foam) cells.

In healthy arteries, shear stress from blood flow, acetylcholine, and other chemicals stimulate endothelial cells to produce nitric oxide from L-arginine by increasing the activity of the enzyme nitric oxide synthase.[22-25] Nitric oxide diffuses to the adjacent smooth muscle and causes vasodilation of the artery. Experimental studies have shown that nitric oxide carries out other functions that regulate inflammation, including inhibiting the expression of monocyte chemoattractant protein-1 and macrophage colony stimulating factor on the luminal surface of the endothelial cell, reducing the endothelial expression of VCAM-1 and inhibiting NF-κB activity.[17,26–28]

The endothelium, however, is dysfunctional at sites of atherosclerosis,[29] and the availability of nitric oxide is reduced by a combination of decreased production and increased degradation of this compound. Oxidized LDL and lysophosphatidylcholine may activate protein kinase C in endothelial cells,[30] which inhibits the production of nitric oxide in experimental studies by several mechanisms. These mechanisms include disabling the receptor-effector coupling system of the nitric oxide pathway,[30] downregulating nitric oxide synthase mRNA and protein levels,[31] and decreasing the activity of endothelial nitric oxide synthase.[32] Increased oxidant stress within the atherosclerotic plaque can also inactivate nitric oxide by its oxidation.[33] These events create a vicious cycle within the intima that promotes the expression of cellular adhesion molecules, chemoattractants, and the activation of inflammatory cells, which leads to a further reduction in nitric oxide availability.

Activated macrophages, leukocytes, and smooth muscle cells are most prevalent at the shoulders of plaques and at sites of plaque rupture.[6,34] T lymphocytes secrete the cytokine γ-interferon, which inhibits the production of collagen by intimal smooth muscle cells[35] and which may also lead to apoptosis (programmed death) of smooth muscle cells.[6] Oxidized LDL also activates vascular smooth muscle and macrophages that have migrated into the intima to produce matrix metalloproteinases that can degrade the fibrous caps of plaques and increase the likelihood of plaque disruption.[6]

The expression of cellular adhesion molecules and chemoattractants on the luminal surface of endothelial cells, and the subsequent development of inflammation within the plaque, reveal the potential for the endothelium to play a critical role in the development of the acute coronary syndromes. However, most of these insights have been derived from tissue culture and animal models and, because of the need to obtain tissue for study, relatively little is known about the expression of cellular adhesion molecules on the surface of cardiac endothelial cells in living humans.

Most information pertaining to the expression of cardiac endothelial leukocyte adhesion molecules in living humans is derived from patients who have had cardiac transplantation and have regular tissue biopsies performed for clinical reasons. These studies have shown that the expression of cellular adhesion molecules on the endothelial surface of microvessels is dynamic, with upregulation and downregulation of these molecules from week to week.[36,37] In patients who have received organ transplants, the expression of cellular adhesion molecules plays an important role in the migration of leucocytes that occurs as part of the rejection process, and precedes the histologic features of transplant rejection.[36] Their expression may also be related to the development of transplant coronary arteriosclerosis.[38]

Human studies of native atherosclerosis have been confined to postmortem studies, and antemortem findings may not reflect the dynamic temporal sequence of events that appears to be a feature of endothelial activation, inflammation, and subsequent derangements that cause clinical events. However, the findings of these studies are consistent with the conclusions from the animal and tissue models and the transplant data.

The expression of cellular adhesion molecules has been examined in the coronary arteries of explanted hearts from patients undergoing cardiac transplantation.[39] Whereas the expression of these molecules was very rare in normal coronary artery segments, intercellular adhesion molecule 1 (ICAM-1), VCAM-1, platelet-endothelial cell adhesion molecule (PECAM), and E-selectin were variably expressed in 20% to 70% of fibrous atherosclerotic lesions. Higher rates of expression were found over lipid-rich plaques.[39]

In another postmortem study,[40] the expression of ICAM-1, E-selectin, and major histocompatibility complex II antigens was higher on endothelial cells adjacent to subendothelial infiltrates with T-lymphocytes and macrophages.[40] Although these studies cannot determine whether the cellular inflammation preceded or was a result of the expression of cellular adhesion molecules, the association demonstrates the close relationship between changes in the endothelium and intimal inflammation.

More recently, several soluble markers of inflammation were identified in patients with sepsis, collagen vascular disease, and malignancy.[41] Increased levels of soluble adhesion molecules and selectins that appear to be shed from activated endothelium are also found in patients with dyslipidemia,[42] diabetes,[43] hypertension,[44] and ischemic heart disease.[45-47] These soluble markers probably reflect a more generalized activation of endothelium at many sites throughout the body, rather than the more localized activation of one particular occult lesion. Other soluble markers of inflammation such as C-reactive protein and interleukin-6 are also associated with the acute coronary syndromes.[46,48-52]

Thus, inflammation within the intima is a major determinant of the vulnerable plaque and risk of acute coronary syndromes. The endothelium plays an important role in determining inflammation in atherosclerotic plaques, and this is likely to have a bearing on the structural qualities of the plaque that predispose to rupture.[53,54]

Endothelium-Dependent Control of Vascular Tone

The last decade has brought increases in our understanding of the role the endothelium in the control of vascular tone. Early experiments demonstrated the presence of an endothelial relaxing factor that is lost in de-endothelialized arteries.[22] Subsequent studies showed that one of the endothelial relaxing factors is nitric oxide[23–25] generated in the endothelium from the action of nitric oxide synthase on L-arginine. The production of nitric oxide is stimulated by several factors including acetylcholine, serotonin, and thrombin.[55] In the cardiac catheterization laboratory, provocative testing of coronary arteries with acetylcholine has revealed that the stimulation of nitric oxide production and subsequent vasodilation in normal coronary arteries is absent and even reversed to constriction in arteries with atherosclerosis.[29] Later studies showed that dyslipidemias and other risk factors for the acute coronary syndromes are also associated with endothelial dysfunction, even in those with angiographically normal coronary arteries or in those with stable angina.[56]

Endothelial vasomotor dysfunction and resultant vasoconstriction may contribute to the clinical manifestation of the acute coronary syndromes by restricting flow at sites of coronary narrowing to critical levels. Several studies performed during cardiac catheterization have shown that vasospasm is more pronounced in culprit coronary segments associated with a recent myocardial infarct or unstable angina.[57–59] These include studies that used pharmacological provocation with intracoronary acetylcholine or methergine, which showed more vasoconstriction in infarct-related arteries compared to non–infarct-related arteries in the same individual,[57] and more coronary vasospasm in those recently after myocardial infarction compared to those with stable syndromes.[58] Endothelial vasomotor function elicited by the more physiological stimuli of the cold pressor test and exercise has also revealed greater coronary vasoconstriction of culprit lesions in unstable angina compared to uninvolved coronary segments.[59]

Although these studies cannot determine the temporal relationship of increased vasoconstrictive responses and plaque disruption, one prospective study[60] suggests that segmental abnormal endothelium-dependent vasomotion and vasoconstriction precede the development of a culprit lesion that causes an acute coronary syndrome. Of 239 patients who had coronary angiograms on two occasions over a median 1 to 2 years, coronary vasoconstriction to intra-aortic ergonovine at the initial angiogram was the strongest factor associated with the subsequent development of myocardial infarction.[60]

Increased vasoreactivity may be related to the risk of acute coronary syndromes by direct and indirect means. It may contribute directly by increasing the likelihood of occlusion in myocardial infarction or increasing the severity of the impairment in blood flow in unstable angina. In the early stages of myocardial infarction treated with thrombolytics, coronary occlusion is intermittent, and vasodilators can assist recanalization.[61] Coronary occlusion is most likely a combination of coronary thrombosis and vasoconstriction at sites of plaque disruption. These two events are closely related because activated platelets at the sites of coronary thrombosis release vasoactive substances, such as serotonin and thromboxane, that can increase vasoconstriction.[62] In the porcine model, the degree of vasoconstriction in injured arterial sites is directly related to the degree of platelet deposition; pretreatment with aspirin can reduce the degree of platelet deposition and vasoconstriction associated with injury.[63] During conventional coronary angioplasty in humans, thrombus formation on the guidewire is also associated with increased vasoconstriction at sites related to the thrombus and distal to the guidewire.[64]

Increased vasoconstriction may also be a more indirect marker of other cellular dysfunctions of the vulnerable plaque that increase the likelihood of plaque disruption and acute coronary syndromes. Impaired nitric oxide generation in the endothelium in response to various stimuli, such as acetylcholine, permits vasoconstriction instead of the normal vasodilatory response.[29] However, the reduced availability of endothelial nitric oxide is also a feature of vulnerable plaques that have increased expression of adhesion molecules and cytokines, including VCAM-1, ICAM-1, E-selectin, and MCP-1, on the endothelial surface, as described earlier. Under this hypothesis, impaired endothelium-dependent vasomotion is only one effect of decreased nitric oxide in the intima of vulnerable plaques, and is a marker for the other plaque features, which include decreased strength of the fibrous cap[6,65] and changes in the structural properties of the plaques[53,54] that may have a more direct bearing on plaque disruption and the development of acute coronary syndromes.

The direct vasoconstrictor effects and indirect relationship of vasoconstriction to inflammation and plaque disruption appear to be closely inter-related. It is therefore difficult to consider them in isolation. Recent studies have found that the powerful vasoconstrictor endothelin-1 is produced primarily by macrophages and vascular smooth muscle cells that are present in atherosclerotic plaques,[66,67] especially at sites of previous plaque hemorrhage.[66,68] These studies, in which tissue obtained by coronary atherectomy was used, suggest that the inflammatory infiltrates may also increase the propensity for vasoconstriction by releasing endothelin-1 in vulnerable plaques, and contribute to the development of plaque disruption and the severity of occlusion in the acute coronary syndromes.

The Endothelium Modulating the Consequences of Plaque Disruption

The acute coronary syndromes most often arise from the disruption of relatively minor plaques. Coronary angiograms shortly after thrombolysis in patients presenting with myocardial infarction revealed that many of the thrombotic occlusions occurred at sites without high-grade stenoses.[69] The majority of culprit lesions were also mild (<50% diameter stenosis) in several series of patients who presented with acute coronary syndromes and had recent angiograms prior to their presentation.[60,70–73] Furthermore, plaque rupture without occlusion and clinical sequela is a relatively common finding in some autopsy series.[74–77] The factors that determine whether a disrupted plaque will develop a flow-limiting narrowing or occlusion depend on the geography of the vessel narrowing and the balance of platelet aggregation and inhibition, thrombosis and thrombolysis, and the presence of vasospasm.

Disruption of the endothelium over a plaque exposes the lipid core and cellular contents of the plaque to the blood. The plaque contents are highly thrombogenic due to the presence of collagen and the production of the procoagulant tissue factor by foam cells.[78,79] Theoretically, a plaque with less inflammation and a smaller necrotic lipid core should present a less thrombogenic stimulus to blood and should decrease the likelihood of a large thrombus causing clinical symptoms.

The endothelium-derived nitric oxide also plays an important role in determining whether disruption of an atherosclerotic plaque is likely to lead to a flow-limiting or occluding lesion. Platelet adhesion and aggregation are reduced by endothelium-derived nitric oxide[80,81] that is released into the lumen.[82–85] A lack of constitutive nitric oxide at sites of disrupted plaque permits platelet activation and extension of thrombus.

The endothelium also modulates thrombosis and thrombolysis by producing tissue plasminogen activator and plasminogen activator inhibitors (PAI-1, PAI-2) that promote or inhibit fibrinolysis.[86] An increased level of PAI-1 is a risk factor for cardiac death in young men who have recently survived a myocardial infarct,[87] and hyperlipidemia, which is also associated with endothelial vasomotor dysfunction, is related to higher levels of plasma PAI-1.[88–90] Atherosclerotic vessels have higher concentrations of mRNA for PAI-1, and secrete more PAI-1 from endothelial cells than do normal vessels.[91,92] Thus, endothelial dysfunction from a variety of causes may decrease the thrombolytic action that limits the size of a thrombus at the site of plaque disruption.

The degree of dysfunction of the endothelium adjacent to a disrupted plaque may play a critical role in modulating the amount of platelet aggregation and adhesion, thrombus formation, and vasospasm that will determine whether an acute coronary syndrome develops.

Conclusions

The endothelium has several functions that can contribute to plaque disruption and the development of the acute coronary syndromes. Although it is uncertain whether changes in vasomotor tone can precipitate plaque rupture, the endothelium does appear to contribute to the recruitment of inflammatory cells in the arterial wall in response to oxidized LDL and changes in the structure of the plaque that can increase its vulnerability. Furthermore, the endothelium adjacent to a disrupted plaque is likely to exert an influence on the consequences of plaque rupture by modulating platelet aggregation, the size of the associated thrombus, and focal vasospasm. The optimal management of acute coronary syndromes will come from an understanding of the complex interactions of these functional aspects of the endothelium in such syndromes.

References

1. Davies MJ. A macro and micro view of coronary vascular insult in ischemic heart disease. *Circulation* 1990;82:II38–II46.
2. Davies MJ, Richardson PD, Woolf N, et al. Risk of thrombosis in human atherosclerotic plaques: Role of extracellular lipid, macrophage, and smooth muscle content. *Br Heart J* 1993;69:377–381.
3. Falk E. Why do plaques rupture? *Circulation* 1992;86(suppl III):30–42.
4. Falk E, Shah PK, Fuster V. Coronary plaque disruption. *Circulation* 1995; 92:657–671.
5. Burke AP, Farb A, Malcom GT, et al. Coronary risk factors and plaque morphology in men with coronary disease who died suddenly. *N Engl J Med* 1997;336:1276–1282.
6. Libby P. Molecular bases of the acute coronary syndromes. *Circulation* 1995; 2844–2850.
7. Selwyn AP, Kinlay S, Creager M, et al. Cell dysfunction in atherosclerosis and the ischemic manifestations of coronary artery disease. *Am J Cardiol* 1997;79(suppl 5a):17–23.
8. Steinbrecher UP, Parthasarathy S, Leake DS, et al. Modification of low

density lipoprotein by endothelial cells involves lipid peroxidation and degradation of low density lipoprotein phospholipids. *Proc Natl Acad Sci U S A* 1984;81:3883–3887.

9. Morel DW, DiCorleto PE, Chisolm CM. Endothelial and smooth muscle cells alter low density lipoprotein in vitro by free radical oxidation. *Arteriosclerosis* 1984;4:357–364.

10. Zang HF, Basra HJ, Steinbrecher UP. Effects of oxidatively modified LDL on cholesterol esterification in cultured macrophages. *J Lipid Res* 1990:31: 1361–1369.

11. Steinbrecher UP. Oxidation of human low density lipoprotein results in esterification of lysine residues of apolipoprotein B by lipid peroxide decomposition products. *J Biol Chem* 1987;262:3605–3608.

12. Fruebis J, Parthasarathy S, Steinberg D. Evidence for concerted reaction between lipid hydroperoxides and polypeptides. *Proc Natl Acad Sci U S A* 1992;89:10588–10592.

13. Berliner JA, Territo MC, Sevanian A, et al. Minimally modified low density lipoprotein stimulates monocyte endothelial interactions. *J Clin Invest* 1990; 85:1260–1266.

14. Cushing SD, Berliner JA, Valente AJ, et al. Minimally modified low density lipoprotein induces monocyte chemotactic protein 1 in human endothelial cells and vascular smooth muscle cells. *Proc Natl Acad Sci U S A* 1990;87: 5134–5138.

15. Rajavashisth TB, Andalibi A, Territo MC, et al. Induction of endothelial cell expression of granulocyte and macrophage colony-stimulating factors by modified low-density lipoproteins. *Nature* 1990;344:254–257.

16. Parhami F, Fang ZT, Fogelman AM, et al. Minimally modified low density lipoprotein- induced inflammatory responses in endothelial cells are mediated by cyclic adenosine monophosphate. *J Clin Invest* 1993;92:471–478.

17. Peng HB, Rajavashisth TB, Libby P, Liao JK. Nitric oxide inhibits macrophage-colony stimulating factor gene transcription in vascular endothelial cells. *J Biol Chem* 1995;270:17050–17055.

18. Collins T, Read MA, Neish AS, et al. Transcriptional regulation of endothelial cell adhesion molecules: NF-kappa B and cytokine-inducible enhancers. *FASEB J* 1995;9:899–909.

19. Marui N, Offermann MK, Swerlick R, et al. Vascular cell adhesion molecule-1 (VCAM-1) gene transcription and expression are regulated through an antioxidant-sensitive mechanism in human vascular endothelial cells. *J Clin Invest* 1993;92:1866–1874.

20. Kume N, Cybulsky MI, Gimbrone MA Jr. Lysophosphatidylcholine, a component of atherogenic lipoproteins, induces mononuclear leukocyte adhesion molecules in cultured human and rabbit arterial endothelial cells. *J Clin Invest* 1992;90:1138–1144.

21. Sugiyama S, Kugiyama K, Ohgushi M, et al. Lysophosphatidylcholine in oxidized low- density lipoprotein increases endothelial susceptibility to polymorphonuclear leukocyte-induced endothelial dysfunction in porcine coronary arteries: Role of Protein kinase C. *Circ Res* 1994;74:565–575.

22. Furchgott RF, Zawadzki JV. The obligatory role of endothelial cells in the relaxation of arterial smooth muscle by acetylcholine. *Nature* 1980;288: 373–376.

23. Palmer RM, Ferrige AG, Moncada S. Nitric oxide release accounts for the biological activity of endothelium-derived relaxing factor. *Nature* 1987;327: 524–526.

24. Palmer RM, Ashton DS, Moncada S. Vascular endothelial cells synthesize nitric oxide from L-arginine. *Nature* 1988;333:664–666.
25. Lamas S, Marsden PA, Li GK, et al. Endothelial nitric oxide synthase: Molecular cloning and characterization of a distinct constitutive enzyme isoform. *Proc Natl Acad Sci U S A* 1992;89:6348–6352.
26. Zeiher AM, Fisslthaler B, Schray-Utz B, Busse R. Nitric oxide modulates the expression of monocyte chemoattractant protein 1 in cultured human endothelial cells. *Circ Res* 1995;76:980–986.
27. Tsao PS, Wang B, Buitrago R, et al. Nitric oxide regulates monocyte chemotactic protein- 1. *Circulation* 1997;96:934–940.
28. DeCaterina R, Libby P, Peng H-B, et al. Nitric oxide decreases cytokine-induced endothelial activation. *J Clin Invest* 1995;96:60–68.
29. Ludmer PL, Selwyn AP, Shook TL, et al. Paradoxical vasoconstriction induced by acetylcholine in atherosclerotic coronary arteries. *N Engl J Med* 1986;315:1046–1051.
30. Kugiyama K, Ohgushi M, Sugiyama S, et al. Lysophosphatidylcholine inhibits surface receptor mediated intracellular signals in endothelial cells by a pathway involving protein kinase C activation. *Circ Res* 1992;71: 1422–1428.
31. Ohara Y, Sayegh HS, Yamin JJ, Harrison DG. Regulation of endothelial constitutive nitric oxide synthase by protein kinase C. *Hypertension* 1995; 25:415–420.
32. Bredt DS, Ferris CD, Snyder SH. Nitric oxide synthase regulatory sites: Phosphorylation by cyclic AMP-dependent protein kinase, protein kinase C, and calcium/calmodulin protein kinase: Identification of flavin and calmodulin binding sites. *J Biol Chem* 1992;267:10976–10981.
33. Ohara Y, Peterson TE, Harrison DG. Hypercholesterolemia increases endothelial superoxide anion production. *J Clin Invest* 1993;91:2546–1551.
34. van der Wal AC, Becker AE, Van der Loos CM, Das PK. Site of intimal rupture or erosion of thrombosed coronary atherosclerotic plaques is characterized by an inflammatory process irrespective of the dominant plaque morphology. *Circulation* 1994;89:36–44.
35. Amento EP, Ehsani N, Palmer H, Libby P. Cytokines positively and negatively regulate interstitial collagen gene expression in human vascular smooth muscle cells. *Arterioscler Thromb* 1991;11:1223–1230.
36. Briscoe DM, Yeung AC, Schoen FJ, et al. Predictive value of inducible endothelial cell adhesion molecule expression for acute rejection of human cardiac allografts. *Transplantation* 1995;59:204–211.
37. Taylor PM, Rose ML, Yacoub MH, Pigott R. Induction of vascular adhesion molecules during rejection of human cardiac allografts. *Transplantation* 1992;54:451–457.
38. Davis SF, Baum MA, Anderson TJ, et al. Chronic low-grade rejection and VCAM-1 induction on serial endomyocardial biopsies predicts transplant coronary artery disease. *Circulation* 1995;92:I–39.
39. Davies MJ, Gordon JL, Gearing AJH, et al. The expression of the adhesion molecules ICAM-1, VCAM-1, PECAM, and E-Selectin in human atherosclerosis. *J Pathol* 1993:171:223–229.
40. van der Wal AC, Das PK, Tigges AJ, Becker AE. Adhesion molecules on the endothelium and mononuclear cells in human atherosclerotic lesions. *Am J Pathol* 1992;141:1427–1433.
41. Gearing AJH, Newman W. Circulating adhesion molecules in disease. *Immunol Today* 1993;14:506–512.

42. Hackman A, Abe Y, Insull W, et al. Levels of soluble adhesion molecules in patients with dyslipidemia. *Circulation* 1996;93:1334–1338.
43. Steiner M, Reinhardt KM, Krammer B, et al. Increased levels of soluble adhesion molecules in type 2 (non-insulin dependent) diabetes mellitus are independent of glycaemic control. *Thromb Haemost* 1994;72:979–984.
44. Blann AD, Tse W, Maxwell SRJ, Waite MA. Increased levels of the soluble adhesion molecule E-selectin in essential hypertension. *J Hypertension* 1994; 12:925–928.
45. Blann AD, Amiral J, McCollum CM. Circulating endothelial cell/leucocyte molecules in ischemic heart disease. *Br J Haematol* 1996;95:263–265.
46. Ikeda H, Takajo Y, Ichiki K, et al. Increased soluble form of P-selectin in patients with unstable angina. *Circulation* 1995;92:1693–1696.
47. Gebuhrer V, Murphy JF, Bordet JC, et al. Oxidized low-density lipoprotein induces the expression of P-selectin (GMP140/ PADGEM/ CD62) on human endothelial cells. *Biochem J* 1995;306:293–298.
48. Berk BC, Weintraub WS, Alexander RW. Elevation of C-reactive protein in "active" coronary artery disease. *Am J Cardiol* 1990;65:168–172.
49. Thompson S, Kienast J, Pyke S, et al. Hemostatic factors and the risk of myocardial infarction or sudden death in patients with angina pectoris. *N Engl J Med* 1995;332:635–641.
50. Liuzzo G, Biasucci LM, Gallimore R, et al. The prognostic value of C-reactive protein and serum amyloid A Protein in severe unstable angina. *N Engl J Med* 1994;331:417–424.
51. Biasucci LM, Vitelli A, Liuzzo G, et al. Elevated levels of interleukin-6 in unstable angina. *Circulation* 1996;94:874–877.
52. Ridker PM, Cushman M, Stampfer MJ, et al. Inflammation, aspirin, and the risk of cardiovascular disease in apparently healthy men. *N Engl J Med* 1997;336:973–979.
53. Richardson PD, Davies MJ, Born GVR. Influence of plaque configuration and stress distribution on fissuring of coronary atherosclerotic plaques. *Lancet* 1989;2:941–944.
54. Cheng GC, Loree HM, Kamm RD, et al. Distribution of circumferential stress in ruptured and stable atherosclerotic lesions: A structural analysis with histopathological correlation. *Circulation* 1993;87;1179–1187.
55. Meredith IT, Yeung AC, Weidinger FF, et al. Role of impaired endothelium-dependent vasodilation in ischemic manifestations of coronary artery disease. *Circulation* 1993;87(suppl V):V56–V66.
56. Vita JA, Treasure CB, Nabel EG, et al. The coronary vasomotor response to acetylcholine relates to risk factors for coronary artery disease. *Circulation* 1990;81:491–497.
57. Okumura K, Yasue H, Matsuyama K, et al. Effect of acetylcholine on the highly stenotic coronary artery: Difference between the constrictor response of the infarct-related coronary artery and that of the noninfarct-related artery. *J Am Coll Cardiol* 1992;19:752–758.
58. Bertrand ME, LaBlanche JM, Tilmant PY, et al. Frequency of provoked coronary arterial spasm in 1089 consecutive patients undergoing coronary arteriography. *Circulation* 1982;65:1299–1306.
59. Bogaty P, Hackett D, Davies G, Maseri A. Vasoreactivity of the culprit lesion in unstable angina. *Circulation* 1994;90:5–11.
60. Nobuyoshi M, Tanaka M, Nosaka H, et al. Progression of coronary atherosclerosis: Is coronary spasm related to progression? *J Am Coll Cardiol* 1991; 18:904–910.

61. Hackett D, Davies G, Chierchia S, Maseri A. Intermittent coronary occlusion in acute myocardial infarction. Value of combined thrombolytic and vaso-dilator therapy. *N Engl J Med* 1987;317:1055–1059.
62. Golino P, Ashton JH, Buja LM, et al. Local platelet activation causes vaso-constriction of large epicardial canine coronary arteries in vivo. Thrombox-ane A2 and serotonin are possible mediators. *Circulation* 1989;79:154–166.
63. Lam JY, Chesebro JH, Steele PM, et al. Is vasospasm related to platelet deposition? Relationship in a porcine preparation of arterial injury in vivo. *Circulation* 1987;75:243–248.
64. Zeiher AM, Schächinger V, Weitzel SH, et al. Intracoronary thrombus for-mation causes focal vasoconstriction of epicardial arteries in patients with coronary artery disease. *Circulation* 1991;83:1519–1525.
65. Kinlay S, Selwyn AP, Delagrange D, et al. Biological mechanisms for the clinical success of lipid-lowering in coronary artery disease and the use of surrogate end-points. *Curr Opin Lipid* 1996;7:389–397.
66. Ihling C, Göbel HR, Lippoldt A, et al. Endothelin-1-like immunoreactivity in human atherosclerotic coronary tissue: A detailed analysis of the cellular distribution of endothelin-1. *J Pathol* 1996;179:303–308.
67. Zeiher AM, Goebel H, Schächinger V, Ihling C. Tissue endothelin-1 immu-noreactivity in the active coronary atherosclerotic plaque: A clue to the mechanism of increased vasoreactivity of the culprit lesion in unstable angina. *Circulation* 1995;91:941–947.
68. Zeiher AM, Ihling C, Pistorius K, et al. Increased tissue endothelin immuno-reactivity in atherosclerotic lesions associated with acute coronary syn-dromes. *Lancet* 1994;344:1405–1406.
69. Gruppo Italiano per lo Studio della Streptochinasi nell'Infarcto Miocardico (GISSI). Effectiveness of intravenous thrombolytic treatment in acute myo-cardial infarction. *Lancet* 1986;1:397–402.
70. Hackett D, Davies G, Maseri A. Pre-existing coronary stenoses in patients with first myocardial infarction are not necessarily severe. *Eur Heart J* 1988; 9:1317–1323.
71. Ambrose JA, Tannenbaum MA, Alexopoulos D, et al. Angiographic pro-gression of coronary artery disease and the development of myocardial infarction. *J Am Coll Cardiol* 1988;12:56–62.
72. Little WC, Constantinescu M, Applegate RJ, et al. Can coronary angiogra-phy predict the site of a subsequent myocardial infarction in patients with mild-to-moderate coronary artery disease? *Circulation* 1988;78:1157–1166
73. Giroud D, Li JM, Urban P, et al. Relation of the site of acute myocardial infarction to the most severe coronary arterial stenosis at prior angiogra-phy. *Am J Cardiol* 1992;69:729–732.
74. Davies MJ, Thomas A. Thrombosis and acute coronary-artery lesions in sudden cardiac ischemic death. *N Engl J Med* 1984;310:1137–1140.
75. Davies MJ, Bland JM, Hangartner JRW, et al. Factors influencing the pres-ence or absence of acute coronary artery thrombi in sudden ischaemic death. *Eur Heart J* 1989:10:203–208.
76. el Fawal MA, Berg GA, Wheatley DJ, Jarland WA. Sudden coronary death in Glasgow: Nature and frequency of acute coronary lesions. *Br Heart J* 1987;57:329–335.
77. Qiao JH, Fishbein MC. The severity of coronary atherosclerosis at sites of plaque rupture with occlusive thrombosis. *J Am Coll Cardiol* 1991;17: 1138–1142.
78. Wilcox JN, Smith KM, Schwartz SM, Gordon D. Localization of tissue factor

in the normal vessel wall and in the atherosclerotic plaque. *Proc Natl Acad Sci U S A* 1989;86:2839–2843.

79. Moreno PR, Bernardi VH, López-Cuéllar J, et al. Macrophages, smooth muscles cells, and tissue factor in unstable angina: Implications for cell-mediated thrombogenicity in acute coronary syndromes. *Circulation* 1996; 94:3090–3097.

80. Moncada S, Gryglewski R, Bunting S, Bane JR. An enzyme isolated from arteries transforms prostaglandin endoperoxidase to an unstable substance that inhibits platelet aggregation. *Nature* 1976;263:663–665.

81. Ubatuba FB, Moncada S, Bane JR. The effect of prostacyclin (PGI2) on platelet behaviour, thrombus formation in vivo and bleeding time. *Thromb Diath Haemorrh* 1979;41:425–434.

82. Azuma H, Ishikawa M, Sekizaki S. Endothelium-dependent inhibition of platelet aggregation. *Br J Pharmacol* 1986;88:411–415.

83. Hogan JC, Lewis MJ, Henderson AH. In vivo EDRF activity influences platelet function. *Br J Pharmacol* 1988;94:1020–1022.

84. Yao S-K, Ober JC, Krishnaswami A, et al. Endogenous nitric oxide protects against platelet aggregation and cyclic flow variations in stenosed and endothelium-injured arteries. *Circulation* 1992;86:1302–1309.

85. Bassenge E. Antiplatelet effects of endothelium-derived relaxing factor and nitric oxide donors. *Eur Heart J* 1991;12(suppl E):12–15.

86. Lijnen HR, Coilen D. Endothelium in hemostasis and thrombosis. *Prog Cardiovasc Dis* 1997;4:343–350.

87. Malmberg K, Bavenholm P, Hamsten A. Clinical and biochemical factors associated with prognosis after myocardial infarction at a young age. *J Am Coll Cardiol* 1994;24:592–599.

88. Cigolini M, Targher G, Seidell JC, et al. Relationships of plasminogen activator inhibitor- 1 to anthropometry, serum insulin, triglycerides and adipose tissue fatty acids in healthy men. *Atherosclerosis* 1994;106:139–147.

89. Crutchley DJ, McPhee GV, Terris MF, Canossa-Terris MA. Levels of three hemostatic factors in relation to serum lipids. Monocyte procoagulant activity, tissue plasminogen activator, and type-1 plasminogen activator inhibitor. *Arteriosclerosis* 1989;9:934–939.

90. Asplund-Carlson A, Hamsten A, Wiman B, Carlson LA. Relationship between plasma plasminogen activator inhibitor-1 activity and VLDL triglyceride concentration, insulin levels and insulin sensitivity: Studies in randomly selected normo- and hypertriglyceridaemic men. *Diabetologia* 1993; 36:817–825.

91. Robbie LA, Booth NA, Brown AJ, Bennett B. Inhibitors of fibrinolysis are elevated in atherosclerotic plaque. *Arterioscler Thromb Vasc Biol* 1996;16: 539–545.

92. Shireman PK, McCarthy WJ, Pearce WH, et al. Elevated levels of plasminogen-activator inhibitor type 1 in atherosclerotic aorta. *J Vasc Surg* 1996;23: 810–817.

Mechanical Forces in Plaque Disruption

Dr. Fuster: I'd like to ask Dr. Wagner about the pharmacological or genetic alteration of the extracellular matrix. I can imagine all the possibilities in the future. It's one of the most exciting things one can think about. Do you think you will ever have anything that can get deep inside the vessel wall where the extracellular matrix is? We are talking about local delivery, obviously I'm talking about 10 years from now.

Dr. Wagner: I don't think you'd have to worry about getting it inside the vessel wall. I think that those genes are there in the vessel wall. It would be just a matter of determining which genes to regulate. Whether it's the metalloproteinases or the enzymes that add sulphate groups to a particular oligosaccharide which would then inhibit a particular factor in the vessel wall, I think the key to the whole issue is regulating what's left there. There may be a difficult task because we've got a paucity of smooth muscle cells in some situations and we've got an excess of macrophages in others. I believe that's really the key to the issue.

Dr. Fuster: But do you think you will be able to regulate the genes inside the vessel wall that are responsible for that. I'm just trying to get a sense of how you take a few cells out, you inject the HDL, and the HDL goes to the sky. I understand all that. But really we are talking about moving muscle cells into the vessel wall and I'd just like to understand if you can tell us what alternatives you see in the future to get there?

Dr. Wagner: Well I think that if you could figure out what targets to attack, then those specific genes could be regulated. If you could figure out exactly what probes to use. I think that's a possibility.

Dr. Libby: I think we have a long way to understand biology before we can use appropriately the genetic technology. I want to know what gene would be an appropriate target. I want to know when, and

I want to know where. I have concerns with systemic antiproliferative therapies. We might be able to think we are producing a beneficial effect for a culprit lesion, perhaps to prevent or minimize restenosis, but actually destabilize the greater number of vulnerable plaques. Let's talk specifically about whether I see metalloproteinases as a therapeutic target. I think that we don't know enough about the biology in the late 1990s. I think first of all we have to consider that metalloproteinases may have many other actions other than merely degrading matrix components. We might have to ask which metalloproteinases would be appropriate targets and which would be inappropriate targets. I'd like to back up one step. I'd like to understand more about the stimuli for inflammation because that's the more proximal mediator. That's the stimulus, as we'll talk about this afternoon for the proteinase expression. In a large number of our patients, we have the hypothesis that lipoproteins and perhaps modified lipoproteins, as Dr. Witztum will talk to us about later, could be the triggers for the local cytokine release, which would then upregulate the proteinase genes. I think that it's a very interesting concept that lipid lowering may be acting as an anti-inflammatory. So that takes care of the patients who have hyperlipoproteinemia, but what about the majority of our coronary patients who have a normal lipid profile. That's where I think the opportunity is to learn more biology to identify new therapeutic targets that could be proinflammatory. We need to unravel the path of biology and identify new targets.

Discussant from the Audience: I'd like to ask the mechanical people, Dr. Ku, have you performed any pulsatile studies with your flow model and I'd like to ask Dr. Lee what effect do you think the shape of the vessel will have. Many of the histology sections you showed were nice and circular, but I'd looked at many which have a lot of sectioning artifact and oblique shapes and what effect will that have on your models?

Dr. Ku: I guess I'll start. Yes, we have done pulsatile studies through these models, both computational as well as experimental. It's essentially the same behavior that I've showed here. The higher the flow, let's say systole in carotids, diastole in coronaries, you get this type of compression phenomenon.

Discussant from the Audience: I have a very brief comment about animal model of plaque rupture. We've just spent a year in collaboration with a pharmaceutical company trying to create such model. I think we're pretty close to a successful end, so the concept is very simple. We have designed a new catheter which allows growth of atherosclerotic lesion around the balloon so then we can expand this balloon and rupture plaque at will. We understand the limitations of this approach, because evidently it may say a lot more about plaque vulnerability.

Dr. Fuster: I'd think you'd have to be very careful about the model and how you extrapolate it, because when you inflate a balloon, you bring the vessel to a very different level of behavior than spontaneously. The pathology of balloon inflation is very different from spontaneous plaque rupture. When you blow up a balloon you get a lot more sheer forces, and certain things, like calcification, start to play a very important role that under normal circumstances they probably don't. It's an interesting model, but you have to probably be careful with how closely you extrapolate.

Dr. Libby: Especially we're talking about where the behavior is coming from. If it's from the lumen or from the adventitia. You are going to do an experiment from inside the plaque.

Dr. Insull: I'm a bit puzzled by the seeming paradox, namely the clinical observation that culprit lesions occur in nonstenotic areas. Yet in the presentation here this morning, Dr. Ku and Dr. Lee emphasized the great forces of tension and compression that occur or are associated with the stenotic lesions. Could you two gentlemen comment on whether or not the effects of those stenoses may actually be carried downstream? Do the oscillations and the mechanical effects influence the culprit or vulnerable lesions downstream and not down the stenotic site.

Dr. Lee: I think actually the scheme I presented is less important when the lesion is very, very severely stenosed and more important when the radius of the lumen is larger. David and I have talked over the years that there's different mechanisms that can be used depending on the lesions. Different lesions can both be playing a role on various points in time. In some lesions like these that rupture—40- or 50-percent lesions or even less—there doesn't have to be any pressure gradient across the stenosis. Other things like turbulence require much larger stenoses and they come into play for different lesions.

Dr. Ku: We have been focusing on high-grades stenosis, and these effects would happen much more on the high-grade stenosis. It wouldn't be so much in a 50 percent stenosis; the effects that Dr. Lee was talking about are more dominant there. We tried to look at carotid stenoses that are very vulnerable. When you have a high-grade carotid stenosis, about 1 out of 4 is going to rupture or the patient is going to have some neurological sequelae. That's a lot better than looking at 1 out of 100 in the much lower grade stenoses.

Dr. Cornhill: There is a downstream effect. Not only is the compression occurring right at the throat of the stenosis, but there is a large amount of turbulence that is generated downstream. That the may have an effect on endothelial cells. Turbulence by itself is not particularly good for endothelial cells but those are more subtle effects.

Dr. Badimon: Bill, I think you brought up a very good point and one that I wanted to come to. If you do have an 80- or 90 percent stenosis at the throat, we start at each end at zero percent so we go from what, in effect, would be zero up through 90 and then back to zero. So I think one of the things that we have to do is stop thinking about lesions in two dimensions. Think of them in three dimensions, both in terms of our imaging strategy and also in terms of our computational fluid and mechanical studies. So I think it's really important that the rupture may in fact start proximally on the axial side and then move into the wall as opposed to our two dimensional approach of looking at it just at the shoulder. So I think that we need to look at it in a more complex way and realize that the 90 percent stenosis that we look at somewhere, upstream or downstream, goes to 30 or 40 percent or it may be down to zero. So I think it's a much more complex approach and we need to adapt, as I said, our imaging computational and also our mechanical testing strategies to three dimensions.

Dr. Fuster: I have a question actually for Dr. Ganz. Peter, I have a problem and I wonder if you had the same problem, of really saying that vasoconstriction leads to plaque rupture. My problem has to do with the realities of the patients that we see. Very rarely actually in your patient population, you can attach vasoconstriction to plaque rupture in the clinical setting. It may happen but I suspect that it's more an exception than a rule.

Dr. Ganz: I agree with you. I could not find any scientific data supporting that the vasoconstriction can contribute to plaque rupture, providing a significant mechanical force to induce it. But when I heard Dr. Ku's talk, I tried to think of mild lesions which start below 80 percent, but you get some superimposed constriction to bring it up to the more severe luminal narrowing so some of these oscillations could then take over.

Discussant from the Audience: I just want to raise the issue of permeability of plaque tissue as the cause of plaque rupture. There is data from the 60s on animal models that hypercholesterolemic animals when injected with, say for example, radiolabeled fibrinogen, have higher intake of the plaque tissue versus normal arterial tissue. There was a recent model of hypercholesterolemia in rabbits where they used fluorescein uptake in the iris of the eye and hypercholesterolemic animals had much higher uptake through that iridic vessel, suggesting higher permeability. We have some data recently with radiolabeled antibodies that plaque is permeable to pretty much whatever you inject, and I'm wondering if anybody has looked at some of the mechanical forces that you have been describing and whether the increased permeability of platelets or fibrinogen or other factors in circulation that may cause plaque rupture.

Dr. Fuster: Dr. Cornhill I think you had done some work in this area, isn't it?

Dr. Cornhill: Yes we did some work years ago with Don Frye and others and had similar observations with regard to the increased permeability of the plaque and also of some increased internal pressures associated with that. One of those forces would be large enough to be an important mechanism other than in terms of its concentration. So I think it gets back, really almost certainly, to the increased concentration of types of materials in the plaque itself which may contribute to it.

Dr. Fuster: This morning, aside of the importance of the inflammatory component and the extracellular matrix, the adventitia came into light, which I like very much. And when we talk about mechanical forces, really it's a very complex issue. Collapsing, bending, sheer stress, sheer rate, and thromobogenicity of plaque are all very fascinating factors. But certainly, these inflammatory, extracellular matrix, and sheer forces or mechanical forces all have been covered in an outstanding way this morning and I hope there is a lot to learn in the near future. So let's get ready for lunch.

Chapter 22

Regulation of Metalloproteinases and Their Inhibitors in Atheroma

Rosalind P. Fabunmi, PhD and
Peter Libby, MD

Introduction

Rupture of atherosclerotic plaque commonly causes the thrombosis that leads to complications such as unstable angina pectoris or acute myocardial infarction.[1,2] The stability of an atherosclerotic plaque depends largely on the structural integrity of its fibrous cap, which is composed mainly of extracellular matrix (ECM) components that are rich in collagen.[3] The deposition of ECM proteins by intimal smooth muscle cells (SMCs) probably provides the atherosclerotic plaque with its tensile strength, rendering it resistant to rupture. Thus, excessive dissolution of the ECM of the collagenous matrix of the plaque's fibrous cap provides a likely mechanism that contributes to plaque rupture. Much recent evidence[29,73–76] supports the involvement of a specialized family of matrix-degrading enzymes, known as matrix metalloproteinases (MMPs), in the catabolism of the structural macromolecules that weaken the plaque's fibrous cap.

Matrix-Degrading Metalloproteinases: Classification and Primary Structure

The MMP family includes 19 structurally related, zinc-dependent enzymes that function at physiological pH in the extracellular space.

From: Fuster, V (ed). *The Vulnerable Atherosclerotic Plaque: Understanding, Identification, and Modification.* Armonk, NY: Futura Publishing Company, Inc.; © 1999.

Recent work[4-7] has defined four integral membrane proteins that differ from the other MMPs in that they associate with the plasma membrane through specific interactions with a hydrophobic transmembrane domain that is lacking in the other MMPs. These membrane-type (MT) metalloproteinases bear the designation MT1-MMP through MT4-MMP. Each MMP has been assigned a number roughly in the sequence of its discovery.[8]

MMPs have been broadly classified into three main groups on the basis of substrate specificity. They include the collagenases (MMP-1, -8, and -13), which degrade intact fibrillar collagens; the gelatinases (MMP-2 and -9), which hydrolyze the denatured collagen fibril and basement membrane collagen type IV; and the stromelysins (MMP-3, -7, -10, and -11), which have the broadest substrate specificity. Table 1 summarizes the classification of MMPs and their individual substrate requirements. Little is known of the substrate requirements for each of the MT-MMPs, but recently it has been demonstrated that MT1-MMP has gelatinolytic activity[9] and degrades collagens of type I, II, and III, as well as proteoglycan, fibronectin, vitronectin, and laminin-1, exhibiting a substrate specificity similar to that of MMP-1.[10] In addition, MT3-MMP can degrade gelatin and casein.[6] The substrate requirements for MMP-18 and MMP-19 are presently unknown. Collectively, the MMPs can degrade all of the major protein components of the ECM.

The MMPs share a similar five-domain structure (Fig. 1). The leader sequence targets the enzyme for secretion and is cleaved during secretion from the cells. The N-terminal domain contains a highly conserved PRCGVPD sequence which maintains latency of the proenzyme through interactions with its unpaired cysteine residue and the active-site zinc in the catalytic domain.[11,12] MT-MMPs 1 through 4, and MMP-11 contain a furin cleavage domain with a RRKR recognition motif between the N-terminus and catalytic domain. Furin belongs to a family of proteolytic enzymes, called *subtilisin-like convertases*, which process a wide variety of precursor proteins to their active forms.[13] In addition to a zinc-binding site, the catalytic domain of all MMPs contains two calcium-binding sites[14] and, in the case of MMP-2 and MMP-9, an additional insert consisting of three fibronectin-like repeats.[15,16] The C-terminal domain shares homology with the plasma protein hemopexin, and is considered important for determining substrate specificity. Although MMP-7 lacks the C-terminal domain, it still retains all of the other characteristics of an MMP.

Not all metalloproteinases of interest in vascular biology belong to the MMP family. The zinc- dependent peptidase known as angiotensin converting enzyme (ACE) is one such example. A family of metalloproteinases known as "the ADAMs" (a disintegrin and metalloproteinase) has recently burgeoned. First recognized in snake venoms and in mam-

Table 1

Classification of MMPs

Enzyme names	MMP-#	Size (kDa)	ECM substrates
Collagenase, interstitial (fibroblast-type)	MMP-1	55	Collagens I, II, III, VII, VIII, X; gelatin: PG core protein
PMN collagenase (neutrophil)	MMP-8	75	Same as above
Collagenase-3	MMP-13	54	Collagen II, aggrecan
Stromelysin-1 Transin-1	MMP-3	57	PG core protein; fibronectin; laminin; collagen IV, V, IX, X; elastin'oCL
Stromelysin-2 Transin-2	MMP-10	57	Same as above
Stromelysin-3	MMP-11		Fibronectin, laminin, gelatin, PG
Putative metalloproteinase-1 (Pump-1), matrilysin	MMP-7	28	Fibronectin, laminin, collagen IV, gelatin, procollagenase, PG core protein
Gelatinase, 72 kDa (A) Type IV collagenase	MMP-2	72	Gelatin; collagens IV, V, VII, X, XI; elastin; fibronectin; PG core protein, laminin
Gelatinase, 92 kDa (B) Type IV collagenase	MMP-9	92	Gelatin; collagens IV, V; elastin; PG core protein
Macrophage metalloelastase	MMP-12	53	Elastin
MT1-MMP	MMP-14	66	Interstitial collagens, gelatin, cartilage PG, fibronectin, vitronectin, laminin
MT2-MMP	MMP-15	66	n.d.
MT3-MMP	MMP-16	69	Gelatin, casein
MT4-MMP	MMP-17	57	n.d.
	MMP-18		n.d.
	MMP-19	56	n.d.

MMP = matrix metalloproteinase; MMP- = MMP numbering according to Reference 8; n.d. = not determined. Modified and updated from Reference 69.

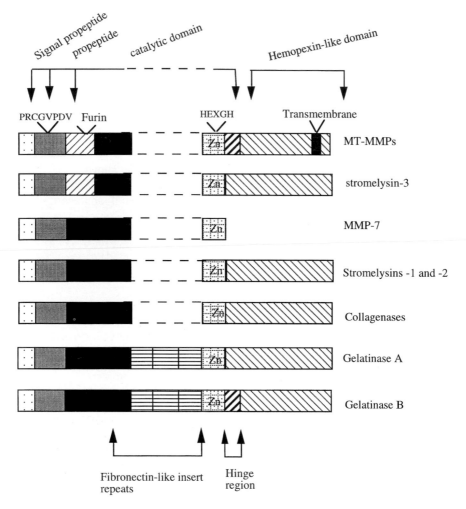

Figure 1. Domain structure of the matrix metalloproteinases.

malian sperm, this family now consists of 18 members. In the vessel wall, ADAM 17, also known as tumor necrosis factor-converting enzyme (TACE), may have special significance, as it cleaves the membrane-bound precursor of this proinflammatory vasoactive cytokine into its soluble form.[17,18]

Regulation of Matrix Metalloproteinases

The regulation of MMPs occurs principally at three levels which include: (1) control of the rate of gene transcription; (2) conversion of

Table 2

Tissue Inhibitors of Matrix Metalloproteinases (TIMPs)

Designation	Enzyme preference	Comments
TIMP-1	proMMP-9	Soluble
TIMP-2	proMMP-2	Soluble
TIMP-3	all	Matrix bound
TIMP-4	nd	Soluble

the initial translational product, an inactive zymogen precursor, to the active form; and (3) inactivation by a family of endogenous inhibitors known as tissue inhibitors of metalloproteinases (TIMPs) (Table 2). Each of these levels of control is discussed in turn, with the emphasis on vascular cells involved in atherogenesis.

Transcriptional Regulation

MMPs are secreted by a number of lesion-associated cells in vitro. For example, SMCs from a variety of species secrete MMP-2 constitutively. Under basal conditions, SMCs, like most connective tissue cells, secrete scant MMP-1, -3, and -9; but a variety of stimuli can induce the expression of these enzymes (Table 3). For example, platelet-derived growth factor (PDGF) and basic fibroblast growth factor (bFGF) induce MMP-1,[19,20] and linoleic acid hydroperoxide increases MMP-1 and MMP-3 expression in human SMC.[21] We have shown induction of MMP-1, MMP-3, and MMP-9 following exposure of SMC to stimuli such as interleukin-1 (IL-1) and tumor necrosis factor (TNF).[22] Interestingly, this induction can be enhanced in the presence of growth factors such as PDGF or bFGF.[23] Phorbol myristyl acetate (PMA), an agonist of protein kinase C, induces MMP-1, -3, and -9 in primate SMC. Heparin inhibits this effect,[24,25] suggesting that heparin may mediate its inhibitory effects on SMC accumulation in the intima of injured arteries in part by inhibiting MMP expression. Human endothelial cells (EC) elaborate MMP-2 and secrete MMP-1, -3, and -9 following exposure to TNF.[26,27] A protein in the membranes of tumors and other cells, known as extracellular matrix metalloproteinase inducer (EMMPRIN),[28] also stimulates expression of MMP-1, -2, and -3 in EC. Other cell types in the plaque, such as T- lymphocytes, secrete MMP-9, which can be further increased in the presence of cytokine.[29,30]

Human peripheral blood-derived monocytes produce little MMP, but differentiation into macrophages yields higher levels of MMP-9

Table 3

Modulators of MMP Expression Relevant to Atherogenesis

Mediator	Abbreviation	Relevant sources	Effect on MMP expression
Platelet-derived growth factor	PDGF	Platelets endothelial cells SMC macrophages	Induces MMP-1 in SMC
Interleukin 1	IL-1	macrophages EC SMC platelets	Induces MMPs-1, 3 and -9 in SMC Induces MMPs-1 & 3 in monocytes
Tumor necrosis factor alpha	TNF-α	macrophages SMC (not EC) lymphocytes	Induces MMPs-1, 3 and -9 in SMC and EC Induces MMP-9 in macrophages
CD40 Ligand (gp 39)	T-lymphocytes EC SMC	Induces MMPs-1 and -3 in macrophages	
Basic fibroblast growth factor	bFGF	endothelial cells SMC macrophages	Induces MMP-1 in SMC
ECM MMP inducer	EMMPR IN	endothelial cells	Induces MMPs-1, -2 and -3

MMP = matrix metalloproteinase; SMC = smooth muscle cells; EC = endothelial cells.

than MMP-1 and MMP-3.[31,32] Secretion of MMP-9 in macrophages can be further induced by TNF-α, IL-1β, and CD40.[33,34] Expression of collagenase (MMP-1) and stromelysin (MMP-3) in macrophages is regulated by microbial products such as bacterial lipopolysaccharide (LPS) and yeast zymosan.[35] T lymphocytes can induce collagenase and stromelysin expression in human monocyte-derived macrophages via ligation of the TNF-receptor–like CD40 molecule.[35a] Interferon γ, dexamethasone, IL-4, and IL-10 suppress the LPS-induced production of MMP-1 and MMP-3 and the constitutive expression of MMP-9 in human macrophages.[34,36-39] The ECM protein laminin augments the synthesis of MMP-9 and urokinase-type plasminogen activator (uPA) in macrophage cell lines and, to a lesser extent, in bone marrow–derived macrophages.[40]

We isolated macrophages from the lesions of cholesterol-fed rabbits and compared their profile of enzymatic activity to that of rabbit alveolar macrophages.[41] The foam cells displayed constitutive levels of expression of MMP-1, -3, and -9. By contrast, the alveolar macrophages did not display expression of these MMPs unless exposed to phorbol ester, indicating that the stimuli responsible for MMP induction in macrophages are present in the microenvironment of the lesion.

Little is known about the transcription factors and consensus-binding motifs responsible for the induction of MMPs in vascular cells. The activator protein-1(AP-1) site in the promoter of MMP-1, -3, -7, and -9 appears to be functional in many cell types, but by itself is insufficient to direct the transcription of MMPs. The AP-1 site confers PMA inducibility on genes by acting as a binding site for the transcription factor AP-1.[42] Transcriptional regulation of MMPs appears to involve an essential interaction with other cis-acting elements in the promoters and transcription factors. For example, the MMP-9 gene requires a complex interaction between AP-1, NF-κB, and Sp1 for maximal levels of transcriptional activation,[43] and appears to be transcriptionally regulated in a cell-specific–type manner. The NF-κB site in the MMP-9 promoter is in keeping with the fact that MMP-9 is a candidate gene in the inflammatory response to atherosclerosis and angioplasty restenosis. Induction of MMP-1 by LPS treatment in human (U937) and murine (J774) monocytic cell lines depends upon the AP-1 site, whereas induction with PMA requires interaction with upstream elements including the polyoma enhancer a-binding protein-3 site (PEA 3) and TTCA sequence.[44] In contrast to other MMP genes, the AP-1 site in the MMP-13 gene, encoding a form of interstitial collagenase, appears to be sufficient for induction by PMA.[45]

Activation of Matrix Metalloproteinases

MMPs are secreted from cells as inactive zymogens and require activation in the extracellular milieu before they attain the capacity to degrade ECM molecules. Activation of MMPs occurs in vitro by organomercurials such as 4 aminophenylmercuric acetate (APMA) and in vivo by proteolytic enzymes such as plasmin and cathepsins B and G. Recently, it has been shown that macrophage-derived reactive oxygen species such as peroxynitrite and hydrogen peroxide activate MMP-2 and MMP-9[46] and thrombin activates MMP-2.[47] MMPs themselves, once processed from the zymogen to the active form, can trigger activation of other members of the MMP family. For example, the active form of stromelysin-1 (MMP-3) and stromelysin-2 (MMP-10) can activate interstitial collagenase (MMP-1)[48] and neutrophil collagenase (MMP-8),[49,50] while active MMP-2 and MMP-3 activate MMP-9 and MMP-13.[49,51,52] Mast cells within atheroma, while far outnumbered by macrophages, can elaborate serine proteinases which may activate MMPs.[53]

MMP-2 differs from the other members of the MMP family in that it is not activated by endopeptidases such as trypsin, plasmin, and stromelysin. Rather, its activation depends on the action of the membrane-bound members of the MMP family, MT1-MMP and MT2-MMP. Formation of a trimolecular MT-1MMP/TIMP-2/MMP-2 complex is required at the cell surface through interactions between the catalytic domain of MT1-MMP and the N-terminal domain of TIMP-2 and the C-terminal domain of TIMP-2 with MMP-2. MMP-2 is then activated by a second molecule of free MT1-MMP.[54,55] Thus, activation of MMP-2 through MT1-MMP requires relatively small amounts of TIMP, as this activation mechanism is inhibited in the presence of large quantities of TIMP-2. Thus, TIMP-2 may have opposing effects, depending on its local concentration. The activation of cell-bound MT1-MMP, itself, remains to be elucidated.

Another special aspect of MMP-2 that is relevant to vascular biology is the ability of the integrin $\alpha_v\beta_3$ (the vitronectin receptor) to bind this proteinase to cell surfaces. This interaction promotes the activation of pro-MMP-2.[56] SMCs express $\alpha_v\beta_3$ integrin after injury or in the atherosclerotic intima, providing another potential pathway of activation of the latent form of the proteinase, constitutively expressed by human SMCs in vitro and in vivo.

Tissue Inhibitors of Metalloproteinases

Endogenous inhibitors known as TIMPs counterbalance MMP activities under usual circumstances. The TIMP family consists of TIMP-1,[57] TIMP-2,[58] and TIMP-3,[59] and a more recently described TIMP-4 (Table 2).[60] TIMP-1 and TIMP-2 are the better characterized members of the group and are secreted in a soluble form by cultured cells. TIMP-3, however, once secreted, binds to and forms an insoluble complex with constituents of the ECM.[61] TIMP-1, -2, and -3 all have similar inhibitory activities against MMPs.[62]

The TIMPs exhibit sequence homology and share domains of identical protein structures that consist of a highly conserved N-terminal region, considered critical for inhibition of the enzymes and a more diverse C-terminal domain of unknown function. In addition to binding active MMPs, TIMP-1 and TIMP-2 also bind the proforms of MMP-9 and MMP-2, respectively, through interaction of the C-terminal domain of each molecule.[63] This process is thought to contribute to maintaining the stability of the enzymes. TIMP-2 is also secreted from cells as a complex with MT1-MMP.[9] The TIMPs have also been shown to have other important functions. For example, mutations in the TIMP-3 gene cause Sorsby's fundus dystrophy, a dominantly inherited form of blindness.[64] TIMP-3 is also involved in cell cycle progression[65] and inhibits bFGF-induced angiogenesis in vitro and in vivo.[66] TIMP-1 and TIMP-2 have growth factor action in some cultured cells[67] and also have erythroid potentiation.[57,68]

The balance between MMP activities and their inhibition by TIMPs is considered critical in the maintenance of ECM homeostasis. Excessive MMP activity occurs in a number of disease states including cancer invasion and metastasis, rheumatoid arthritis, glomerulosclerosis, and gingival disease.[69] Moreover, substantial evidence implicates MMPs in the pathogenesis of accelerated connective tissue turnover associated with other degenerative diseases of the vessel, such as aortic aneurysms and vein graft stenosis, and in the migration of SMC from the media to the intima following arterial injury.[70]

The regulation of TIMP-1, -2, and -3 has been studied in SMC by us and others. In general, the expression of TIMP-1 and TIMP-3 undergoes regulation, whereas TIMP-2 is secreted constitutively with little variation, consistent with most other cell types.[22,23,25] Growth factors such as PDGF and TGFβ can induce TIMP-3 in rabbit and human SMC, and PDGF increases TIMP-1, suggesting possible mechanisms for induction of TIMPs 1 and 3 in SMC in vivo[23,] (Fabunmi RP, unpublished observations). Interestingly, expression of TIMP-1 and TIMP-2 does not appear to be modulated by cytokines such as IL-1 or TNF, which increase MMP activities in SMC. A role for TIMP-1 in arterial injury has been tested with use of a rat model of balloon injury. Local retroviral-mediated gene transfer of rat SMCs overexpressing TIMP-1 into balloon- injured rat carotid arteries resulted in a reduction in intimal hyperplasia.[71] In addition, arterial injury in rats increases expression of TIMP-2, as well as plasminogen activator inhibitor type 1.[72] These various studies suggest an important counterregulatory role for TIMP-1 and TIMP-2 in the arterial response to injury.

Expression of Matrix Metalloproteinases and Tissue Inhibitors of Metalloproteinases in Human and Rabbit Atheroma

As an initial test of the hypothesis that MMPs may be involved in atherosclerosis, we and others have examined uninvolved tissue and atheromatous lesions for the presence and distribution of MMPs. Consistent with in vitro data, both normal and atherosclerotic arteries constitutively express MMP-2. By contrast, little to moderate expression of MMP-1, -3, -7, and -9 were found in normal tissue, but levels were augmented in atheroma.[29,73–76] Interestingly, in all of these studies, expression was localized primarily to macrophages in rupture-prone areas of the lesion. Interstitial collagenase (MMP-1), gelatinase B (MMP-9), and stromelysin-1 (MMP-3) are expressed in the fibrous cap, the lesion's shoulders, and the base of the lipid core,[29,73–75] and matrilysin (MMP-7) is predominantly expressed in macrophages overlying the lipid core.[76] Expression was also observed in SMC, T-lymphocytes, and endothelial cells of microvessels, establishing these cells as an in vivo source of MMPs.[29] Moreover, high expression of MMPs was detected in lipid-laden macrophages from the experimental lesions of cholesterol-fed rabbits but not in alveolar macrophages,[29] and increased secretion of gelatinases A and B has been observed in the aortas of rabbits fed a cholesterol-rich diet, with highest levels of expression correlating with those of lesion severity.[77]

We and others have found constitutive expression of TIMP-1 and -2 in both normal and diseased arteries,[29,75] and more recently, we have found that the ECM-associated TIMP-3 localizes in atheromatous tissue as well (Fabunmi RP, unpublished observations). Interestingly, the spatial distribution of all three TIMPs within atheroma correlates with that previously reported for MMP expression.[29,73–75] Most of the expression of MMPs and TIMPs in atheroma is in macrophages, suggesting that the balance between the synthesis and degradation of the ECM macromolecules in the atherosclerotic plaque may largely depend on the macrophage. The close proximity of enzyme and inhibitor in the plaque supports the hypothesis that the TIMPs serve as an important counter-regulatory mechanism limiting excessive MMP activity in vivo.

However, SMC may also play an important role in regulating the balance between matrix biosynthesis and catabolism in both normal and atherosclerotic arteries. Immunoprecipitation of SMC-conditioned media with use of an anti–TIMP-2 antibody coprecipitated the 72-kDa gelatinase (MMP-2),[22] providing biochemical evidence that the majority of TIMP-2 secreted by SMC is complexed with MMP-2. We can speculate that MMP-2 also binds to TIMP-2 in vivo, where the enzyme and its inhibitor colocalize, as shown by immunohistochemical study.[29] Thus, the constitutive expression of MMP-2 in the media of normal arteries probably does not result in net proteolytic activity.

Because MMPs are secreted as zymogens and the presence of TIMPs may block activity, we tested directly whether atherosclerotic lesions contain active forms of MMP-1 and -9. For this purpose we developed a method to detect enzymatic activity directly in tissue sections, known as in situ zymography.[78] Our results revealed an excess of gelatinolytic (MMP-2 and -9) and caseinolytic (MMP-3) activities in tissue sections that colocalized with areas of immunostaining.[29,78] Together these data demonstrate excessive MMP activities in atherosclerotic plaques, supporting the hypothesis that MMPs favor destruction of ECM components in the plaque and thus render it more susceptible to rupture and other complications.

Conclusions and Therapeutic Implications

Considerable evidence supports the involvement of MMPs in the regulation of the vulnerability of atheroma. These enzymes localize at sites prone to rupture, and possess proteolytic capacity, as shown by the in situ zymographic studies cited above. The macrophage, the leading candidate for the source of MMPs in the context of plaque rupture, and the T cell, a source of inducers of MMP expression such as TNF and CD40 ligand, predominate at sites of clinical plaque rupture, leading to fatal thromboses. Activated macrophages elaborate proteolytic activity that can degrade collagen in human fibrous caps in vitro. All of these findings support the role of MMP in the regulation of features of plaques related to stability.

One may then ask if it would be appropriate to attempt therapeutic inhibition of MMPs as a measure to stabilize plaques. A number of drugs are under investigation in other diseases (eg, tumor metastases, arthritides) that effectively inhibit MMPs. While trials in unstable coronary syndromes seem inevitable, a number of limitations should be borne in mind. First, not all of the proteinases in plaques are metalloenzymes. Increasing evidence implicates serine (eg, uPA) and cysteine proteinases (eg, cathepsins S and K) in catabolism of components of the plaque's ECM.[79] These nonmetalloenzymes would not be inhibited by currently available MMP inhibitors. Therefore, one might envisage targeting more proximal steps in the inflammatory pathway of atherogenesis that could interrupt the induction of expression of a number of nocent stimuli elaborated locally, including proteinases. Examples of such anti-inflammatory agents might include cytokine antagonists, inhibitors of cyclooxygenase 2 (COX-2), nitric oxide donors, inhibitors of NF-κB activation, or antioxidants. The practicability and efficacy of these strategies awaits further work.

There is, however, one proven strategy for stabilizing atherosclerotic lesions that remains insufficiently implemented in practice, and that may act as an anti-inflammatory in the plaque—namely lipid-lowering therapy. Numerous clinical studies have shown decreased acute coronary events in patients undergoing lipid lowering by a variety of interventions, ranging from diet to drugs.[80-83] By lowering ambient lipoprotein levels, such therapies may limit the induction of cytokines and oxidant species by products of lipoprotein modification within the artery wall. We know from experimental studies that hypercholesterolemia can induce MMP expression in lesional macrophages.

Whether or not lipid lowering actually can reduce MMP expression remains under investigation. Certainly, atherosclerosis and the acute coronary syndromes involve many more factors than hyperlipidemia alone. However, it is likely that improved understanding of the molecular pathogenesis of the acute coronary syndromes will enhance our ability to prevent lesion destabilization in patients by design of rational strategies in the future.

References

1. Davies MJ, Thomas AC. Plaque fissuring: The cause of acute myocardial infarction, sudden ischemic death, and crescendo angina. *Br Heart J* 1985; 53:363–373.
2. Fuster V, Badimon I, Badimon J, Chesebro J. The pathogenesis of coronary artery disease and the acute coronary syndromes. *N Engl J Med* 1992;326: 242–250.
3. Richardson P, Davies M, Born G. Influence of plaque configuration and stress distribution on fissuring of coronary atherosclerotic plaques. *Lancet* 1989;2:941–944.
4. Sato H, Takino T, Okada Y, et al. A matrix metalloproteinase expressed on the surface of invasive tumour cells. *Nature* 1994;370:61–65.
5. Takino T, Sato H, Shinagawa A, Seiki M. Identification of the second membrane-type matrix metalloproteinase (MT-MMP-2) gene from a human placenta cDNA library. MT-MMPs form a unique membrane-type subclass in the MMP family. *J Biol Chem* 1995;270:23013–23020.
6. Shofuda K, Yasumitsu H, Nishihashi A, et al. Expression of three membrane-type matrix metalloproteinases (MT-MMPs) in rat vascular smooth muscle cells and characterization of MT3-MMPs with and without transmembrane domain. *J Biol Chem* 1997;272:9749–9754.
7. Puente X, Pendas A, Llano E, et al. Molecular cloning of a novel membrane-type matrix metalloproteinase from a human breast carcinoma. *Cancer Res* 1996;56:944–949.
8. Nagase H, Barrett A, Woessner F. Nomenclature and glossary of the matrix metalloproteinases. *Matrix* 1992;(suppl 1):421–424.
9. Imai K, Ohuchi E, Aoki T, et al. Membrane-type matrix metalloproteinase 1 is a gelatinolytic enzyme and is secreted in a complex with tissue inhibitor of metalloproteinases 2. *J Cancer Res* 1996;56:2707–2710.
10. Ohuchi E, Imai K, Fujii Y, et al. Membrane type 1 matrix metalloproteinase digests interstitial collagens and other extracellular matrix macromolecules. *J Biol Chem* 1997;272:2446–2451.
11. Springman EB, Angleton EL, Birkedal-Hansen H, Van Wart HE. Multiple modes of activation of latent human fibroblast collagenase: Evidence for the role of a Cys-73 active-site zinc complex in latency and a "cysteine switch" mechanism for activation. *Proc Natl Acad Sci U S A* 1990;87:364–368.
12. Van Wart HE, Birkedal-Hansen H. The cysteine switch: A principle of regulation of metalloproteinase activity with potential applicability to the entire matrix metalloproteinase gene family. *Proc Natl Acad Sci U S A* 1990;87: 5578–5582.
13. Denault J, Leduc R. Furin/PACE/SPC1: A convertase involved in exocytic

and endocytic processing of precursor proteins. *FEBS Lett* 1996;379: 113–116.

14. Vallee BL, Auld DS. New perspective on zinc biochemistry: Cocatalytic sites in multi-zinc enzymes. *Biochemistry* 1993;32:6493–6500.
15. Collier IE, Wilhelm SM, Eisen AZ, et al. H-ras oncogene-transformed human bronchial epithelial cells (TBE-1) secrete a single metalloprotease capable of degrading basement membrane collagen. *J Biol Chem* 1988;263: 6579–6587.
16. Wilhelm SM, Collier IE, Marmer BL, et al. SV40-transformed human lung fibroblasts secrete a 92-KDa type 1V collagenase which is identical to that secreted by normal human macrophages. *J Biol Chem* 1989;264:17213–17221.
17. Black RA, Rauch CT, Kozlosky CJ, et al. A metalloproteinase disintegrin that releases tumour-necrosis factor-alpha from cells. *Nature* 1997;385: 729–733.
18. Moss M, Jin S, Milla M, et al. Cloning of a disintegrin metalloproteinase that processes precursor tumour-necrosis factor-alpha. *Nature* 1997;385: 733–736.
19. Yanagi H, Sasaguri Y, Sugama K, et al. Production of tissue collagenase (matrix metalloproteinase 1) by human aortic smooth muscle cells in response to platelet-derived growth factor. *Atherosclerosis* 1991;91:207–216.
20. Kennedy S, Rouda S, Qin H, et al. Basic FGF regulates interstitial collagenase gene expression in human smooth muscle cells. *J Cell Biochem* 1997;65: 32–41.
21. Sasaguri Y, Kakita N, Murahashi N, et al. Effect of linoleic acid hydroperoxide on production of matrix metalloproteinases by human aortic endothelial and smooth muscle cells. *Atherosclerosis* 1993;100:189–196.
22. Galis ZS, Muszynski M, Sukhova GK, et al. Cytokine-stimulated human vascular smooth muscle cells synthesize a complement of enzymes required for extracellular matrix digestion. *Circ Res* 1994;75:181–189.
23. Fabunmi R, Baker A, Murray E, et al. Divergent regulation by growth factors and cytokines of 95-kDa and 72-Da gelatinases and tissue inhibitors of metalloproteinases-1, -2 and -3 in rabbit aortic smooth muscle cells. *Bio chem J* 1996;315:335–342.
24. Au YP, Montgomery KF, Clowes AW. Heparin inhibits collagenase gene expression mediated by phorbol ester-responsive element in primate arterial smooth muscle cells. *Circ Res* 1992;70:1062–1069.
25. Kenagy RD, Nikkari ST, Welgus HG, Clowes AW. Heparin inhibits the induction of three matrix metalloproteinases (stromelysin, 92-kD gelatinase and collagenase) in primate arterial smooth muscle cells. *J Clin Invest* 1994; 93:1987–1993.
26. Hanemaaijer R, Koolwijk P, Le Clercq L, et al. Regulation of matrix metalloproteinase expression in human vein and microvascular endothelial cells: Effects of tumour necrosis factor- a, interleukin 1 and phorbol ester. *Biochem J* 1993;296:803–809.
27. Okamura K, Sato Y, Matsuda T, et al. Endogenous basic fibroblast growth factor-dependent induction of collagenase and interleukin-6 in tumor necrosis factor-treated human microvascular endothelial cells. *J Biol Chem* 1991;266:19162–19165.
28. Kataoka H, Decastro R, Zucker S, Biswas C. Tumor cell-derived collagenase-stimulatory factor increases expression of interstitial collagenase, stromelysin, and 72-kDa gelatinase. *Cancer Res* 1993;53:3154–3158.
29. Galis ZS, Sukhova GK, Lark MW, Libby P. Increased expression of matrix

metalloproteinases and matrix degrading activity in vulnerable regions of human atherosclerotic plaques. *J Clin Invest* 1994;94:2493–2503.

30. Johnatty R, Taub D, Reeder S, et al. Cytokine and chemokine regulation of proMMP-9 and TIMP-1 production by human peripheral blood lymphocytes. *J Immunol* 1997;158:2327–2333.

31. Welgus H, Campbell E, Cury J, et al. Neutral metalloproteinases produced by human mononuclear phagocytes. Enzyme profile, regulation, and expression during cellular development. *J Clin Invest* 1990;86(5):1496–1502.

32. Campbell EJ, Cury JD, Shapiro SD, et al. Neutral proteinases of human mononuclear phagocytes: Cellular differentiation markedly alters cell phenotype for serine proteinases, metalloproteinases, and tissue inhibitor of metalloproteinases. *J Immunol* 1991;146:1286–1293.

33. Malik N, Greenfield B, Wahl A, Kiener P. Activation of human monocytes through CD40 induces matrix metalloproteinases. *J Immunol* 1996;156: 3952–3960.

34. Sarén P, Welgus HG, Kovanen PT. TNF-α and IL-1β selectively induce expression of 92-kDa gelatinase by human macrophages. *J Immunol* 1996; 157:4159–4165.

35. Shapiro S, Kobayashi D, Welgus H. Identification of TIMP-2 in human alveolar macrophages. Regulation of biosynthesis is opposite to that of metalloproteinases and TIMP-1. *J Biol Chem* 1992;267:13890–13894.

35a. Mach F, Schonbeck U, Bonnefoy J, et al. Activation of monocyte/ macrophage functions related to acute atheroma complication by ligation of CD40: Induction of collagenase, stromelysin, and tissue factor. *Circulation* 1997;96:396–399

36. Shapiro SD, Campbell EJ, Kobayashi DK, Welgus HG. Dexamethasone selectively modulates basal and lipopolysaccharide-induced metalloproteinase and tissue inhibitor of metalloproteinase production by human alveolar macrophages. *J Immunol* 1991;146:2724–2729.

37. Shapiro SD, Campbell EJ, Kobayashi DK, Welgus HG. Immune modulation of metalloproteinase production in human macrophages. Selective pretranslational suppression of interstitital collagenase and stromelysin biosynthesis by interferon-g. *J Clin Invest* 1990;86:1204–1210.

38. Lacraz S, Nicod L, Galve-de Rochemonteix B, et al. Suppression of metalloproteinase biosynthesis in human alveolar macrophages by interleukin-4. *J Clin Invest* 1992;90:382–388.

39. Lacraz S, Nicod L, Chicheportiche R, et al. IL-10 inhibits metalloproteinase and stimulates TIMP-1 production in human mononuclear phagocytes. *J Clin Invest* 1995;96:2304–2310.

40. Khan K, Falcone D. Role of laminin in matrix induction of macrophage urokinase-type plasminogenactivator and 92-kDa metalloproteinase expression. *J Biol Chem* 1997;272:8270–8275.

41. Galis ZS, Sukhova GK, Kranzhöffer R, et al. Macrophage foam cells from experimental atheroma constitutively produce matrix-degrading proteinases. *Proc Natl Acad Sci U S A* 1995;92:402–406.

42. Angel P, Karin M. The role of jun, fos and the AP-1 complex in cell proliferation and transformation. *Biochim Biophys Acta* 1991;1072:129–157.

43. Sato H, Seiki M. Regulatory mechanism of 92-kDa Type-IV collagenase gene expression which is associated with invasiveness of tumor cells. *Oncogene* 1993;8:395–405.

44. Pierce R, Sandefur S, Doyle G, Welgus H. Monocytic cell type-specific transcriptional induction of collagenase. *J Clin Invest* 1996;97(8):1890–1899.

45. Pendas A, Balbin M, Llano E, et al. Structural analysis and promoter characterization of the human collagenase-3 gene (MMP13). *Genomics* 1997;40: 222–233.
46. Rajagopalan S, Meng X, Ramasamy S, et al. Reactive oxygen species produced by macrophage-derived foam cells regulate the activity of vascular matrix metalloproteinases in vitro. Implications for atherosclerotic plaque stability. *J Clin Invest* 1996;98:2572–2579.
47. Galis Z, Kranzhofer R, Fenton JW, Libby P. Thrombin promotes activation of matrix metalloproteinase-2 produced by cultured vascular smooth muscle cells. *Arterioscler Thromb Vasc Biol* 1997;17:483–489.
48. Murphy G, Cockett MI, Stephens PE, et al. Stromelysin is an activator of procollagenase: A study with natural and recombinant enzymes. *Biochem J* 1987;248:265–268.
49. Knauper V, Wilhelm S, Seperack P, et al. Direct activation of human neutrophil procollagenase by recombinant stromelysin. *Biochem J* 1993;581–586.
50. Knauper V, Will H, Lopez-Otin C, et al. Cellular mechanisms for human procollagenase-3 (MMP-13) activation. Evidence that MT1-MMP (MMP-14) and gelatinase a (MMP-2) are able to generate active enzyme. *J Biol Chem* 1996;271:17124–17131.
51. Desrivières S, He L, Peyri N, et al. Activation of the 92-kDa type-IV collagenase by tissue kallikrein. *J Cell Physiol* 1993;157:587–593.
52. Fridman R, Bird RE, Hoyhtya M, et al. Expression of human recombinant 72 kDa gelatinase and tissue inhibitor of metalloproteinase-2 (TIMP-2): Characterization of complex and free enzyme complex. *Biochem J* 1993;289: 411–416.
53. Kaartinen M, Penttila A, Kovanen, P. Mast cells of two types differing in neutral proteasecomposition in the human aortic intima. Demonstration of tryptase- and tryptase/chymase-containing mast cells in normal intimas, fatty streaks, and the shoulder region of atheromas. *Arterioscler Thromb* 1994;14:966–972.
54. Strongin A, Collier I, Bannikov G, et al.Mechanism of cell surface activation of 72-kDa type IV collagenase. Isolation of the activated form of the membrane metalloprotease. *J Biol Chem* 1995;270:5331–5338.
55. Kolkenbrock H, Hecker-Kia A, Orgel D, et al. Activation of progelatinase A and progelatinaseA/TIMP-2 complex by membrane type 2-matrix metalloproteinase. *Biol Chem* 1997;378:71–76.
56. Kubota S, Ito H, Ishibashi Y, Seyama Y. Anti-alpha 3 integrin antibody induces the activated form of matrix metalloprotease-2 (MMP-2) with concomitant stimulation of invasion through matrigel by human rhabdomyosarcoma cells. *Int J Cancer* 1997;70:106–111.
57. Docherty AJP, Lyons A, Smith BJ, et al. Sequence of human tissue inhibitor of metalloproteinases and its identity to erythroid-potentiating activity. *Nature* 1985;318:66–69.
58. Stetler-Stevenson WG, Brown PD, Onisto M, et al. Tissue inhibitor of metalloproteinases-2 (TIMP-2) mRNA expression in tumor cell lines and human tumor tissues. *J Biol Chem* 1990;265:13933–13938.
59. Uría JA, Ferrando AA, Velasco G, et al. Structure and expression in breast tumors of human TIMP-3, a new member of the metalloproteinase inhibitor family. *Cancer Res* 1994;54:2091–2094.
60. Greene J, Wang M, Liu Y, et al. Molecular cloning and characterization of human tissue inhibitor of metalloproteinase 4. *J Biol Chem* 1996;271(48): 30375–30380.

61. Pavloff N, Staskus PW, Kishnani NS, Hawkes SP. A new inhibitor of metal-loproteinases from chicken: ChIMP-3; A third member of the TIMP family. *J Biol Chem* 1992;267:17321–17326.
62. Apte S, Olsen B, Murphy G. The gene structure of tissue inhibitor of metal-loproteinases (Timp)-3 and its inhibitory activities define the distinct TIMP gene family. *J Biol Chem* 1995;270:14313–14318.
63. Willenbrock F, Murphy G. Structure-function relationships in the tissue inhibitors of metalloproteinases. *Am J Respir Crit Care Med* 1994;150: S165–S170.
64. Weber B, Vogt G, Pruett R, et al. Mutations in the tissue inhibitor of metallo-proteinases-3 (TIMP3) in patients with Sorsby's fundus dystrophy. *Nat Genet* 1994;8:352–356.
65. Wick M, Bürger C, Brüsselbach S, et al. A novel member of human tissue inhibitor of metalloproteinases (TIMP) gene family is regulated during G1 progression, mitogenic stimulation, differentiation and senescence. *J Biol Chem* 1994;29:18953–18960.
66. Anand-Apte B, Pepper M, Voest E, et al. Inhibition of angiogenesis by tissue inhibitor of metalloproteinase-3. *J Invest Ophthalmol Vis Sci* 1997;38: 817–823.
67. Yamashita K, Suzuki M, Iwata H, et al. Tyrosine phosporylation is crucial for growth signaling by tissue inhibitors of metalloproteinases (TIMP-1 and TIMP-2). *FEBS Lett* 1996;396:103–107.
68. Stetler-Stevenson W, Bersch N, Golde D. Tissue inhibitor of metalloprotei-nase-2 (TIMP-2) has erythroid-potentiating activity. *FEBS Lett* 1992;296: 231–234.
69. Birkedal-Hansen H, Moore WGI, Bodden MK, et al. Matrix metalloprotei-nases: A review. *Crit Rev Oral Biol Med* 1993;4:197–250.
70. Dollery C, McEwan J, Henney A. Matrix metalloproteinases and cardiovas-cular disease. *Circ Res* 1995;77:863–868.
71. Forough R, Koyama N, Hasenstab D, et al. Overexpression of tissue inhibi-tor of matrix metalloproteinase-1 inhibits vascular smooth muscle cell func-tions in vitro and in vivo. *Circ Res* 1996;79(4):812–820.
72. Hasenstab D, Forough R, Clowes A. Plasminogen activator inhibitor type 1 and tissue inhibitor of metalloproteinases-2 increase after arterial injury in rats. *Circ Res* 1997;80(4):490–496.
73. Henney AM, Wakely PR, Davies MJ, et al. Localization of stromelysin gene expression in atherosclerotic plaques by in-situ hybridization. *Proc Natl Acad Sci U S A* 1991;88:8154–8158.
74. Brown DL, Hibbs MS, Kearney M, et al. Identification of 92-kD gelatinase in human coronary atherosclerotic lesions: Association of active enzyme synthesis with unstable angina. *Circulation* 1995;91:2125–2131.
75. Nikkari S, Geary R, Hatsukami T, et al. Expression of collagen, interstitial collagenase, and tissue inhibitor of metalloproteinases-1 in restenosis after carotid endarterectomy. *Am J Pathol* 1996;148(3):777–783.
76. Halpert I, Sires U, Roby J, et al. Matrilysin is expressed by lipid-laden macrophages at sites of potential rupture in atherosclerotic lesions and localizes to areas of versican deposition, a proteoglycansubstrate for the enzyme. *Proc Natl Acad Sci U S A* 1996;18:9748–9753.
77. Zaltsman A, Newby A. Increased secretion of gelatinases A and B from the aortas of cholesterol fed rabbits: Relationship to lesion severity. *Athero-sclerosis* 1997;130:61–70.
78. Galis Z, Sukhova G, Libby P. Microscopic localization of active proteases

by in situ zymography. Detection of matrix metalloproteinase activity in vascular tissue. *FASEB J* 1995;9:974–980.

79. Sukhova G, Simon D, Chapman H, Libby P. Cytokines regulate the expression by vascular smooth muscle cells of cathepsin S, an elastase found in human atheroma. *J Invest Med* 1995;43:311A.

80. Blankenhorn DH, Hodis HN. Arterial imaging and atherosclerosis reversal. *Arterioscler Thromb* 1994;14:177–192.

81. Brown BG, Zhao XQ, Sacco DE, Albers JJ. Lipid lowering and plaque regression. New insights into prevention of plaque disruption and clinical events in coronary disease. [Review]. *Circulation* 1993;87:1781–1791.

82. Group SSSS. Randomised trial of cholesterol lowering in 4444 patients with coronary heart disease: The Scandanavian Simvastatin Survival Study (4S). *Lancet* 1994;344:1383–1389.

83. Sheperd J, Cobbe S, Ford I, et al. Prevention of coronary heart disease with pravastatin in men with hypercholesterolemia. *N Engl J Med* 1995; 333:1301–1307.

Chapter 23

New Concepts in Regulation of Vascular Calcification

Farhad Parhami, PhD and
Linda L. Demer MD, PhD

Significance of Vascular Calcification

With the advent of new and more sensitive vascular imaging techniques such as intravascular ultrasound (IVUS) and electron beam computed tomography (EBCT), it has become evident that vascular calcification occurs early during the development of atherosclerotic lesions.[1] In fact, calcification is considered a common feature of atherosclerotic lesions and a sensitive marker for their detection,[2] especially in the younger individuals in whom its specificity with respect to association with atherosclerotic lesions reaches 80% to 90%.[3] The deposition of calcium minerals has several consequences which impair the proper functioning of the vessel wall.[4] Such complications include impaired vascular tone and distensibility, impaired compensatory enlargement, coronary insufficiency due to lack of aortic recoil, dissection in angioplasty, increased chance of plaque rupture, and higher susceptibility to restenosis following balloon angioplasty (Fig. 1).

Acute coronary events that lead to myocardial infarction and sudden death are strongly associated with plaque rupture and subsequent thrombosis and embolism.[5,6] Although the role of calcium deposits in this process is not yet clear, several reports have indicated that their presence aggravates the ongoing pathology. Demer et al[7,8] have reported that calcified human vessels are less distensible in vivo and ex vivo than noncalcified vessels. Elegant works by Richardson et al,[9] based on computer modeling, as well as by Lee et al,[10] with use of computer-assisted analysis of tensile stress on excised plaques, have

From: Fuster, V (ed). *The Vulnerable Atherosclerotic Plaque: Understanding, Identification, and Modification.* Armonk, NY: Futura Publishing Company, Inc.; © 1999.

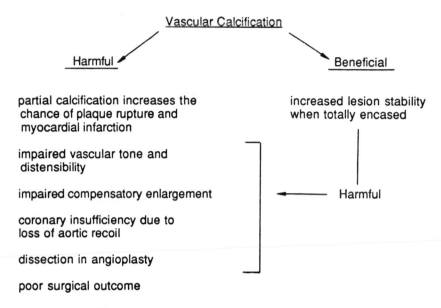

Figure 1. Significance of vascular calcification.

shown that sites prone to rupture are often associated with greatest tensile stress in the vessel wall, which occurs at the interphases between two tissues with differing elastic properties. Such interphases occur in regions of transition between plaque and normal wall or between areas of soft and calcified plaque. Fitzgerald et al[11] and Leon et al[12] have shown by IVUS postangioplasty that most dissections occur adjacent to the calcified portion of the vessel wall. In addition, Fitzgerald et al noted a significant correlation between the presence of intraplaque calcium and the size, as well as site, of dissection. Although plaque fracture and dissection are considered necessary for immediate success of balloon angioplasty and lumen enlargement, the control of the extent of dissection is still difficult, and larger than necessary dissections may cause plaque detachment and embolization, as well as extensive medial damage, which has been associated with accelerated restenosis.[13] Several histologic studies of autopsy specimens have indicated the presence of calcium deposits in ruptured plaques. Farb et al[14] have reported that 69% of the ruptured plaques studied were calcified. Although most of these studies were done on a relatively small number of specimens, collectively they show a positive correlation between plaque rupture and presence of calcification.

Despite the above attributions of harmful effects of calcification on vessel wall and plaque rupture, the possible contribution of calcification to plaque stabilization requires consideration (Fig. 1). Doherty and Detrano[15] have suggested that encasement of the plaque by a calcium shield may protect the plaque from mechanical forces, which normally weaken the fibrous cap and lead to its breakage. In fact, symptoms of stable, as opposed to unstable, angina are often correlated with older, more fibrocalcified, and thus more stable lesions.[16] Although the new concept of promoting plaque stabilization with the possible contribution of calcification is of utmost importance, it must also be recognized that the extent of calcification required for achieving plaque encasement and stability would inevitably result in impairment of vascular wall mechanical function, which is important for maintenance of adequate hemodynamics and circulation.

Whether future assessments of vascular calcification in the atherosclerotic process point toward a beneficial or harmful role, its control will not be possible without detailed understanding of the mechanisms involved in its formation and regulation.

Vascular Calcification: An Active Process

Vascular calcification has only recently become a target of active study. Calcification was once considered a passive inevitable process associated with end-stage atherosclerosis. However, with the identification of factors in the artery wall that are known to be associated with the regulation of bone metabolism (Table 1), we hypothesized that vascular calcification is an actively regulated process similar to osteogenesis. This is supported by the old observations of pathologists who noted that calcification in the artery wall is "ossification" that may advance to fully formed bone with trabeculae and marrow.[17] Indeed, artery wall is noted as the most frequent site of ectopic bone formation. The active

---

Table 1

Bone and Cartilage Associated Factors in Calcified Vessel Wall

Bone morphogenetic protein-2[20]
Collagens I and II[26,27]
Osteopontin[28]
Osteocalcin[29]
Osteonectin[30]
Matrix GLA protein[24]
Matrix vesicles[31]
Hydroxyapatite[32]

nature of vascular calcification renders it more accessible to control than a passive unregulated process. However such control requires in-depth understanding of the underlying cellular and molecular mechanisms.

A Developmental Process Revisited

The mechanism of ectopic bone formation, ie, bone forming in a tissue other than the skeleton, is known to resemble embryonic osteogenesis. This involves the interaction between two tissue layers, the epithelium and underlying mesenchymal tissue, a process called *inductive interaction*. Osteogenic factors such as bone morphogenetic proteins released from the epithelial cells signal osteoprogenitor cells of the underlying mesenchyme to migrate to the site of future bone formation. An aggregation or *condensation* of these cells forms the site of further differentiation of the precursor cells into mature osteoblasts and the subsequent formation of a matrix, osteoid, which is permissive for calcification. We hypothesize that ectopic mineralization in the atherosclerotic vessel wall follows that same pattern of events. The arterial simple squamous epithelium, the endothelium, is activated by local inflammatory mediators present in the atherosclerotic vessel wall, to produce osteogenic factors which then signal precursor mesenchymal cells in the arterial media to differentiate along an osteoblastic pathway leading to the formation of a matrix susceptible to calcification. We are currently testing the validity of this hypothesis, and the following observations are in its support.

Calcifying Vascular Cells

The first line of evidence for the presence of a preosteoblastic cell in the artery wall was the identification of calcifying vascular cells (CVC) in the artery wall that spontaneously undergo osteoblastic differentiation and form a calcified matrix in vitro. These calcifying vascular cells have osteoblast-associated markers including bone-liver-kidney isozyme of alkaline phosphatase, osteopontin, osteocalcin, osteonectin, and collagen I. (Table 2).[18] In vitro, CVC form cellular condensations that are immunoreactive with peanut agglutinin lectin (PNA), which is commonly used to identify condensing mesenchymal cells during bone formation.[19] These condensations are the site of abundant matrix formation which serves as a nidus for calcification. They are also immunoreactive with a pericyte-specific monoclonal antibody, 3G5. By immunohistochemistry, 3G5 identified the CVC as a subpopulation of

Table 2

Calcifying Vascular Cells (CVC)

Constitute a subpopulation of artery wall cells
Form calcified nodules in vitro
Express osteoblast markers including osteopontin, osteocalcin, osteonectin, alkaline phosphatase, and collagen I
Form matrix—vesicle-like structures
May be responsible for in vivo vascular calcification

cells sporadically located in the intima and media of artery wall.[18] The calcium mineral formed in the CVC cultures was characterized as hydroxyapatite, the same mineral found in bone as well as in the calcified vessel wall.[20] Therefore, CVC may serve as the preosteoblastic cell that responds to osteogenic factors in the atherosclerotic vessel wall.

Bone Morphogenetic Protein in the Artery Wall

In an important tie to developmental biology, we reported in 1993 that bone morphogenetic protein-2 (BMP-2) is expressed in human calcified vessel wall.[20] Members of the BMP family are potent osteogenic factors that drive embryonic bone formation, and BMP-2 is known to induce ectopic bone formation in animal models. We have also found that cultured human aortic endothelial cells express BMP-2 and BMP-4, as well as insulin-like growth factor-2, another known osteogenic factor. Presence of these osteogenic factors suggests that as in embryonic osteogenesis, inductive interactions between endothelial and mesenchymal layers of the artery wall coordinate vascular calcification.

Homeobox Genes in the Artery Wall

We recently found that a member of the homeobox family of genes is expressed in the calcified human arteries but not in normal arteries (Bostrom et al, unpublished observations, 1997). Homeobox genes are known to be involved in development of tissue identity during embryogenesis, and their expression is regulated by BMPs. The homeobox gene products are transcription factors, which ultimately regulate the expression of genes that are important during developmental processes. The expression of homeobox genes in the calcified vessel wall again supports recapitulation of embryonic inductive interactions that contribute to the pathogenesis of ectopic mineralization and bone formation in the artery wall.

Induction of In Vitro Vascular Cell Calcification by Factors Present in Atherosclerotic Plaque

The role of oxidized lipids in atherogenesis is well established.[21] Oxidized low-density lipoprotein (Ox-LDL) and its constituents have been shown to induce inflammatory reactions by activating the cellular constituents of the artery wall. As a result, a sequence of events including endothelial activation, leukocyte adhesion to the endothelium and transmigration into the subendothelial space, formation of chemotactic and differentiation factors for monocytes, and foam cell formation lead to the development of the fatty streaks in the artery wall. It is known that calcification also occurs at an early stage during atherogenesis, and that the calcium deposits are closely associated with lipids.[22] Thus, as oxidized lipids are one of the first inducers of the atherosclerotic lesion formation, we tested the effect of several oxidized lipids and lipoproteins on the induction of in vitro calcification in the CVC model. We found that 25-hydroxycholesterol, an abundant oxysterol in the atherosclerotic lesion, exacerbates calcification in CVC cultures.[18] More recently, we reported that minimally oxidized LDL (MM-LDL) and 8-isoprostaglandin E_2, an oxidation product of arachidonic acid present in oxidized LDL, caused significant induction of osteoblastic differentiation in CVC.[23] This induction was marked by cessation of proliferative activity as well as increased expression of several osteoblastic markers, including collagen I and alkaline phosphatase.[23] In addition to the oxidized lipids, transforming growth factor β (TGF-β)[18] and tumor necrosis factor α (TNF-α) (Patel et al, unpublished observations, 1997) are other components of the diseased vessel wall that are capable of inducing osteoblastic differentiation of CVC. Increased collagen I formation is a hallmark of increased matrix synthesis in the atherosclerotic plaque and plays an important role in differentiation and calcification of osteoblastic cells, including CVC. Therefore it is apparent that the atherosclerotic vessel wall possesses factors which make it a permissive milieu for calcification to take place (Table 1).

Future Directions

It is evident that the understanding of vascular calcification has recently come a long way, from being considered a passive, unregulated process to an actively regulated process which may be similar to osteogenesis. The identification of CVC and their use as an in vitro model of vascular calcification has allowed investigators to begin identifying mechanisms involved in that process. In parallel, the identification of bone-associated factors in the atherosclerotic vessel wall has given more support to the similarities between vascular calcification and osteogenesis. An exciting new development in elucidating the mechanism of vascular calcification has been the use of genetically engineered mice that lack expression of different factors. A recent report by Ducy et al[24] showed spontaneous arterial calcification developing in mice lacking matrix GLA protein. In that report, the authors noted that chondrocytes, which synthesize a typical cartilage matrix, can be seen in the calcified arteries of these Mgp-null mice. This observation suggests that the vascular calcification process is similar to endochondral bone formation, whereby a cartilaginous matrix mineralizes to form bone. This demonstration that inhibition of calcification in the artery wall requires the product of a specific gene further supports the notion that arterial calcification is a genetically regulated process.[25] With a better understanding of the mechanism of arterial calcification, we will be able to identify targets for its therapeutic regulation, provide animal models of vascular calcification, and more definitively address such questions as whether calcification plays a role in vascular pathophysiology, such as impaired vasomotion and plaque rupture.

References

1. Guyton JR, Klemp KF. Transitional features in human atherosclerosis. *Am J Pathol* 1993;143:1444–1457.
2. Breen JF, Sheedy PF, Schwartz RS, et al. Coronary artery calcification detected with ultrafast CT as an indication of coronary artery disease. *Radiology* 1992;185:435–439.
3. Stanford W, Thompson BH, Weiss RM. Coronary artery calcification: Clinical significance and current methods of detection. *AJR* 1993;161:1139–1146.
4. Demer LL. A skeleton in the atherosclerosis closet. *Circulation* 1995;92:2029–2032.
5. Shah PK. Pathophysiology of plaque rupture and the concept of plaque stabilization. *Cardiol Clin* 1996;14:17–29.
6. Boyle JJ. Association of coronary plaque rupture and atherosclerotic inflammation. *J Pathol* 1997;181:93–99.
7. Demer LL. Effect of calcification on in vivo mechanical response of rabbit arteries to balloon dilatation. *Circulation* 1991;83:2083–2093.
8. Park JC, Siegel RJ, Demer LL. Effect of calcification and formalin fixation on in vitro distensibility of human femoral arteries. *Am Heart J* 1993;125:344–349.
9. Richardson PD, Davies MJ, Born GVR. Influence of plaque configuration and stress distribution on fissuring of coronary atherosclerotic plaques. *Lancet* 1989;2:941–944.
10. Lee RT, Grodzinsky AJ, Frank EH, et al. Structure-dependent dynamic

mechanical behavior of fibrous caps from human atherosclerotic plaques. *Circulation* 1991;83:1764–1770.

11. Fitzgerald PJ, Ports TA, Yock PG. Contribution of localized calcium deposits to dissection after angioplasty. *Circulation* 1992;86:64–70.

12. Leon M, Karen G, Pichard A, et al. Intravascular ultrasound assessment of plaque responses to PTCA helps explain angiographic findings. *J Am Coll Cardiol* 1991;17:47A. Abstract.

13. Nobuyoshi M, Kimura T, Ohishi H, et al. Restenosis after percutaneous transluminal coronary angioplasty: Pathologic observation in 20 patients. *J Am Coll Cardiol* 1991;17:433–439.

14. Farb A, Burke AP, Tang AL, et al. Coronary plaque erosion without rupture into a lipid core: A frequent cause of coronary thrombosis in sudden coronary death. *Circulation* 1996;93:1354–1363.

15. Doherty TM, Detrano RC. Coronary arterial calcification as an active process: A new perspective on an old problem. *Calcif Tissue Int* 1994;54: 224–230.

16. Fuster V. Elucidation of the role of plaque instability and rupture in acute coronary events. *Am J Cardiol* 1995;76:24C–33C.

17. Virchow R. *Cellular Pathology: As Based Upon Physiological and Pathological Histology. 1863.* unabridged reprinting 1971. Dover, New York. 404–408.

18. Watson KE, Bostrom K, Ravindranathan R, et al. TGF-b and 25-hydroxycholesterol stimulate osteoblast-like vascular cells to calcify. *J Clin Invest* 1994; 93:2106–2113.

19. Dunlop LLT, Hall B. Relationships between cellular condensation, preosteoblast formation and epithelial-mesenchymal interactions in initiation of osteogenesis. *Int J Dev Biol* 1995;39:357–371.

20. Bostrom K, Watson KE, Horn S, et al. Bone morphogenetic protein expression in human atherosclerotic lesions. *J Clin Invest* 1993;91:1800–1809.

21. Witztum JL, Steinberg D. Role of oxidized low density lipoprotein in atherogenesis. *J Clin Invest* 1991;88:1785–1792.

22. Hirsch D, Azoury R, Sarig S, et al. Colocalization of cholesterol and hydroxyapatite in human atherosclerotic lesions. *Calcif Tissue Int* 1993;52: 94–98.

23. Parhami F, Morrow AD, Balucan JP, et al. Lipid oxidation products have opposite effects on calcifying vascular cell and bone cell differentiation: A possible explanation for the paradox of arterial calcification in osteoporotic patients. *Arterioscler Thromb Vasc Biol* 1997;17:680–687.

24. Luo G, Ducy P, McKee MD, et al. Spontaneous calcification of arteries and cartilage in mice lacking matrix GLA protein. *Nature* 1997;386:78–81.

25. Qiao J, Xie P, Fishbein MC, et al. Pathology of atheromatous lesions in inbred and genetically engineered mice: Genetic determination of arterial calcification. *Arterioscler Thromb* 1994;14:1480–1497.

26. Kastuda S, Okada Y, Minamoto T, et al. Collagens in human atherosclerotic plaques. *Arterioscler Thromb* 1992;12:494–502.

27. Qiao JH, Fishbein MC, Demer LL, et al. Genetic determination of cartilagenous metaplasia in mouse aorta. *Arterioscler Thromb Vasc Biol* 1995;15: 2265–2272.

28. Giachelli CM, Bae N, Almeida N, et al. Osteopontin is elevated during neointima formation in rat arteries and is a novel component of human atherosclerotic plaques. *J Clin Invest* 1993;92:1686–1696.

29. Ginsberg B, van Haarlem LJM, Soute BAM, et al. Characterization of a GLA-containing protein from calcified human atherosclerotic plaques. *Arteriosclerosis* 1990;10:991–995.

30. Hirota S, Imakita M, Kohri K, et al. Expression of osteopontin messenger RNA by macrophages in atherosclerotic plaques. A possible association with calcification. *Am J Pathol* 1993;143:1003–1008.
31. Tanimura A, McGregor DH, Anderson HC. Matrix vesicles in atherosclerotic calcification. *Proc Soc Exp Biol Med* 1983;172:173–177.
32. Schmid K, McSharry WO, Pameijer CH, et al. Chemical and physicochemical studies on the mineral deposits of the human atherosclerotic aorta. *Atherosclerosis* 1980;37:199–210.

Chapter 24

Plaque Stabilization:
Present and Future Trends

Valentin Fuster, MD, PhD

Our understanding of the pathophysiology of coronary atherosclerosis has dramatically changed in the last few years. The types of atherosclerotic lesions, the mechanisms of progression of coronary atherosclerosis with plaque instability and rupture, and the subsequent thrombotic phenomenon leading to acute coronary syndromes are now much better understood.[1-3] Therapeutic strategies leading to atherosclerotic lesion stabilization and even regression, as well as improvement in vascular function, are being pursued.

The Lesions of Atherosclerosis-Thrombosis

According to the criteria set by the American Heart Association Committee on Vascular Lesions, plaque progression can be subdivided into five phases, as shown in Figure 1.[3,4]

Phase 1 consists of a small lesion of the kind commonly present in people under the age of 30. Such lesions may progress over a period of years and are categorized into three types: type I lesions consist of macrophage-derived foam cells that contain lipid droplets, type II lesions consist of both macrophages and smooth muscle cells with extracellular lipid deposits, and type III lesions consist of smooth muscle cells surrounded by extracellular connective tissue, fibrils, and lipid deposits.

Phase 2 consists of a plaque that, although not necessarily stenotic, may be prone to disruption because of its high lipid content. The lesion is categorized morphologically as one of two variants. Type IV plaques

Parts of this chapter modified from recent reviews by V. Fuster et al in two publications: *Lancet* 1996;348(suppl):s7–s10 and *Thromb Haemost* 1997;78(1):247–255.

From: Fuster, V (ed). *The Vulnerable Atherosclerotic Plaque: Understanding, Identification, and Modification.* Armonk, NY: Futura Publishing Company, Inc.; © 1999.

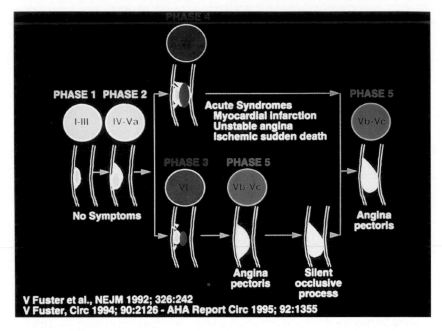

Figure 1. Schematic of staging (phases and lesion morphology of the progression of coronary atherosclerosis according to gross pathological and clinical findings). See text for more details. Modified from Reference 3, with permission.

consist of confluent cellular lesions with a great deal of extracellular lipid, intermixed with fibrous tissue, whereas type Va plaques possess an extracellular lipid core covered by a thin fibrous cap. Phase 2 can evolve into acute phases 3 and 4, and either of these can evolve into fibrotic phase 5.

Phase 3 consists of the acute "complicated" type VI lesions; disruption of a type IV or Va lesion leads to the formation of a mural thrombus, which does not completely occlude the artery. Changes in geometry of the disrupted plaque, and organization of the mural thrombus by connective tissue, can lead to the more occlusive and fibrotic type Vb or Vc lesions of phase 5. Such type Vb or Vc lesions may cause angina. A final occlusion may be silent or clinically inapparent, however, because the preceding stenosis and ischemia can give rise to a protective collateral circulation.

The acute "complicated" type VI lesion of phase 4, rather than being characterized by a small mural thrombus (as in phase 3), consists of an occlusive thrombus and may result in an acute coronary syndrome.

Both phase 3 and phase 4 can develop into the occlusive and fibrotic type Vb or Vc lesions of Phase 5.

Vulnerable Lipid-Rich Plaques

Entry and Exit of Lipoproteins in Plaque Formation: A Dynamic Process[5]

The type III lesion or fatty streak (Fig. 1) is the earliest grossly detectable lesion of atherosclerosis. By age 25 years, almost everyone has fatty streaks,[4] which consist of an accumulation of lipid (mainly oxidized low-density lipoproteins (LDL) within macrophages or foam cells and mostly in the extracellular space of the intima. Increased density of smooth muscle cells and extracellular fibrils is also observed. Based on observations made in humans and in experimental animals, the development of type III lesions is described below.

Chronic minimal injury to the arterial endothelium is physiological and is often the result of a disturbance in the pattern of blood flow in certain parts of the arterial tree, such as bending points and areas near bifurcations (Fig. 2).[1,2,5] In addition to local shear forces, which are

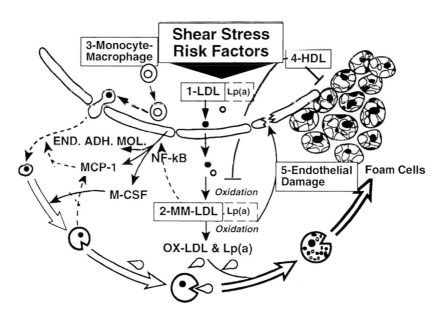

Figure 2. Schematic of pathogenesis of phase I of progression: chronic endothelial injury and risk factors—influx, accumulation, and fate of lipids and monocyte-macrophages. ENDOT = endothelial; END.ADH.MOL = endothelial adhesion molecule; HDL = high-density lipoprotein; LDL = low-density lipoprotein; Lp(a) = lipoprotein (a); MCP-1 = monocyte chemotactic protein-1; M-CSF = monocyte-colony stimulating factor; MM = minimally modified; NF-κB = necrosis factor-κB; OX = oxidized. Modified from Reference 6 and from Steinberg D, *Circulation* 1991;84:1420, with permission.

probably enhanced in hypertension, several other factors may poten-tiate chronic minimal endothelial injury or dysfunction, leading to accu-mulation of lipids and monocytes (macrophages) at these sites.[1] These factors include hypercholesterolemia, advanced glycation end products in diabetes (particularly insulin-dependent diabetes mellitus (IDDM), chemical irritants in tobacco smoke, circulating vasoactive amines, im-mune complexes, and infection.

During atherogenesis, the entry, accumulation, and fate of lipids and monocyte-macrophages can be divided into five stages[5,6,7] (Fig. 2): (1) Most lipids deposited in the atherosclerotic lesions are derived from plasma LDL that enter the vessel wall through the injured or dysfunc-tional endothelium. (2) All major cell types within the vessel wall and atherosclerotic lesions can oxidize LDL, but the endothelial cell is prob-ably critical in these very early stages of atherogenesis, as it mildly oxidizes LDL. (3) Mildly oxidized LDL (or minimally modified LDL) and the regional low shear and turbulent flow may play an initial role in monocyte recruitment by inducing the expression of adhesive cell-surface glycoproteins intracellular adhesion molecule (ICAM-1) and vascular cell adhesion molecule-1 (VCAM-1) on the endothelium.[6] After monocytes adhere to the surface of the vessel wall, other specific molecules, such as a specific chemotactic protein (monocyte chemotac-tic protein-1 or MPC-1) and colony-stimulating factor (M-CSF), may attract and modify monocytes within the subendothelial space.[6] After entering the vessel wall, monocytes differentiate into macrophages. They may be responsible for converting mildly oxidized LDL into highly oxidized LDL, which binds to the scavenger receptors of macro-phages and enters the cells, converting them into foam cells. (4) High-density lipoproteins (HDL) may protect against excess lipid accumula-tion in the vessel wall by inhibiting the oxidation of LDL or its subse-quent effects.[6] The HDL may also contribute to "reverse cholesterol transport" or active LDL removal from the vessel wall and from the macrophage foam cells.[8] (5) Macrophages or foam cells, after saturation with lipid and before or after their deaths, can liberate a large number of products, including cholesterol (esterified and oxidized), that can further damage the endothelium and so participate in the evolution of the atherosclerotic lesion. Such alteration of the endothelium in early atherosclerosis may lead to local vasoconstriction, as well as to platelet-vessel wall interaction with release of platelet-derived growth factor (PDGF), subsequent smooth muscle cell activation, and synthesis of extracellular matrix.[7] The endothelium can profoundly affect vascular tone by releasing relaxing factors such as prostacyclin[9] and endothelial-derived relaxing factor (EDRF), now known to be nitric oxide (NO),[10] and contracting factors such as endothelin-1.[11] Under physiological conditions, EDRF appears to predominate. However, as indicated above, there is now significant evidence that an alteration in the endo-thelium occurs in early atherogenesis, particularly under the effect of atherogenic risk factors, as shown in humans.[12] This alteration may cause endothelial cells to generate more mediators that enhance con-striction and fewer mediators that enhance dilation.[1,3] Recent work in humans has also revealed that the cardiovascular risk factors known to affect the epicardial coronary arteries also affect coronary microcircu-latory function, with a tendency for vasoconstriction that may contrib-ute to anginal pain.[13]

The fatty streak, or type III lesion, represents a balance between limited intimal deposition of fat and smooth muscle cells with extracel-lular fibrils.[4,5] Specifically, such a lesion represents the above-men-tioned dynamic processes of entry and exit of lipoproteins, as well as extracellular matrix development. It is reasonable to assume that a decrease in lipoprotein entry (such as by modifying risk factors and thus endothelial injury) will result in a predominance of lipoprotein exit and final scarring. However, if risk factor profile remains significant, an increase of lipoprotein entry will predominate over the efflux and scarring, resulting in the vulnerable type IV and Va lesions, which are prone to disruption (Fig. 1).[3–5]

Disruption of the Vulnerable Plaque[5]

Over the last few years, pathological studies have revealed that such type IV and Va lesions are commonly composed of an abundant crescentic mass of lipids, intermixed or separated from the vessel lumen by a discrete component of extracellular matrix (Figs. 3 and 4).[3,14,15] Interestingly, it has become apparent that arteriographically mild coro-nary lesions may be associated with significant progression to severe stenosis or total occlusion.[15–17] These lesions may be accountable in up to two thirds of the patients in whom unstable angina or other acute coronary syndromes develop (Fig. 5).[14,15] This unpredictable and epi-sodic progression is most likely caused by disruption of type IV and type V lesions with subsequent thrombus formation, which changes the plaque geometry and leads to intermittent plaque growth and acute occlusive coronary syndromes.[15,18]

Plaques that undergo disruption tend to be relatively soft and have a high concentration of cholesteryl esters, rather than of free cholesterol monohydrate crystals. In addition to this rather "passive" phenomenon of plaque disruption, a better understanding of an "active" phenome-non related to macrophage activity is evolving.

"Passive" plaque disruption related to physical forces occurs most frequently where the fibrous cap is thinnest, most heavily infiltrated

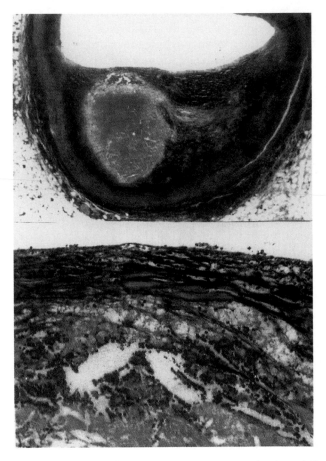

Figure 3. Photomicrographs illustrating composition and vulnerability of coronary plaques. A vulnerable plaque containing a core of soft atheromatous gruel (devoid of blue-stained collagen) that is separated from the vascular lumen by a thin cap of fibrous tissue. The fibrous cap is infiltrated by foam cells that can be clearly seen at high magnification, indicating ongoing disease activity. Such a thin and macrophage-infiltrated cap is probably weak and vulnerable, and it was indeed disrupted nearby, explaining why erythrocytes (red) can be seen in the gruel just beneath the macrophage-infiltrated cap. From Reference 15, with permission.

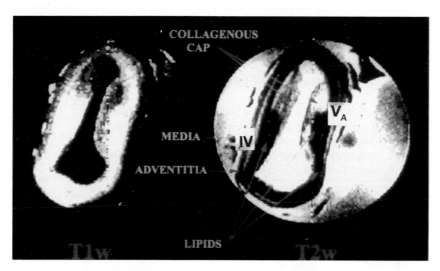

Figure 4. Nuclear magnetic resonance images of vulnerable or unstable lesions. I2w image identifies a collagenous cap on both plaques. In the type V lesions (right), the cap completely covers the lipid core. In the type IV lesions (left), the plaque is only partially covered, and infiltration of fat is more diffuse. Modified from Reference 3, with permission.

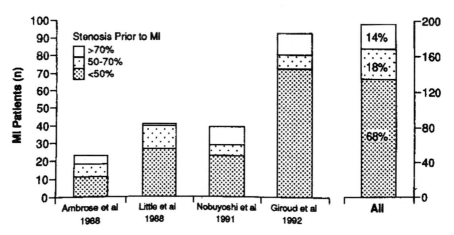

Figure 5. Bar graph showing stenosis severity and associated risk of myocardial infarction (MI). MI evolves most frequently from plaques that are only mildly to moderately obstructive months to years before infarction. The bar graph is constructed from data in References 16, 17, and from Nobuyoshi et al in *J Am Coll Cardiol* 1991;18:904–910 and Giroud et al in *Am J Cardiol* 1988;12:56–62.

- Mild to Medium Size - Not Severely Stenotic
- Significant Lipid Core and Fibrous Cap
- Inflamation (Macrophages)
- Wall Stress:
  1. Circumferential Wall Stress $(\sigma) = \dfrac{\text{Pressure (P) x Radium (r)}}{\text{Cap Thickness (h)}}$

  2. Localized Wall Stress - Structural Configuration
  3. Blood Flow Rheology - External Configuration
     Degree of Stenosis (Shear Stress)
     Angulation (Flow Separation or Oscillatory Flow)
  4. Lipid Density (Crystals) - Regression

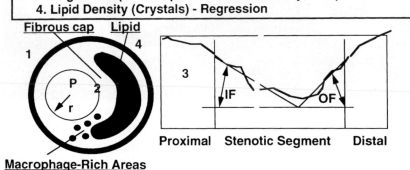

Fibrous cap   Lipid

Proximal   Stenotic Segment   Distal

Macrophage-Rich Areas

Figure 6. Pathogenesis of vulnerable or unstable lipid-rich lesion types IV and Va. Composite modified from References 14 and 19 and from Loree et al, *Circ Res* 1992;71:850 and Taeymans et al, *Circulation* 1992;85:78. IF = inflow angle; OF = outflow angle.

by foam cells and, therefore, weakest. For eccentric plaques, this is often the shoulder or between the plaque and the adjacent vessel wall.[14] Pathoanatomic examination of intact and disrupted plaques and in vitro mechanical testing of isolated fibrous caps from aorta indicate that vulnerability to rupture depends on four factors[3,15] (Fig. 6): (1) circumferential wall stress or cap "fatigue," which in part relates to a combination of the thickness and collagen content of the fibrous cap covering the core, blood pressure, and the radius of the lumen;[19] thus, long-term repetitive cyclic stresses may weaken a material and increase its vulnerability to fracture, ultimately leading to sudden and unprovoked (ie, untriggered) mechanical failure; (2) location, size, and consistency of the atheromatous core; and (3) blood flow characteristics, particularly impact of flow on the proximal aspect of the plaque (ie, configuration and angulation of the plaque, etc); and (4) lipid density (fluid vs crystals).

As mentioned, an active phenomenon of plaque disruption is probably important. Thus, atherectomy specimens from patients with acute coronary syndromes revealed macrophage-rich areas.[20] Macrophages can degrade extracellular matrix by phagocytosis or by secreting proteolytic enzymes such as plasminogen activators and a family of matrix metalloproteinases (MMPs): collagenases, gelatinases, and stromelysins) that may weaken the fibrous cap, predisposing it to rupture. Indeed, the MMPs and their cosecreted tissue inhibitors of metalloproteinases (TIMP-1 and TIMP-2) are critical for vascular remodeling. Moreover, we have observed that human monocyte-derived macrophages grown in culture are capable of degrading cap collagen, while expressing MMP-1 (interstitial collagenase) and inducing MMP-2 (gelatinolytic) activity in the culture medium that can be prevented by MMP inhibitors (Fig. 7).[15,21] Several studies[22,23] have now identified MMPs in human coronary plaques and lipid-filled macrophages (foam cells) that may be particularly active in destabilizing plaques, thus predisposing them to rupture.

Acute Thrombosis

As recently reviewed,[24] disruption of a vulnerable or unstable plaque with a subsequent change in plaque geometry and thrombosis

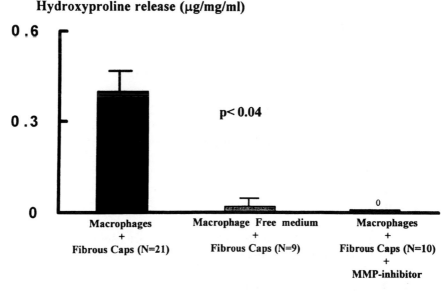

Figure 7. Data supporting the role of monocyte-derived macrophages and matrix-degradng metalloproteinases (MMPs) in inducing collagen breakdown in fibrous caps of human atherosclerotic plaques. Bar graph showing that incu bation of fibrous caps with macrophages results in hydroxyproline release into the supernatant (indicative of collagen breakdown), a process inhibited by an MMP inhibitor. From Reference 15, with permission.

results in a type VI or complicated lesion (Fig. 1). Such a rapid change in atherosclerotic plaque may result in acute occlusion or subocclusion with clinical manifestations of unstable angina or other acute coronary syndromes.[3,4] More frequently, however, such rapid changes appear to result in mural thrombus without evident clinical symptoms which, by self-organization, may be a main contributor to the progression of atherosclerosis.[3,4] More specifically, at the time of coronary plaque disruption, a number of local and thrombogenic factors may influence the degree and the duration of thrombus deposition[1,3,25] (Table 1); such a thrombus may then either be partially lysed or become replaced in the process of organization by the vascular repair response.[4,26]

Substrate-Dependent Thrombosis[24]

In regard to the composition of human atherosclerotic plaques, there is a significant heterogeneity, even in the same individual, and plaque disruption exposes various vessel wall components to blood. Data on the thrombogenicity of disrupted atherosclerotic lesions are

---

Table 1

Thrombotic Complications of Plaque Disruption: Local and Systemic Thrombogenic Risk Factors

---

Local Factors
  Degree of plaque disruption (ie, fissure, ulcer)
  Degree of stenosis (ie, change in geometry)
  Tissue substrate (ie, lipid-rich plaque)
  Surface of residual thrombus (ie, recurrence)
  Vasoconstriction (ie, platelets, thrombin)
Systemic Factors
  Catecholamines (ie, smoking, stress, cocaine)
  Renin-angiotensin (ie, DD genotype)
  Cholesterol, lipoprotein(a) and other metabolic states (ie, homocystinemia, diabetes)
  Fibrinogen, impaired fibrinolysis (ie, plasminogen activator inhibitor-1), activated platelets, and clotting (ie, Factor VII, thrombin generation [fragment 1 + 2] or activity [fibrinopeptide A])

High risk: presumably by the presence of several local or systemic thrombogenic risk factors at the time of plaque disruption, indicates acute occlusive labile thrombus versus fixed mural thrombus (unstable angina and non-Q wave and Q wave myocardial infarction). Low risk: presumably by the paucity of thrombogenic risk factors at the time of plaque disruption, indicates only mural thrombus (progressive atherogenesis). From Reference 3, With permission.

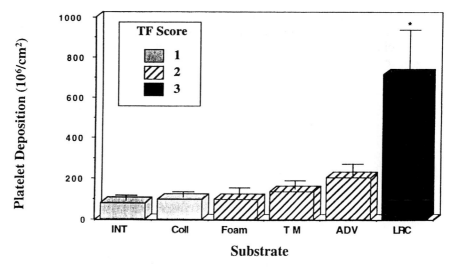

Figure 8. Platelet deposition and tissue factor activity. Platelet deposition data are expressed as Mean ± SEM; TF staining intensity is expressed as the average of the independent observers. Note the positive correlation between platelet-thrombus formation and TF score on the exposed human substrates ($P<0.01$). INT = normal intima; COLL = collagen-rich matrix; FOAM = foam cell-rich matrix; TM = normal tunica media; ADV − adventitia; LRC = lipid-rich core (*$P=0.0002$), ANOVA). From Reference 27, with permission.

limited. The thrombogenicity of human atherosclerotic plaques was evaluated by exposure to flowing blood at high shear rate. The evaluated aortic plaques included normal intima (disease- free), fatty streaks, sclerotic plaques, fibrolipid plaques, and atheromatous lipid-rich core. The lipid core abundant in cholesterol ester displayed the highest thrombogenicity (Fig. 8).[26,27]

Tissue Factor-Dependent Thrombosis[24]

Tissue factor (TF), a small-molecular–weight glycoprotein, initiates the extrinsic clotting cascade and is considered a major regulator of coagulation, hemostasis, and thrombosis. TF forms a high-affinity complex with coagulation factors VII/VIIa; TF-VIIa complex activates factors IX and X, thereby leading to thrombin generation.[28] TF antigen is normally present only in the arterial adventitia. However, each of the major cell types in plaques (smooth muscle cells, macrophages, and endothelial cells) is capable of TF expression. TF antigen is found in the cells of atherosclerotic plaques and, extracellularly, in the lipid-rich core and fibrous matrix as well.[29] We examined the role of TF in the

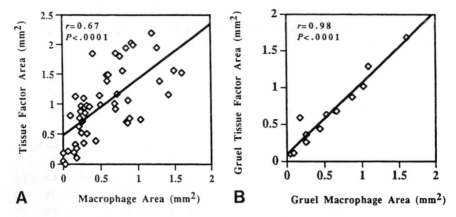

Figure 9. **A.** scatterplot showing association of macrophage area (mm²) identified with KP1 immunostaining, and tissue factor area (mm²) identified with a polyclonal antibody in coronary atherectomy specimens from 50 patients with acute coronary syndromes. **B.** scatterplot showing association of lipid-rich macrophage area (mm²) identified with trichrome staining, and lipid-rich tissue factor area (mm²) identified with a polyclonal antibody in coronary atherectomy specimens from 50 patients with acute coronary syndromes. From Reference 30, with permission.

thrombogenicity of various types of atherosclerotic plaques and their components. As in previous studies,[26] in vitro examination revealed that platelet deposition was significantly greater on lipid-rich atheromatous core than on all other substrates (Fig. 8).[27] The lipid-rich core also exhibits the most intense TF staining when compared to other arterial components. This observation suggests that TF is an important determinant of the thrombogenicity of human atherosclerotic lesions after spontaneous or mechanical plaque disruption. Colocalization of directional coronary atherectomy specimens from patients with unstable angina demonstrated a strong relationship between TF and macrophages (Fig. 9).[30] Finally, a positive relationship was also observed between TF antigen content and activity in human coronary artery plaque tissue.[31] As a result of these recent observations, it appears that TF content and activity in the atheromatous gruel is mediated by macrophages, thus suggesting a cell-mediated thrombogenicity in patients with acute coronary syndromes following plaque disruption.

Lipid-Modifying Approaches to Prevention[5]

Clinical Observations

An approach to retarding or even reversing atherosclerotic lesion development in humans in order to prevent acute coronary events is the better control of risk factors, such as by the reduction of plasma cholesterol levels. Thus, it might be possible to modify the lipid-rich atherosclerotic plaques that are more prone to rupture, thereby preventing progression and even inducing regression by removal of lipid. In published trials that compared a more aggressive with a more conservative treatment of lipid abnormalities in patients with coronary disease identified at arteriography, three important observations were made.[32] (1) More aggressive approaches significantly decreased disease progression, but, overall, only minimal regression of atherosclerosis has been shown (1% to 2% decrease in degree of stenosis). (2) There was a substantial reduction (over 50%) in the incidence of acute cardiac events in most trials despite marginal impact on arteriographic regression. The Scandinavian 4S study of a well-identified large group of patients with coronary disease and significant dyslipoproteinemia; the CARE study, in which the patients with coronary disease had only mild dyslipoproteinemia; and the West of Scotland Coronary Prevention Study in a large group of men with hypercholesterolemia but without obvious evidence of coronary disease, all showed a decrease in mortality and coronary events with the use of statins.[33–36] These landmark studies, with the use of an aggressive pharmacological approach, support and go beyond the data of the regression and stabilization studies. (3) It appears that the impact on coronary disease progression and coronary events, aside from lipid lowering, was also observed by modification of other risk factors.

Beneficial Effects on the Vulnerable Lipid-Rich Plaques[5]

According to these three clinical observations, the following interpretation of the data is evolving with regard to the atherosclerotic lesions[32,37]: (1) The lack of significant regression observed in the atherosclerotic lesions seen on arteriography is probably because such lesions tend to be already advanced, fibrotic, and less lipid-rich; therefore, they are less prone to reabsorption or to favorable remodeling. (2) The substantial reduction in coronary events is probably related to favorable dynamics of influx and efflux of lipoproteins in the smaller lipid-rich plaques—those not necessarily visualized at arteriography, but prone to disruption and to acute events. Specifically, when high LDL cholesterol is substantially reduced therapeutically, efflux from the plaques of the liquid or esterified cholesterol, and also deposition in the vessel wall as cholesterol crystals, predominate over the influx of LDL choles-

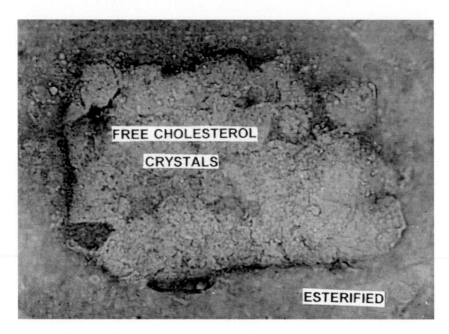

Figure 10. When high cholesterol is substantially reduced therapeutically, two processes take place: (1) efflux from the plaques of the lipid or sterified cholesterol and (2) its hydrolysis into cholesterol crystals, which precipitate and deposit in the vessel wall. From Fuster et al, *Thromb Haemost* 1997;78(1): 247–255, with permission.

terol (Fig. 10).[38–41] Consequently, there is a decrease in the softness of the plaque and so, presumably, in the passive phenomenon of plaque disruption previously described. Whether there is also a partial decrease in the number and activity of the macrophages and in the active phenomenon of plaque disruption is under investigation. Other effects of lipid-modifying strategies on endothelial function and in thrombogenicity (whether related to the plasma levels of LDL cholesterol or to the specific agents used) are also under investigation. (3) Finally, the beneficial effects exerted by modification of risk factors other than LDL or HDL cholesterol are probably because of their influence on the entry of LDL cholesterol into the vessel wall, as well as their influence on the thrombogenic complication of plaque disruption.

Antithrombotic Approaches to Prevention

As previously mentioned, approaches toward retardation or even reversal of atherosclerotic lesions in humans for the prevention of plaque disruption and acute coronary events include the better control of risk factors, such as reducing plasma cholesterol levels. Nevertheless, if atherosclerotic plaque disruption cannot be prevented, a beneficial effect of antiplatelet and anticoagulant agents has been observed in the prevention of acute coronary events. The best-suited, least toxic, and most widely used antithrombotic agent in acute and chronic coronary artery disease is aspirin. It has been shown to be effective in unstable angina and acute myocardial infarction during and after coronary revascularization, in the secondary prevention of chronic coronary and cerebrovascular disease, and in primary prevention, particularly in high-risk groups.[5,24] Aspirin interferes with only one of the three pathways of platelet activation—the one dependent on thromboxane A_2. The other two pathways—one dependent on ADP and collagen and the other on thrombin—remain unaffected, as does the coagulation system. On the other hand, current anticoagulant agents interfere only partially with the coagulation system and do not affect platelet activation. It is not surprising, therefore, that aspirin or anticoagulants cannot completely prevent coronary thrombotic events, although the relative antithrombotic effectiveness of both types of antithrombotic agents is clinically similar.

Combination therapy with a platelet inhibitor (aspirin or ticlopidine) and an anticoagulant agent (intravenous heparin, subcutaneous low-molecular–weight heparin, or oral warfarin) may have an additive effect. Thus far, such therapy (aspirin and heparin/warfarin) is being considered only for the short term (<1 week to 3 months) in patients at high risk for thrombotic events, such as those with acute myocardial infarction or unstable angina. The long-term (3 years) postmyocardial study, CHAMP, is randomizing patients to receive either 160 mg/day of aspirin or 80 mg of aspirin plus Coumadin to achieve an international normalized ratio (INR) of 1.5 to 2.5. Results of this study may settle some of the unanswered questions regarding the use of anticoagulants and antiplatelet agents for long-term secondary prevention of acute myocardial infarction. As we have reported, the combination of fixed very low dose anticoagulants and antiplatelet agents in the long-term secondary prevention of acute myocardial infarction has been discouraging in the CARS study, involving 9000 patients.[42] Similar discouraging results with very low dose anticoagulants have been reported by the SPAF III investigators on atrial fibrillation[43] and by the study group on coronary artery bypass grafts for the prevention of graft disease and occlusion.[44]

Table 2 outlines some of the newer antithrombotic approaches that are being investigated for the treatment of acute coronary syndromes or at the time of percutaneous transluminal coronary angioplasty (PTCA).[24] These antithrombotics are used intravenously and act by

Table 2

Antithrombins and IIb/IIIa Blockers-Clinical Trials, 1998

Agents	Unst angina	Myoc infarction	PTCA-occlusion
Hirudin	GUSTO IIB[1] *OASIS I*[4] OASIS II	HIT-III[2] GUSTO-IIB, TIMI-9B[5] *OASIS I*[4]-OASIS II	HELVETICA[3]
Hirulog	TIMI-8	*HERO (SK)*[6]	
IIb/IIIa Block.	*CANADIAN (Pilot)*[7] *PRISM*[9] *(EARLY)* PRISM PLUS[9] *(INTERV.)* PURSUIT[16] PARAGON	PARADIGM II	IMPACT-II PTCA[8] RAPPORT[11] RESTORE[10] CAPTURE[14] EPIC[12]-EPISTENT[15] EPILOG (Resten)[13] ERASER (Stent)

Questionable; *Definitive—Benefit*, Ongoing.

either blocking the early stage of thrombin-related platelet activation, such as the specific antithrombins hirudin and hirulog, or by blocking the late stage of receptor glycoprotein IIb/IIIa-related platelet activation. Other intravenous agents such as TF inhibitors[45] as well as subcutaneous and oral antithrombins and receptor glycoproteins IIB/IIIa blockers are new exploratory antithrombotic strategies for the prevention of coronary thrombosis.

References

1. Fuster V, Badimon L, Badimon JJ, Chesebro JH. The pathogenesis of coronary artery disease and the acute coronary syndromes. *N Engl J Med* 1992; 326(5):310–318.
2. Ross R. The pathogenesis of atherosclerosis: A perspective for the 1990s. *Nature* 1993;362:801–809.
3. Fuster V, Lewis A. Conner Memorial Lecture. Mechanisms leading to myocardial infarction: Insights from studies of vascular biology. *Circulation* 1994;90(4):2126–2146.
4. Stary HC, Chandler AB, Dinsmore RE, et al. A definition of advanced types of atherosclerotic lesions and a histological classification of atherosclerosis: A report from the Committee on Vascular Lesions of the Council on Arteriosclerosis, American Heart Association. *Circulation* 1995;92:1355–1374.
5. Fuster V. Human lesion studies. *Ann N Y Acad Sci* 1997;811:207–225.
6. Steinberg D. Oxidative modification of LDL and atherogenesis. Lewis A. Conner Memorial Lecture. *Circulation* 1997;95:1062–1071.
7. Ross R, Fuster V. The pathogenesis of atherosclerosis. In: Fuster V, Ross R, Topol E eds: *Arteriosclerosis and Coronary Artery Disease*. Philadelphia, PA: Lippincott-Raven; 1996:Vol.1:441–460.

8. Badimon L, Badimin JJ, Fuster V. Regression of atherosclerotic lesions by high density lipoprotein plasma fractions in the cholesterol-fed rabbit. *J Clin Invest* 1990;85:1234–1241.

9. Moncada S, Gryglewski R, Bunting S, Vane JR. An enzyme isolated from arteries transforms prostaglandin endoperoxides to an unstable substance that inhibits platelet aggregation. *Nature* 1976;263(5579):663–665.

10. Furchgott RF, Zawadzki JV. The obligatory role of endothelial cells in the relaxation of arterial smooth muscle by acetylcholine. *Nature* 1980; 288(5789):373–376.

11. Yanagisawa M, Kurihara H, Chimaera S, et al. A novel potent vasoconstrictor peptide produced by vascular endothelial cells. *Nature* 1988;332(6163): 411–415.

12. Selwyn AP, Kinlay S, Libby P, Ganz P. Atherogenic lipids, vascular dysfunction, and clinical signs of ischemic heart disease. *Circulation* 1997;95: 5–7.

13. Reddy KG, Nair RN, Sheehan HM, Hodgson JM. Evidence that selective endothelial dysfunction may occur in the absence of angiographic or ultrasound atherosclerosis in patients with risk factors for atherosclerosis. *J Am Coll Cardiol* 1994;25(4):833–843.

14. Richardson PD, Davies MJ, Born GV. Influence of plaque configuration and stress distribution on fissuring of coronary atherosclerotic plaques. *Lancet* 1989;2(8669):1462–1463.

15. Falk E, Shah PK, Fuster V. Coronary plaque disruption. *Circulation* 1995; 92:657–671.

16. Ambrose JA, Tannenbaum M, Alexpoulos D, et al. Angiographic progression of coronary artery disease and the development of myocardial infarction. *J Am Coll Cardiol* 1988;12:56–62.

17. Little WC, Constantinescu M, Applegate RJ, et al. Can coronary angiography predict the site of a subsequent myocardial infarction in patients with mild-to-moderate coronary artery disease? *Circulation* 188;78(5 Pt.1): 1157–1166.

18. Davies MJ. Stability and instability: Two faces of coronary atherosclerosis. The Paul Dudley White Lecture 1995. *Circulation* 1996;94(8):2013–2020.

19. MacIssac AL, Thomas JD, Topol EJ. Toward the quiescent coronary plaque. *J Am Coll Cardiol* 1993;22:1228–1241.

20. Moreno PR, Falk E, Palacios IF, et al. Macrophage infiltration in acute coronary syndromes. Implications for plaque rupture. *Circulation* 1994;90(2): 775–778.

21. Shah PK, Falk E, Badimon JJ, et al. Human monocyte-derived macrophages induce collagen breakdown in fibrous caps of atherosclerotic plaques. Potential role of matrix-degrading metalloproteinases and implications for plaque rupture. *Circulation* 1995;92:1565–1569.

22. Galis ZS, Sukhova GK, Lark MW, Libby P. Increased expression of matrix metalloproteinase and matrix degrading activity in vulnerable regions of human atherosclerotic plaques. *J Clin Invest* 1994;94(6):2493–2503.

23. Galis ZS, Sukhova GK, Kranzhofer R, et al. Macrophage foam cells from experimental atheroma constitutively produce matrix-degrading proteinases. *Proc Natl Acad Sci U S A* 1995;92(2):402–406.

24. Fuster V, Fallon JT, Nemerson Y. Coronary thrombosis. *Lancet* 1996; 348(suppl):s7–s10.

25. Burke AP, Farb A, Malcolm GT, et al. Coronary risk factors and plaque morphology in men with coronary disease who died suddenly. *N Engl J Med* 1997;336(18):1276–1281.

26. Fernandez-Ortiz A, Badimon JJ, Falk E, et al. Characterization of the relative thrombogenicity of atherosclerotic plaque components: Implications for consequences of plaque rupture. *J Am Coll Cardiol* 1994;23:1562–1569.
27. Toschi V, Gallo R, Lettino M, et al. Tissue factor predicts the thrombogenicity of human atherosclerotic plaque components. *Circulation* 1997;95: 594–599.
28. Banner DW, D'Arcy A, Chene C, et al. The crystal structure of the complex of blood coagulation factor VIIa with soluble tissue factor. *Nature* 1996; 380(6569):41–46.
29. Thiruvikraman SV, Guha A, Roboz J, et al. In situ localization of tissue factor in human atherosclerotic plaques by binding of digoxigenin labeled factors VIIa and X. *Lab Invest* 1996;75:451–461.
30. Moreno PR, Bernardi VH, Lopez-Cuellar J, et al. Macrophages, smooth muscle cells and tissue factor in unstable angina: Implications for cell mediated thrombogenicity in acute coronary syndromes. *Circulation* 1996;94: 3090–3097.
31. Marmur JDE, Thiruvikraman SV, Fyfe BS, et al. The identification of active tissue factor in human coronary atheroma. *Circulation* 1996;94:1226–1232.
32. Fuster V, Badimon JJ. Regression or stabilization of atherosclerosis means regression or stabilization of what we don't see in the arteriogram. *Eur Heart J* 1995;16:6–12.
33. Blankenhorn DH, Hodis HN. George Lyman Duff Memorial Lecture. Arterial imaging and atherosclerotic reversal. *Arterioscler Thromb* 1994;14(2): 177–192.
34. Scandinavian Simvastatin Survival Study Group. Randomised trial of cholesterol lowering in 4,444 patients with coronary heart disease: The Scandinavian Simvastatin Survival Study (4S). *Lancet* 1994;344(8934):1383–1389.
35. The Cholesterol And Recurrent Events (CARE) Trial Investigators. The effect of pravastatin on coronary events after myocardial infarction in patients with average cholesterol levels. *N Engl J Med* 1996;335:1001–1009.
36. Shepard J, Cobbe SM, Ford I, et al. Prevention of coronary heart disease with pravastatin in men with hypercholesterolemia. *N Engl J Med* 1995; 333:1301–1307.
37. Brown BG, Zhao XO, Sacco DE, Albers JJ. Lipid lowering and plaque regression. New insights into prevention of plaque disruption and clinical events in coronary disease. *Circulation* 1993;87(6):1781–1791.
38. Small DM. Progression and regression of atherosclerotic lesions. Insights from Lipid-Physical Biochemistry. *Arteriosclerosis* 1988;8:103–129.
39. Loree HM, Tobias BJ, Gibson LJ, et al. Mechanical properties of model atherosclerotic lesion lipid pool. *Atheroscler Thromb* 1994;14:230–234.
40. Guyton JR, Klemp KF. Development of the atherosclerotic core region. Chemical and ultrastructure analysis of microdissected atherosclerotic lesions from human aorta. *Arterioscler Thromb* 1994;14:1305–1314.
41. Toussaint J-F, Southern JF, Fuster V, Kantor HL. 13C-NMR spectroscopy of human atherosclerotic lesions: Relation between fatty acid saturation, cholesteryl ester contents, and luminal obstruction. *Arterioscler Thromb* 1994;14:1951–1957.
42. Coumadin Aspirin Reinfarction Study (CARS) Investigators (Fuster V, Investigator). Randomised, double-blind trial of fixed low-dose warfarin plus aspirin after myocardial infarction. *Lancet* 1997;350:389–396.
43. Stroke Prevention in Atrial Fibrillation Investigators. Adjusted-dose warfarin versus low- intensity, fixed-dose warfarin plus aspirin for high-risk

patients with atrial fibrillation: Stroke Prevention in Atrial Fibrillation III randomised clinical trial. *Lancet* 1996;348:633–638.

44. The Post Coronary Artery Bypass Graft Trial Investigators. The effect of aggressive lowering of low-density lipoprotein cholesterol levels and low-dose anticoagulation on obstructive changes in saphenous-vein coronary artery bypass grafts. *N Engl J Med* 1997;336:152–162.

45. Badimon JJ, Lettino M, Toschi V, et al. Inhibitory effects of TFPA on thrombus formation triggered by lipid-rich human atherosclerotic plaques. *Circulation* 1995;92(suppl I):I-693.

Bibliography for Table 2

1. The Global Use of Strategies to Open Occluded Coronary Arteries (GUSTO) IIb Investigators. A comparison of recombinant hirudin with heparin for the treatment of acute coronary syndromes. *N Engl J Med* 1996;335:775–782.

2. Neuhaus KL, von Essen R, Tebbe U, et al. Safety observations from the pilot phase of the randomized r-Hirudin for Improvement of Thrombolysis (HIT-III) study. *Circulation* 1994;90:1638–1642.

3. Serruys PW, Herrman JP, Simon R, et al. A comparison of hirudin with heparin in the prevention of restenosis after coronary angioplasty. Helvetica Investigators. *N Engl J Med* 1995;333:757–763.

4. Organization to Assess Strategies for Ischemic Syndromes (OASIS) Investigators. Comparison of the effects of two doses of recombinant hirudin compared with heparin in patients with acute myocardial ischemia without ST elevation: A pilot study. *Circulation* 1997;96:769–777.

5. Antmann EM for the TIMI 9B Investigators. Hirudin in acute myocardial infarction. Thrombolysis and Thrombin Inhibition in Myocardial Infarction (TIMI) 9B trial. *Circulation* 1996;94:911–921.

6. White HD, Aylward PE, Frey MJ, and the Hirulog Early Reperfusion/Occlusion (HERO) Trial Investigators. Randomized, double-blind comparison of hirulog versus heparin in patients receiving streptokinase and aspirin for acute myocardial infarction. *Circulation* 1997;96:2155–2161.

7. Theroux P, Kouz S, Roy L, et al. Platelet membrane receptor glycoprotein IIb/IIIa antagonism in unstable angina. The Canadian Lamifiban study. *Circulation* 1996;94:899–905.

8. IMPACT-II Investigators. Randomized placebo-controlled trial of effect of eptifibatide on complications of percutaneous coronary intervention: IMPACT-II. Integrilin to minimise Platelet Aggregation and Coronary Thrombosis II. *Lancet* 1997;349:1422–1428.

9. Platelet Receptor Inhibition in Ischemic Syndrome Management in Patients Limited by Unstable Signs and Symptoms (PRISM-PLUS) Study Investigators. Inhibition of the platelet glycoprotein IIb/IIIa with tirofiban in unstable angina and non-Q-wave myocardial infarction. *N Engl J Med* 1998; 338:1488–1497. Platelet Receptor Inhibition in Ischemic Syndrome Management (PRISM) Study Investigators. A comparison of aspirin plus tirofiban with aspirin plus heparin for unstable angina. *N Engl J Med* 1998;338: 1498–1505.

10. The RESTORE Investigators. Effects of platelet glycoprotein IIb/IIIa blockade with tirofiban on adverse cardiac events in patients with unstable angina or acute myocardial infarction undergoing coronary angioplasty. *Circulation* 1997;96:1445–1453.

11. Brener SJ, Barr LA, Burchenal J, et al. A randomized, placebo-controlled trial of abciximab with primary angioplasty for acute MI. The RAPPORT Trial, *Circulation* 1997;96:I473.
12. The EPIC Investigators. Use of a monoclonal antibody directed against the platelet glycoprotein IIb/IIIa receptor in high-risk coronary angioplasty. *N Engl J Med* 1994;330:956–961. Topol EJ, Califf RM, Weisman HF, et al, on behalf of the EPIC Investigators. Randomised trial of coronary intervention with antibody against platelet IIb/IIIa integrin for reduction of clinical restenosis: Results at six months. *Lancet* 1994;343(8902):881–886.
13. The EPILOG Investigators. Platelet glycoprotein IIb/IIIa receptor blockade and low-dose heparin during percutaneous coronary revascularization. *N Engl J Med* 1997;336:1689–1696.
14. The CAPTURE Investigators. Randomised placebo-controlled trial of abciximab before and during coronary intervention in refractory unstable angina: the CAPTURE study. *Lancet* 1997;349:1429–1435.
15. The EPISTENT Investigators. Randomised, placebo-controlled and balloon angioplasty-controlled trial to assess safety of coronary stenting with use of platelet glycoprotein IIb/IIIa blockade. *Lancet* 1998;352:87–92.
16. The PURSUIT Trial Investigators. Inhibition of platelet glycoprotein IIb/IIIa with eptifibatide in patients with acute coronary syndromes. *N Engl J Med* 1998;339:436–443.
17. Yusuf S. OASIS II Trial. Presented at the 20th Congress of the European Society of Cardiology. Vienna, Austria, August 1998.

Panel Discussion VI

Functional Components of the Vulnerable Plaque

Dr. Fuster: I would now like to open the session for discussion.

Dr. Taubman: One comment to your presentation. Just because the statin lowered cholesterol as well as reduced inflammation and prevented thrombogenesis, it should not be assumed that the reduction in cholesterol is the cause of reduced thrombogenicity. The statin has multiple effects, including inhibition of cell proliferation. These effects may be more important than any effect on plasma cholesterol. One of the experiments that remains to be completed is to treat people with the statins and to maintain their plasma cholesterol. I suspect that you might find inhibitory effect as well.

Dr. Fuster: We are doing that study. As I said, I am not sure if this is a direct effect of lipid lowering or statins by themselves on the monocytes or are other mechanisms involved.

Discussant from the Audience: I am interested in the fate of small, lipid-filled lesions about 1 to 2 millimeters in size. Can these lesions grow quickly within a week, and perhaps rupture and continue to grow?

Dr. Fuster: I'm not sure things can grow in a week. Once a plaque ruptures, there is a change in geometry, a thrombus forms, and these changes occur very rapidly. This is all based on angiographic studies. However, I doubt very much that you can make type IVa lesions—the most troublesome lesions with a very high lipid pool—develop very rapidly. Perhaps others can comment.

Dr. Rosenfeld: Based on studies in rabbits and mice, the earliest time following diet-induced hypercholesterolemia before you observe monocyte adhesion and the presence of foam cells is about 3 to 4 weeks.

Dr. Libby: I just wanted to say that several years ago Professor Bruska from Leiden published a study of patients who had undergone three serial angiograms over a period of several years. He showed that the growth of the plaque, by angiography, was discontinuous. So I

413

agree totally with Dr. Fuster that the plaque grows intermittently and that crisis in the life of a plaque leading to progression assessed angiographically might include thrombotic events and healing.

Dr. Fuster: I think that is an important interpretation of that data. The plaque fractures and changes very rapidly, but I'm not entirely sure that the plaque grows as a result of increases in its extracellular material or directly by monocyte recruitment. I think the animal models behave the same way you need 6 months to detect plaque growth in the iliac or femoral arteries for example.

Discussant from the Audience: Do you believe that these inflammatory lesions could be stimulated by a virus or bacteria?

Dr. Fuster: We have people in attendance who are interested in inflammation and I would ask their opinion.

Dr. Libby: I chaired the NHLBI special emphasis panel convened in September to examine this issue. We expect to publish a report of the meeting in *Circulation*. The bottom line is that Koch's postulates are not satisfied. At this time, Koch's traditional postulates for causality are not satisfied by any infectious agent in human beings. My own personal view is that if you have a Chlamydia infection or an active viral arteritis, you can potentiate the traditional modes of atherogenesis and cause a more rapid progression of complications.

Dr. Rosenfeld: I'm involved in studies at University Washington to provide the test of Koch's with regard to Chlamydia. I don't know if many of you are familiar with the association of Chlamydia pneumonia, a respiratory pathogen, with atherosclerosis. Epidemiologic data exist, and the presence of Chlamydia antigen has been detected in a large number of plaques. We are in the process of developing a means for sustaining infection in mice and in rabbits. There was a recent report of Chlamydia infection of 3 to 4 weeks in rabbits, causing endothelial injury. We are in the process testing this in the apoE knockout mouse with a prolonged 16-week infection with Chlamydia.

Dr. Fuster: Thank you. I have a question for Dr. Ward Casscells. Yesterday but Dr. Yasumi Uchida presented a very interesting prospective study on angioscopy of the coronary arteries, and described two types of yellow lesions. One was pure yellow, while the other was a glistening yellow, probably indicating the presence of a very thin capsule. The second type of yellow lesion was predictive of coronary events in the patients Dr. Uchida followed. When you talk about colors and temperature, are you talking about the carotid arteries or other arteries?

Dr. Casscells: It was carotid arteries. We did not look at the color as a predictor of clinical outcome. We determined whether a yellow lesion was warmer than a gray or white lesion, or warmer than a pink or red lesion. There was very little relationship of color to the underlining temperature or to the underlining macrophage density. However, the temperature, rather than color, was a better indicator the location of the macrophages. What that says about outcome is unclear. Since we know macrophages are often attacking a pool of cholesterol in the lesion, we expect a correlation. I'm sorry I missed Dr. Uchida's presentation, but in our opinion, yellow is a bad thing. It indicates cholesterol but it does not seem that you can pick up, by color, the cholesterol pool that has a large inflammatory component. We know there are cholesterol pools that are not very inflamed. We also know there is inflammation without cholesterol.

Dr. Fuster: The yellow Dr. Uchida is talking about appears to represent a very thin capsule where I believe the macrophage component may be more important. I have a question For Dr. Libby. Several years ago, you talked about the lymphocyte playing a very important role in coronary artery disease and later you began very enthusiastically to talk about the monocyte and macrophage. When you look at the plaque, the number of monocytes are much greater than the number of lymphocytes. Nevertheless, the CD40 information you presented in T cell membranes is very exciting data. Do you think that the high concentration that you used is an effective concentration to stimulate the macrophage in vivo?

Dr. Libby: You are eluding to the relatively high concentrations of recombinant CD40 ligand that we used. For natural CD40, a surface molecule, there are stearic constraints that make it quite effective. It is very well known if you talk about multimolecular reactions that a surface reaction is much more powerful than a solution reaction. The recombinant soluble CD40 ligand we used may be much less potent than the surface molecule. This is the reason we did the experiment with T cell membranes. I believe that the CD40 ligands simply allow us to clean up the system biochemically. The important experiment is the experiment with the T cell membranes. So I think that the test of the importance of CD40 will require studies using neutralization of CD40, CD40 ligand, using antibody strategies, or by using knockout mice. These studies are ongoing in several laboratories.

Dr. Rosenfeld: Jonathan Smith recently presented data with the back cross of the RAG1 mouse with the apoE mouse, and indicated that there was very little, if any, effect on atherosclerosis.

Dr. Libby: Yes, so size does not matter. I think that to do a costly experiment to make compound mutant mice and then just measure the lesion size is an enormous waste of resources. I know that Jonathan is completing additional studies. RAG1 is a very complex mutation and knocks out humoral as well as cellular immunity. The reason that we're interested in the cross talk between lymphocytes and monocytes and other lesion-associated cells is because we are interested in very subtle issues like vulnerability, for which we presently do not have an appropriate animal model.

Discussant from the Audience: Valentin, I would like to bring up for discussion the fact that while in primary prevention trials such as WOSCOPS, the statins cause a divergence of the treated versus untreated and in events within 6 to 8, in secondary prevention trials such as the SSS Trial or in the CARE Trial, it took up to 2 to 3 years for significant effects, depending on LDL effects. If these effects, in large part, are driven by the effects on the blood monocyte and the coagulability, etc., you would expect a similar rather than a different time course.

Dr Fuster: I suspect statins work through different mechanisms which may vary depending upon the populations studied. I presented the curves just to say they diverge, but I didn't emphasize the timing. Overall, the drugs reduced coronary events by about 25 percent. This indicates we still have much more to be gained. In the follow-up of 2 or 3 years, the fact of the matter is that we are not achieving much. A person who already has the disease is under a burden even if the plasma cholesterol concentration is low. I suspect it takes time for the plaque to become stabilized, but at least the benefit is continuous. It is my assumption that this is the beginning of a beneficial effect that would, if continued for 15 years, eventually result in a much better clinical outcome.

Discussant from the Audience: Yes but I would also propose that the statins are not the total answer and we can find ways to decrease the time in secondary prevention trials.

Discussant from the Audience: I would like to ask Dr. Libby a question. We are all well aware of the rupture plaque and the occlusive thrombus as to being a very pertinent pathologic lesion, but there are many ulcerated plaques that do not have thrombus. My question is whether the ulcerated plaques without thrombus are pathologic lesions, which we really need to prevent, or are they a physiologic component of the overall defense against accumulating atherosclerotic plaques?

Dr. Libby: By ulcerated plaque I presume you're not talking about a superficial erosion but about an ulcer crater.

Discussant from the Audience: Yes, real ulcer craters.

Dr. Libby: Well you know I think we can learn the answer from the pathophysiology of certain types of cerebral emboli or particularly ophthalmic emboli that originate from the carotid artery. If we see an empty crater, it is probably because something left there. Those of you who have had a chance to examine a patient who has amaurosis fugax and see a plaque of Hollenhorst lodged at the bifurcation with a brightly refractory cholesterol embolus that presumably arose from one of those craters, appreciate the concept that there is the potential for thrombi to form and then leave. So I believe that just because the crater is empty, it may be like the bird that has flown away from the nest. The ulcerative lesion is still the nidus for renewed clotting and perhaps ongoing thrombosis with embolization, which is the natural history of carotid artery disease in many cases.

Dr. Fuster: Studies of pathologic specimens indicate that a number of ulcerated lesions do not have thrombus.

Discussant from the Audience: Yes I agree that they do not have a thrombus, but my question is, is that empty plaque really a defense?

Dr. Fuster: Well I don't think it's a defense. I think that empty plaques, and any ulcerated plaque, indicate a potential for trouble.

Dr. Taubman: I think all of the evidence indicates that virtually every plaque you look at has the components necessary for thrombus formation. They all have a substantial amount of tissue factor and all you need is the right set of circumstances for thrombus formation, even if you don't have a large lipid core. You have plenty of macrophages and muscle cells expressing tissue factor, but presumably there have been a number of mechanisms that have been developed to protect against the development of thrombus. We still do not understand why in an injured vessel wall, where you have tissue factor and where you have fibrinogen, you have factors VII, VIII, and X in that wall, but you do not see fibrin. The implication is that there is a "protector" or "protectors"; whether there are phospholipids associated with platelets or whether there are other factors adhering to the vessel wall is not completely understood. Nevertheless, the ulcerated plaques that don't look thrombogenic are probably below the level at which the critical components are actually able to be exposed.

Discussant from the Audience: What would happen to that ulceration if a thrombus did not form? What is the natural history?

Dr. Taubman: That's a good question.

Dr. Fuster: Yes, there was a paper published in the *American Journal of Cardiology* 2 to 3 years ago which reported that plaques can remain chronically ulcerated and not progress.

Dr. Paterkamp: I have just a question about visualizing the unstable plaque. What is the unstable plaque? In our studies in the femoral arteries and in the coronary arteries, we observed the presence of macrophage infiltration and T lymphocytes. In about 30 percent of all cross sections—those are patients without any previous cardiovascular problems—we found 30 or 40 percent of the section filled with macrophages and T lymphocytes. What difference does it make if we visualize the presence of macrophages or T lymphocytes in the lesion cap?

Dr. Fuster: This is a good way to finish this symposium, because this topic will be covered in the next meeting. The theme of the next meeting to be held April or May 1999 is going to be "what really is an unstable plaque and how can we manage it?" We should learn which lesions are instable and which are not. Today we tried to define the plaques that have ruptured, and once they ruptured we observed specific attributes. There are many plaques that may or may not be vulnerable, and this is something that we should be thinking about for the next meeting.

This is the time to close this symposium. I want to thank all of you for making the meeting a success. I want to also express my sincere appreciation to Mary Winston and the American Heart Association for their help. And certainly, my appreciation to Merck and Co., Inc., who provided the funds to conduct the meeting. Merck has been very, very helpful, not only in making this meeting possible, but also in the preparation of an audiovisual CD-ROM.

Index

Page numbers followed by "t" indicate tables.